MEDICATIONS:

A Guide for the
Health Professions
Second Edition

NORTH SHORE
COMMUNITY COLLEGE

One Ferncroft Road
Danvers, Massachusetts

Learning Resource Center
Lynn Campus

Gift Book

DISCARD
MEDICATIONS:

A Guide for the
Health Professions
Second Edition

Karen Lane, CMA-AC
Senior Clinical Research Coordinator
Division of Neurocritical Care
The Johns Hopkins University School of Medicine
Baltimore, Maryland

Linda Reed, MS, RN, CMA-AC
Program Chairman
Medical Assisting
Indiana Vocational Technical College
Indianapolis, Indiana

 F. A. DAVIS COMPANY • Philadelphia

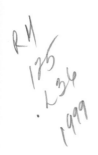

Printed in the United States of America

Last digit indicates print number: 10 9 8 7 6 5 4 3 2 1

Publisher: Jean-François Vilain
Developmental Editor: Marianne Fithian
Cover Designer: Louis J. Forgione

As new scientific information becomes available through basic and clinical research, recommended treatments and drug therapies undergo changes. The author(s) and publisher have done everything possible to make this book accurate, up to date, and in accord with accepted standards at the time of publication. The authors, editors, and publisher are not responsible for errors or omissions or for consequences from application of the book and make no warranty, expressed or implied, in regard to the contents of the book. Any practice described in this book should be applied by the reader in accordance with professional standards of care used in regard to the unique circumstances that may apply in each situation. The reader is advised always to check product information (package inserts) for changes and new information regarding dose and contraindications before administering any drug. Caution is especially urged when using new or infrequently ordered drugs.

Library of Congress Cataloging-in-Publication Data

Lane, Karen
    Medications : a guide for the health professions / Karen Lane
— 2nd ed.
        p.   cm.
    Includes index.
    ISBN 0-8036-0378-9
    1. Drugs—Administration. 2. Pharmacology. 3. Therapeutics. 4. Allied health personnel.
I. Reed, Linda. II. Title.
    [DNLM: 1. Pharmaceutical Preparations—administration & dosage. 2. Drug Therapy—methods. WB 340L265mb 1998]
    RM125.L36 1999
    615'.1—dc21
    DNLM/DLC
    for Library of Congress   98-27995
                                                                                            CIP

Preface to the Second Edition

The most important new feature in this edition is the new approach to dosage calculations. Former methods requiring complex variations of ratio and proportion analysis has been simplified to the use of a *single* mathematical formula for *all* calculations of dosage. This eliminates the need to memorize multiple formulas, makes calculations quick, reduces the possibility of error, and requires only basic arithmetic skills. This technique has been standard in mathematics and engineering departments in the United States and continues to gain acceptance among allied health and nursing educators.

The new edition continues to make the book easy to use. Additional exercises and assignments have been included as homework. Examples and exercises are realistic, using actual labels and dosages for the drugs most commonly administered by the allied health practitioner in the health care setting. To further increase the students' understanding, generic and trade (brand) names as well as therapeutic classifications identify the drugs. Sections have been added to give the student more experience with reconstituting drugs from powdered forms and reading the various parts of a drug's labeling.

As with the last edition, the book is self-contained, supplying conversions and abbreviations necessary for dosage calculations and the listing of the top 50 prescribed drugs. New assignments give the student experience creating drug information cards on the top 50 prescribed drugs for personal use or use in patient teaching. Faculty, students, and members of the health community are encouraged to learn the material by studying the chapters in sequence. This allows the reader to move from the introductory basics of pharmacology through to the more complex activities of teaching patients about the medications they take and of administering medications under the direction of the physician-provider. The overriding theme is to guide new members of the health profession in the safe preparation and administration of medication.

This text also is used by students and health professionals already in the workplace as an introduction to or review of drug dosage calculation and administration. It can be used as part of a review for certification and licensing examinations. It is an excellent professional reference for the physician in private practice or the health maintenance organization. We also encourage the practitioner in the workplace to consider recording and reporting (where applicable) the time spent reading and testing in this textbook as part of continuing education activities. Check the applicable rules with the organization (for example, national medical assisting or pharmacy technician society) that awards these credits.

KAREN LANE, CMA-AC
LINDA REED, MS, RN, CMA-AC

Acknowledgments

My friend, Harry Benson, first listened to my ideas on publishing a condensed pharmacology textbook for medical assistants and other health-related professionals at a time when he was encouraging me and other medical assisting educators to write on topics specifically relevant to our field. He was responsible for my first writing successes. When he convinced Jean-François Vilain, publisher at F.A. Davis, to take on this project in late 1990, the task of writing the first draft was already completed. My first and chief acknowledgment must surely be to him.

My debt to my immediate sponsor, Jean-François Vilain, is a real one, particularly for his work through the revisions of the subsequent drafts and in the final stages of publication. I express my gratitude for the encouragement he has given me and for much practical advice. Marianne Fithian, of the editorial department of F.A. Davis, checked with care all that I had written and sometimes forgotten to write, and Donna King, the production editor, guided the manuscript to a quality finished product. To them I am also grateful.

Apart from my correspondence and stimulating conversation with the four people just mentioned, I have prepared this book with my co-author in some isolation and solitude, during all too brief periods of leisure. I owe the freedom to pursue my writing to my tolerant and sometimes lonely husband, Steve.

Linda Reed reviewed the first edition in typescript through three revisions. As Consulting Editor, she made numerous valuable suggestions adapted from her years of experience with her own students. Ms. Reed now has joined me in revising the text and, as co-author, contributed substantially to all the chapters. Thanks to Ms. Reed, this edition extends the range and scope of the written competencies and practice procedures and includes written assignments to guide the student through the rudiments of the top 50 drugs prescribed in the United States. These improvements are to mention but a few of her contributions. It is a pleasure to have her as my collaborator.

Three reviewers joined Ms. Reed as reviewers of the first edition: Mary Ann Frew, Marcia (Marti) Lewis, and Debbie Odgaard. Perhaps my greatest critics, I knew them to be my friends. I grew very fond of them during the months of rewrite; I detected their occasional exasperation and savored their compliments. Theirs was not a cursory review but a labor of love for the students this book is intended to serve. The hours of work they gave to the book made the finished product possible.

My co-author and reviewers embody the greatest patronage for which any author could hope. My eternal thanks.

KAREN LANE

Thanks to Dave Crume with the DEA for providing information and reviewing text.
Thanks to Connie Bollinger for support and guidance in developing the math instruction.
Thanks to Karen for being a patient teacher as well as my co-author.

LINDA REED

Contents

8 Routes of Administration and Injection Techniques 221

9 Drugs Commonly Administered or Prescribed in the Medical Office 265

1

The Language of Pharmacology

Abbreviations, Systems of Measurement, and Conversions

OBJECTIVES

WRITTEN COMPETENCY 1-1: Identify, write, and use units of measurement and their abbreviations for the metric system.

WRITTEN COMPETENCY 1-2: Identify, write, and use units of measurement and their abbreviations for the apothecary system and household measurements.

WRITTEN COMPETENCY 1-3: Convert medication orders within systems and from one system to another.

TERMINAL PERFORMANCE OBJECTIVE (PROCEDURE 1-1): Measure and convert liquid medications.

1

Using the Basic Written Language and Mathematic Processes of Drug Therapy

The basic terms and arithmetic for administering precise and correct medications form the foundation for the application of drug therapy in the clinical setting. Two fundamental elements are involved in administering correctly measured medications: correctly written and understood orders and the precise use of three systems of measurement used in medicine in the United States.

Although the number and type of medications administered in medical centers and other healthcare settings are usually limited by specialty or patient population, the area of measuring medications can be one in which errors frequently occur. The first way to decrease errors in drug administration is to commit thoroughly to learning the correct techniques of charting and translating drug orders. The basic abbreviations, symbols, and terminology related to making the correct entries on the patient chart are significant to the patient's well-being. Poor or incorrect recording techniques can result in injury to the patient and have legal implications as well. Even a correctly administered medication cannot be defended in a court of law if it is recorded inaccurately.

The second way to decrease errors in drug administration is to perfect one's understanding of how to convert equal quantities of drug from one system to another. Before a dose can be measured or calculated, both the dose ordered and the dose in storage must be expressed in the same system and unit of measure. Although the order for a medication comes from the physician, it is the responsibility of the medical assistant to carry out the order with a conscientious attitude, a knowledge of dosage calculation, and the ability to prepare and deliver a medication accurately.

Although understanding mathematics and working with numbers can be intimidating, the ability to do so is of the utmost importance. Specifically, one must be able to add, subtract, multiply, and divide fractions, decimals, and percentages.

By memorizing the formulas, using the tables, and practicing the exercises in this chapter, one should be able, both verbally and in writing, to use the specific symbols of drug preparation, and to perform accurately the fundamental mathematics necessary to measure (or to convert first and then to measure) the correct dose of a drug for a patient, within any of the three systems of measurement used in drug therapy today.

Commonly Used Pharmacologic Abbreviations

Medication orders and prescriptions are written in a special language, derived from either Latin or English terms. This language is further shortened by using *abbreviations* for each of the Latin or English terms. Pharmacologic abbreviations are used when the physician writes a prescription or a medication order on a patient's chart and when labels are prepared for the stock solutions mixed at the medical facility. These abbreviations are specific and universal and require a strict adherence to precise procedures for writing them on medical records (Table 1–1).

Problem Terms and Misunderstood Abbreviations

Abbreviations of terms and units of measurement are a convenience, but they can be misunderstood. Too often, abbreviated drug orders are misinterpreted or not understood. Each medical practice should formulate an approved list of abbreviations, and every attempt should be made to require all personnel to use the accepted list. There are, however, certain

TABLE 1–1. **Abbreviations for Drug Orders, Labels, and Prescriptions**

Abbreviation	Meaning	Latin Derivative
$\overline{aa}$	Of each	Ana
ac	Before meals	Ante cibum
ad	Up to	Addetur
a.d.	Right ear	aurio dextra
ad lib	As desired	Ad libitum
a.L., a.s.	Left ear	aurio laeva, aurio sinister
AM	Morning	ante meridiem
amp	Ampul	
amt	Amount	
aq	Water	aqua
ASAP	As soon as possible	
a.u.	Each ear	aures uterque
bid	Twice a day	Bis in die
BSA	Body surface area	
$\overline{c}$	With	Cum
cc	Cubic centimeter	
cap	Capsule	
d	Day	Dies
dc, d/c	Discontinue	
dil	Dilute	
disp	Dispense	
dr, ʒ	Dram	
elix	Elixir	
ext	Extract	
fl	Fluid	
gm or g	Gram	
gr	Grain	
gt, gtt	Drop, drops	Gutta
h, hr	Hour	Hora
hs	Hour of sleep	Hora somni
ID	Intradermal	
Kg	Kilogram	
IM	Intramuscular	
IV	Intravenous	
Ⓛ	Left	
L	Liter	
mcg	Microgram	
meq, mEq	Milliequivalent	
♏	Minim	
mg	Milligram	
ml, mL	Milliliter	
NS	Normal saline	
npo	Nothing by mouth	Nulla per os
pt	Pint	
OD	Right eye	Oculus dexter
OS	Left eye	Oculus sinister
OU	Both eyes	Oculi unitas
otic	Ear	
ophthal	Eye	
os	Mouth	Os
ʒ	Ounce	
p	After	Post
pc	After meals	Post cibum
per	By	
PO	By mouth	Per os
prn	When necessary	Pro re nata
q	Every	Quoque
q4h	Every 4 hours	quoque 4 horae
qid	Four times a day	Quarter in die
QS	Quantity sufficient	Quantum satis
Ⓡ	Right	
Rx	To take	Recipe
$\overline{s}$	Without	Sine

Table continued on following page

TABLE 1–1. **Abbreviations for Drug Orders, Labels, and Prescriptions** (*Continued*)

Abbreviation	Meaning	Latin Derivative
SC or subcut	Subcutaneously	
Sig	Write on label	Signetur
SL	Under the tongue	Sublingual
sol	Solution	
sos	Once if necessary	Si opus sit
$\overline{ss}$	One half	Semis
stat	Immediately	Statim
supp	Suppository	Suppositorium
syr	Syrup	Syrupus
Tab	Tablet	Tabella
tbs	Tablespoon	
tid	Three times a day	Ter in die
tsp	Teaspoon	
Tx	Treatment	
Ud	As directed	
ung	Ointment	Unguentum
vo	Verbal order	
x	Times	
#	Number (of tablets to dispense)	

frequently misunderstood abbreviations that should not be approved because of potentially dangerous results (Table 1–2). In addition to misunderstood abbreviations that relate to directions, the following rules should be followed:

1. Do not use symbols for medicinal or chemical names; write out the full medication name.
2. Lettered abbreviations should not be used for drug names; use generic or trade names. The exception is when a brand name contains initials, such as Bicillin L-A (long acting) or Robitussin-DM (dextromethorphan hydrobromide).
3. Apothecary symbols and terms should be used sparingly.
4. Take your time and write every abbreviation clearly and in ink.
5. All unfamiliar abbreviations and units of measurement should be brought to the attention of the physician for clarification and approval. Do not guess at the meaning of any unknown symbol or abbreviation.

TABLE 1–2. **Misunderstood Abbreviations**

Abbreviation	Mistaken For	Write Instead
OD (for once daily)	Right eye	Once daily
qod (for every other day)	Once daily or four times a day	Every other day
qd (for every day)	Four times a day	Once daily
qn (for every night)	Every hour	hs or bedtime
qhs (for every night)	Every hour	HS or bedtime
U (for Unit)	4 or cc	unit
μg (for microgram)	mg	mcg
sq or subq (for subcutaneous)	Every	SC or subcut
PO (for by mouth)	Left eye	Orally, by mouth
H_2O	Not understood	Write full name

Source: Adapted from Davis, NM and Cohen, MR: Medication Errors: Causes and Prevention. Geo. F. Stickley and Co., Philadelphia, 1981.

Number and Decimal Systems Used in Pharmacology

At the very core of medication administration are the measurements that ensure successful and safe drug therapy. Correct measurements are made in terms of arbitrarily defined units. It is important to begin with a brief consideration of numbers and arithmetic.

The origin of numbers predates history, back to a time when fingers and toes or sticks were used. The oldest records indicating the systematic use of written numerals (/, //, ///, ////, ⧾⧾⧾⧾) date back to the Sumerians and Egyptians. *Arabic numerals* (0, 1, 2, 3, 4, 5, 6, 7, 8, 9) were first used in India and then introduced to the West by the Arabs. *Roman numerals*, later developed by the Romans, are based on seven basic symbols: I or i = 1; C or c = 100; V or v = 5; X or x = 10; L or l = 50; D or d = 500; M or m = 1000. In medieval times, the symbol for 1 was J; then in modern times, the lowercase j was changed to a final i, the most common roman numeral used in medical prescription writing today.

Roman numerals are written according to the following rules:

1. A symbol following one of equal or greater value adds to its value (e.g., II = 2).
2. A symbol preceding one of greater value subtracts from its value (e.g., IV = 4).
3. When a symbol stands between two of greater value, its value is subtracted from the second and the remainder is added to the first (e.g., XIV = 14).
4. The symbol of the larger value must be written first (e.g., XIV, not VIX).

For writing the larger numbers, the Babylonians, who followed the Sumerians, invented the same principle that appears in our number system today: the principle of position. The value of a number depends not only on the symbol "2," for example, but also on the position it occupies with respect to the other symbols in a number grouping. The digit "2" has different meaning in the two numbers 482 and 234; in the first example it stands for two and in the second it stands for two one-hundreds.

The Babylonians also invented the idea of using the same base for counting *and* measurement, but the idea was lost and not revived until the metric system was founded by French scientists in 1795. The metric system is based on the meter, which is theoretically 1/10,000,000 of the distance from the equator to the North Pole, as measured on the earth's surface. Our present metric system is a decimal system using a base of 10.

PRACTICE PROBLEMS: Convert the roman numeral notations to arabic numbers; and convert the arabic numbers to roman numerals.

1. xvi   = _____
2. xii   = _____
3. iv   = _____
4. ix   = _____
5. xx   = _____
6. xix   = _____
7. xL   = _____
8. xiv   = _____
9. CD   = _____
10. MLx   = _____
11. 11   = _____
12. 18   = _____
13. 23   = _____

14. 27   = _____

15. 34   = _____

16. 39   = _____

17. 53   = _____

18. 77   = _____

19. 121   = _____

20. 376   = _____

21. vii   = _____

22. xxv   = _____

23. CCix   = _____

24. ix   = _____

25. xvii   = _____

26. xC   = _____

27. xxx   = _____

28. iv + xvii = _____

29. iv + xi   = _____

30. xxv + xiv = _____

See end of chapter for answers.

In pharmacology, ½ is the only fraction assigned a special roman numeral:

$$\overline{ss} \text{ or } ss = ½$$

Arabic decimal numbers are written for most other fractions used with the metric system for prescription writing and the preparation of medications; for example:

Correct	*Incorrect*
0.25	1/4
0.33	1/3
0.75	3/4

Very small fractional quantities are *not* measured in the decimal system, however, as they are more easily understood in the fractional form. For example, "nitroglycerin 1/300 gr" is used rather than "nitroglycerin 0.03 gr."

PRACTICE PROBLEMS: Using Table 1–1 convert the roman numeral notations to arabic numbers and translate the medication orders.

1. tabs iiss once daily: _____

2. i qid: _____

3. ii q4h prn: _____

4. i bid × 10 days: _____

5. disp: tabs #50: _____

6. disp: oz iv: _____

7. Sig: gt i OD hs: _____

8. tabs #40 Sig: ad lib: _____

9. caps i tid ac: _____

10. gtt iii in water QS ℥ii pc: _____

11. 25 mg stat and q4h prn: _____

12. 10 cc in water qid × 10 day: _____

13. 1/6 gr IM q3–4h prn: _____

14. gtt ii OU tid × 3 days: _____

15. i tab ac and hs: _____

16. iss tsp q12h: _____

17. 50 mg IM prn for N/V (nausea/vomiting): _____

18. 2 tsp prn for temp ˆ101°F: _____

19. 8 meq bid: _____

20. 20 U sc before breakfast and @ 4 pm: _____

21. 15 cc qid: _____

22. 5 mg bid × 4 doses then 3 mg bid × 4 doses then 2 mg bid × 4 then 1 mg bid: _____

23. 1 mg daily × 2d and then dc: _____

24. 80 mg stat: _____

25. 4 mg/Kg: _____

26. 2L IV then DC: _____

27. i tab pc prn: _____

28. 1/150 gr for chest pain SL; may repeat q5min × 3: _____

29. 0.1 mg q12h × 10: _____

30. 10 gtt in water q6h: _____

31. 1 ℥ in 8 ℥ juice mix and drink quickly: _____

See end of chapter for answers.

Systems of Measurement

Systems of measurement are uniform and reliable standards for measuring volume, weight, and length. There are three separate systems used in prescribing drugs: *metric, apothecary, and household.* Prescriptions may be written according to any of these three systems, and sometimes they are written using a combination of two or all three. Drugs are conventionally manufactured in the metric system that physicians commonly prescribe or order them according to one or another system depending on individual preference. Therefore, it is necessary to know the components of each system and how to convert from one system to another.

THE METRIC SYSTEM

The metric system is very exact. It has a decimal relationship and is therefore based on powers of 10—that is, each basic unit is multiplied by 10 or divided by 10 to arrive at larger or smaller units, respectively. Each unit of measurement is further self-defined with specific Latin and Greek prefixes (Table 1–3).

TABLE 1–3. **Prefixes Used for the Metric System**

Greek Prefixes			Unit	Latin Prefixes*		
1000	**100**	**10**	**1.0**	**0.1**	**0.01**	**0.001**
(Kilo)	*(Hecto)*	*(Deca)*		*(deci)*	*(centi)*	*(milli)*
Kl	Hl	Dl	L = liter (liquid; volume)	dl	cl	ml‡
Km	Hm	Dm	M = meter (area)	dm	cm	mm
Kg†	Hg	Dg	G = gram (solids; weight; strength)	dg	cg	mg§

*Not included in table: 1 microgram (mcg) = 0.000001 g. The only subdivision of the gram used are the milligram (0.001 g) and the microgram (0.001 mg):

$$1 \text{ kg} = 1000 \text{ g}$$
$$1 \text{ g} = 1000 \text{ mg}$$
$$1 \text{ mg} = 1000 \text{ mcg}$$

†Unit of measurement often used in determining patient weight for the administration of medications.
‡Common prefix used in measuring liquid medications.
§Common prefix used in manufacturing medication strength.

The gram (g) is used to measure the weight or mass of a solid medication. Solid medications are in the form of powders, tablets, topical preparations, and medications dissolved or suspended in liquid medications and injectable medications. Measuring the weight is the same as measuring the *strength* of a particular medication.

The milliliter (ml) is used to measure the volume of a liquid medication, in the form of either oral liquids or fluids for injection. Measuring volume is the same as determining the *amount* of medication to be taken orally or given by injection.

PRACTICE PROBLEMS: For each quantity, enter the **decimal point** in the correct place without changing the value, use the correct **abbreviation** for each quantity, and then **circle strength** or **amount,** depending on which is being measured.

   Example: 1 liter = <u>1.0 liter</u> (amount)

 1. 1000 liters   = _____ (strength, amount)

 2. 100 liters   = _____ (strength, amount)

 3. 10 liters   = _____ (strength, amount)

 4. 1/10 liter   = _____ (strength, amount)

 5. 1/100 liter   = _____ (strength, amount)

 6. 1/1000 liter = _____ (strength, amount)

 7. 1000 g   = _____ (strength, amount)

 8. 100 g   = _____ (strength, amount)

 9. 10 g   = _____ (strength, amount)

10. 1/10 g   = _____ (strength, amount)

11. 1/100 g   = _____ (strength, amount)

12. 1/1000 g   = _____ (strength, amount)

See end of chapter for answers.

Another term used frequently in the preparation of medications is the cubic centimeter (cc). A cubic centimeter (length) is the amount of space (cubed area) occupied by a milliliter (volume) of liquid (Fig. 1–1). Therefore, one milliliter (1 ml) of medication is considered equivalent to one cubic centimeter (1 cc) of medication. The ml can be interchanged with cc at anytime.

PRACTICE PROBLEMS: Convert milliliters to cubic centimeters.

1. 1 ml   = _____ cc
2. 10 ml   = _____ cc
3. 30 cc   = _____ ml
4. 32 cc   = _____ ml
5. 0.5 cc = _____ ml
6. 0.01 ml = _____ cc
7. 500 ml = _____ cc
8. 0.95 cc = _____ ml
9. 750 cc = _____ ml
10. 1.5 ml = _____ cc

See end of chapter for answers.

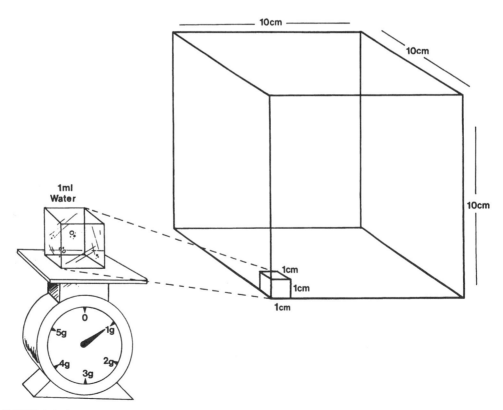

FIGURE 1–1. The equivalency of the metric system is based on 1 cc (cm³) of capacity will hold 1 ml of water at its maximum density and weigh 1 g.

WRITING THE METRIC ORDER

In writing metric orders, arabic numbers are used. The quantity always precedes the abbreviation or written word.

Example: 5 ml or 500 mg; 5 milliliters or 500 milligrams

In the metric system, fractions are not used. Numbers are written as a whole number or as a whole number and decimal part. For example:

Correct	Incorrect
0.25 ml	−1/4 − ml
1.5 cc	1 − 1/2 − cc
0.5 g (500 mg)	1/2 − g

For accuracy and understanding of medication orders involving milliliters and cubic centimeters in quantities less than one, a zero (0) is placed before the decimal point; for example, two tenths of a milliliter would be written as 0.2 ml. For example:

Correct	Incorrect
0.1 ml	.10 − ml
0.5 cc	.5 − − cc
0.01 ml	.01 − ml

Using the decimal point and one zero in this manner ensures that there will be no misunderstanding of the amount of medication. In the first example directly preceding, the order ".1 ml" could be misread as "1 ml," if the decimal point is not obvious.

Rule of Zero: Never add a zero (0) when not necessary. Always add a zero (0) before a decimal point.

CONVERSION WITHIN THE METRIC SYSTEM

Many times a medication order will need to be converted within the metric system. A physician may order 0.25 g, but the medication is labeled "milligrams." Units within the metric system are converted by moving the decimal point in multiples of 10.

Table 1–3 can be used to learn the positions of the 10 and 1/10 multiples. The Latin and Greek prefixes specify the multiples, making calculation within the metric system easy. By visually remembering the prefix positions in the table, you can convert metric measurements without multiplication or division.

Example: The drug on hand is measured in milligrams. The physician orders 0.25 g.

Using Table 1–3, notice that the milligram column is three places to the right of the gram column; so take 0.25 and move the decimal point three places to the right: 0.25 now becomes 250. Gram converts to milligram; therefore,

$$0.25 \text{ g} = 250 \text{ mg}$$

PRACTICE PROBLEMS: Using Table 1–3, convert the following:

1. 1.0 g   = _____ mg

2. 1000 g   = _____ kg

3. 0.025 g   = _____ mg

4. 1000 ml   = _____ liter

5. 0.5 liter   = _____ ml

6. 15 cc   = _____ ml

7. 0.2 mg   = _____ mcg

8. 0.5 g   = _____ mg

9. 125 mcg   = _____ mg

10. 750 mg   = _____ g

11. 2.7 L   = _____ cc

12. 10 mg   = _____ mcg

13. 5 mcg   = _____ g

14. 250 cc   = _____ L

15. 2 Kg   = _____ g

See end of chapter for answers.

THE APOTHECARY SYSTEM

The apothecary system is a very old English system of measurement. The origin of the system is not exactly known. There are two units of measurement in the apothecary system—the *grain* (gr), which measures solids (weight), and the *minim*, which measures liquids (volume). The basic unit, 1 gr, is the weight of 1 gr of wheat; 1 minim is the amount of water that would weigh 1 gr.

In the apothecary system fluid measures closely approximate solid measures, and it is permissible to consider them equal and interchangeable in measuring within the system (Table 1–4).

The grain or dram (gr, dr), is used to measure the weight of a solid medication. Solid medications are in the form of powders, tablets, topical preparations, and medications dissolved or suspended in liquid medications and injectable medications. Measuring the weight is the same as measuring the *strength* of a particular medication.

The minim (m̨), fluid dram (fl dr, f℥), and fluid ounce (fl oz, f℥) are used to measure the volume of a liquid medication, in the form of oral liquids or liquids for injection. Measuring of volume is the same as determining the *amount* of medication to be taken orally or given by injection.

TABLE 1–4. **Apothecary System**

Measurement of Solids *(Weight, Strength)*	*Measurement of Liquids* *(Volume, Amounts)*
60 gr = 1 dr	60 minims = 1 fl dr
8 dr = 1 oz	8 fl dr = 1 fl oz
16 oz = 1 lb	16 fl oz = 1 pt

TABLE 1–5. **Apothecary Abbreviations and Symbols**

Abbreviations	Symbol	Abbreviations	Symbol
grain = gr		minim = minim	℥
dram = dr	ʒ	fluid dram = fl dr	fʒ
ounces = oz	℥	fluid ounce = fl oz	f℥

WRITING THE APOTHECARY ORDER

When using an apothecary abbreviation or symbol, the quantity is usually written as a roman numeral and **follows** the abbreviation or symbol (Table 1–5):

Sig: gr v once daily
(Directions to patient: 5 grains every day)

More Examples		Using Abbreviations	Using Symbols
3 drams	=	dr iii	ʒ iii
1-1/2 ounces	=	oz iss	℥ iss
10 grains	=	gr x	gr x
16 minims	=	minims xvi	℥ xvi
4 fluid ounces	=	fl oz iv	f℥iv
1 fluid dram	=	fl dr i	fʒi

THE HOUSEHOLD UNITS OF MEASUREMENT

Household units of measurement are more difficult to use, and should be avoided in the medical facility, if there is a choice of using either the metric or the apothecary systems. Household units are used in most American households, however, and the system is the most convenient for administering medications at home. Although health professionals work most often in the metric and apothecary systems, it is important to know frequently used household conversions when instructing patients.

Patients also need to be instructed to use proper, standardized measuring equipment. For example, the silverware teaspoon is quite different in size from the standard measuring spoon that is used in cooking. Patients should not use silverware or dinnerware materials for measuring medications (see Chapter 6, Fig. 6–4).

All household measurements are volume (liquid) measurements. The smallest household unit is the drop (gt, gtt). The other household units commonly used in the preparation of medications are the teaspoon (tsp) and tablespoon (tbs) (Table 1–6). Larger units, such as the household ounce (oz), pints (pt), and gallons (gal), occasionally may be used in the medical facility to prepare large quantities of stock solutions. The preparation of stock medications will be covered in Chapter 6.

TABLE 1–6. **Household Units of Measurement Used in the Administration of Medications (With Abbreviations)**

Measurement of Liquids (Volume, Amounts)
60 gtt = 1 tsp
3 tsp = 1 tbs
2 tbs = 1 oz
8 liquid oz = 1 c
2 c = 1 pt
2 pt = 1 qt
4 qt = 1 gal

WRITING THE HOUSEHOLD ORDER

When writing the household order, the quantity always precedes the abbreviation and is written using arabic numbers:

Sig: 1 tsp bid
(Directions to patient: 1 teaspoon two times a day)

Conversions Between Systems of Measurement

Medication orders may need to be converted from one system to another. A medication might be ordered in the apothecary system, but the container is manufactured using the metric system. The conversion of the amount of medication ordered *to* the available form of measurement is the responsibility of the physician ordering the drug; however, the person preparing the medication is legally responsible to *recalculate* the conversion before preparing the drug. This double-checks the process of providing safe dosages of drug.

Table 1–7 lists the most commonly used equivalents. Although it is not necessary to memorize the entire table, the most commonly used equivalents should be learned. With experience, these commonly used equivalents will become committed to memory.

If an equivalent is not listed on a table, the equivalent may be determined by multiplying other listed equivalents. Using the known facts in Table 1–6, one may calculate the number of drops in 1 tbs as follows:

$$60 \text{ gtt} = 1 \text{ tsp}$$

$$3 \text{ tsp} = 1 \text{ tbs}$$

$$60 \text{ gtt} \times 3 \text{ tsp} = 180 \text{ gtt}$$

A conversion is calculated by multiplication or division. For example, to convert 4 fl oz (apothecary) to its metric unit equivalent (using Table 1–7), the known conversion to use is 1 fl oz = 30 ml.

$$1 \text{ fl oz} = 30 \text{ ml}$$

TABLE 1–7. **Conversions Between Systems of Measurement**

Metric	Apothecary	Household
Solids, Mass		
1 g = 1000 mg	15 gr (gr xv)	
60/64/65/66 mg (use what # comes out even)	1 gr (gr i)	
30 mg	1/2 gr (gr iss)	
1 mg = 1000 mcg	1/60 gr (gr 1/60)	
154 g		1.0 lb
1 Kg		2.2 lb
1 g = 1 cc = 1 ml		
Liquids, Volume		
1.0 liter = 1000 ml (or cc)		1 qt (approx)
0.5 liter = 500 ml		1 pt
240 ml	8 fl oz (f℥ viii)	1 c
30–32 ml	1 fl oz (f℥ i)	2 tbs
15–16 ml	4 fl dr (f℥ iv)	1 tbs = 3 tsp
8 ml	2 fl dr (f℥ ii)	2 tsp
4–5 ml	1 fl dr (f℥ i)	1 tsp = 60 gtt
1 ml	15–16 minim (ɱ xv–xvi)	15–16 gtt
0.06 ml	1 minim (ɱ i)	1 gt

$$4 \text{ fl oz} = 4 \times 30 \text{ ml} = 120 \text{ ml}$$

Answer: There are 120 ml in 4 fl oz.

Example: Convert 4 oz to milliliters

To convert from one system to another, we first set up a fraction made up of the units as they are listed on a conversion table. The fraction will have the known units on the bottom and the new units to convert to on the top. Table 1–7 lists **"30–32 ml = 1 fl oz."** Set up the fraction to contain *fl oz* on the *bottom* and *ml* on the *top*. (When converting use the unit of measure that comes out even.)

$$\frac{\text{ml}}{\text{oz}} \qquad \text{(new unit)}$$
$$\phantom{\frac{\text{ml}}{\text{oz}}} \qquad \text{(old unit)}$$

This fraction must always include *equivalent* measures and *equal 1*. Next, we simply multiply the "equivalent fraction" times the *known unit*.

$$\frac{30 \text{ ml}}{1 \text{ oz}} \times 4 \text{ oz}$$

$$\frac{30 \text{ ml}}{1 \text{ o\!\!\!/z}} \times \frac{4 \text{ o\!\!\!/z}}{1} = 120 \text{ ml}$$

Written simply, it becomes the formula:

$$\frac{\text{New Equivalent}}{\text{Known Equivalent}} \times \text{Known Unit} = \text{New unit of measure}$$

Each time a medication is converted from one system to another, the equivalent is *approximate* but safe enough for patient administration. Sometimes, however, a drug is recalculated into another system to provide a more accurate measurement with the equipment on hand. In Chapter 7, syringe preparation examples will demonstrate occasions when equipment calibrations necessitate conversion from the metric system to the apothecary system.

A quick way to remember apothecary-metric conversions is to visualize a clock (see Fig. 1–2).

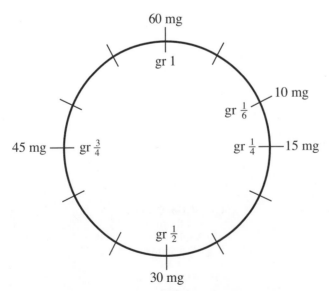

FIGURE 1–2. Apothecary-metric conversion clock.

On this conversion clock, 60 mg (representing 60 min) equals gr 1 (1 hour). Two times around the clock (gr 2) equals 2 hours, or 120 mg; gr 5 = 300, and so on. Other conversions that do not relate exactly to the clock are:

$$gr\ 15 = 1000\ mg\ (1\ G)$$

$$gr\ 5 = 300\ mg\ (approximately)$$

$$1\ oz = 30\ ml$$

$$1\ tbs = 15\ ml$$

$$1\ tsp = 5\ ml$$

THE MILLIEQUIVALENT MEASURE

One other system for measuring fluids is the *milliequivalent*. The milliequivalent is usually abbreviated meq, however, the abbreviation MEQ also is used. The milliequivalent is derived from the concentration of electrolytes in a certain volume of solution, expressed as meq/L (per liter). The most common example of this measurement is the meq/L of potassium; it is the amount of potassium crystalloid in an intravenous fluid replacement (IV fluids). Most solutions measured as milliequivalents are for intravenous use.

PRACTICE PROBLEMS: Using Table 1–7 and the conversion formula, convert the following:

$$\frac{New\ Equivalent}{Old\ Equivalent} \times Known\ unit = New\ unit\ of\ measure$$

1. 150 gr   = _____ g
2. 1/4 gr   = _____ mg
3. 45 minims = _____ ml
4. 2 qt   = _____ liter(s)
5. 10 ml   = _____ tsp
6. 46 kg   = _____ lb
7. 90 ml   = _____ fl oz
8. 90 mg   = _____ gr
9. 2000 mcg   = _____ mg
10. 500 cc   = _____ liter(s)

See end of chapter for answers.

Written Competency 1–1

Performance Competence: Identify, write, and use units of measurement and their abbreviations for the metric system within 15 minutes. Do not give yourself credit for partial or incorrect answers.

1. To express a measurement representing 1/1000, use the prefix _____.

2. The commonly used metric unit of measurement for measuring the *strength* of a solid medication is the _____.

3. The two metric units of measurement commonly used to measure the *amount* of a liquid medication are the _____ and _____.

4. 1 g is _____ (greater than, less than, the same as) 1000 mg.

5. 1 ml is _____ (greater than, less than, the same as) 1 cc.

6. 0.50 g is _____ (greater than, less than, the same as) 50 mg.

7. 150 ml is _____ (greater than, less than, the same as) 1.5 liters.

8. To minimize the danger of an error, a _____ is placed before the decimal point when writing a fraction of a metric unit.

9. Record the verbal order: "One tenth of a milliliter." _____

10. Record the verbal order: "Two cubic centimeters." _____

11. Which is correct 0.10, .1, 0.1? _____

12. The metric units that measure volume are _____, _____, _____.

13. The cubic centimeter measures _____.

14. What is the relationship between cc and ml? _____

15. The metric system is based on multiples of _____.

What is the prefix for

16. 0.001 _____

17. 1000 _____

18. 0.000001 _____

19. 0.01 _____

20. 0.1 _____

Score: _____

See Appendix B for answers.

Written Competency 1–2

Performance Competence: Identify, write, and use units of measurement and their abbreviations for the apothecary system and household measurements within 15 minutes. Do not give yourself credit for partial or incorrect answers.

1. In the apothecary system, the basic unit for measuring the strength of a solid medication is the _____, which is abbreviated _____. The basic unit for measuring the amount of liquid medication to be administered is the _____, which is designated by the symbol _____.

2. _____ gr equal 1 dram. _____ minims equal 1 fl dr. One dr is _____ (greater than, less than, equal to) 1 fl dr.

3. Practice writing the symbol for the dram eight times. _____
   _____

4. Practice writing the symbol for the apothecary ounce eight times. _____
   _____

5. Write the apothecary order for "Dispense four ounces and label: 1-1/2 drams three times a day." _____
   _____

6. In household units, the basic unit for measuring the amount of liquid medication to be administered is the _____, which is abbreviated _____ (singular) and _____ (plural).

7. There are _____ drops in 1 tsp.

8. In household units, the abbreviation for cup is _____, and the abbreviation for gallon is _____.

9. 1 gal equals _____ oz.

10. Write the household order for: "Label 1 teaspoon of liquid Tylenol four times a day."
    _____
    _____

11. In the Apothecary system, the unit of measure comes (before, after) the quantity.
    _____

12. One-half is written with what abbreviation? _____

13. In the apothecary system, quantities are written using (Arabic numbers, Roman numerals).
    _____

14. In the Apothecary system, quantities less than one-half are written correctly as (1/150, 0.15). _____

Write the following using Apothecary abbreviations.

15. two and one-half ounces _____

16. six minims _____

17. one and two-thirds drams _____

18. twenty drops _____

19. five grains _____

20. one tenth grain _____

Score: _____

See Appendix B for answers.

Written Competency 1–3

Performance Competence: Convert medication orders within systems and from one system to another with at least 90 percent accuracy and within 15 minutes. Do not give yourself credit for partial or incorrect answers.

1. 1 ml   = _____ cc

2. 1 liter   = _____ ml

3. 30–32 ml = _____ fl oz

4. 90 ml   = _____ fl oz

5. 1 ml   = _____ minims

6. 1 tbs   = _____ minims

7. 30 minims = _____ ml

8. 120 mg   = _____ gr

9. 1/4 gr   = _____ mg

10. 1 tsp   = _____ ml

11. 30 cc   = _____ dram

12. 3 tsp   = _____ cc

13. gr V   = _____ mg

14. 154 lbs. = _____ Kg

15. gr 1/150 = _____ mg

16. dram iiiss = _____ cc

17. oz viii   = _____ cc

18. 0.1 g   = _____ mg

19. 120 mg   = _____ gr

20. 250 mcg = _____ mg

21. 50 kg   = _____ lbs.

22. 2 tsp   = _____ gtt

23. 10 cc   = _____ minims

24. 16 oz   = _____ cc

25. gr 1/300 = _____ mcg

26. gr ss   = _____ mg

27. 1.25 g   = _____ mg

28. 750 mg   = _____ g

29. 1 L   = _____ oz

30. 1 oz   = _____ minims

Score: _____

See Appendix B for answers.

Terminal Performance Objective/Competency

Procedure 1–1: Measure and Convert Liquid Medications

EQUIPMENT	Three medicine cups	5.0-ml regular syringe ($\bar{s}$ needle)	Mineral oil bottle
	Medicine bottle	3.0-ml regular syringe ($\bar{s}$ needle)	Paper towels
	Measuring spoon	Two medicine droppers	Waste container

Performance Competence: Practice converting liquid units of measurement among the metric, apothecary, and household systems for measurement. Complete each step of this procedure and record your observations with exact accuracy for each measurement and within reasonable job production time as stated by your evaluator.

$\boxed{\text{V}}$ $\boxed{\text{S}}$ $\boxed{\text{U}}$*

PROCEDURAL STEPS

Equipment: Using the medicine bottle, the first medicine cup, and the 5.0-ml syringe:

1. With the medicine cup sitting on a flat surface, pour the water from the medicine bottle with the label toward your palm (to prevent the liquid from dripping onto the label) to measure 4.0 ml in the medicine cup. (Measure on the flat surface, at eye level, and at the bottom of the miniscus.) Is your measurement accurate to 4.0 ml?

   Yes _____ No _____   ☐ ☐ ☐

2. Withdraw all the water from the first medicine cup into the syringe. What does the water measure in the syringe? _____   ☐ ☐ ☐

Equipment: Using the medicine bottle, the second medicine cup, the dropper, and the teaspoon:

3. Dispense 60 gtt of water from the bottle into the second empty medicine cup. The 60 gtt equal how many milliliters? _____   ☐ ☐ ☐

4. Pour the water from the second medicine cup into the teaspoon. Is the medication in the cup greater than, less than, or equal to the teaspoon measure? _____   ☐ ☐ ☐

   How many drops equal 1 tsp? _____   ☐ ☐ ☐

   How many milliliters equal 1 tsp? _____   ☐ ☐ ☐

Equipment: Using the first dropper, the second medicine cup, and water:

5. Dispense 15 to 16 gtt of the water into the medicine cup by holding the dropper vertically and using consistent pressure. How many minims do 15 to 16 gtt equal? _____   ☐ ☐ ☐

---

*V = Value, to be filled in if assigning points or other specific values to each step.
S = Satisfactory completion of the step.
U = Unsatisfactory completion of the step or step incomplete; needs more practice.

Equipment: Using the third medicine cup, a clean dropper, and the mineral oil:

6. Dispense 15 to 16 gtt of the mineral oil into the third clean medicine cup as follows:

   a. Dispense 5 gtt with the dropper held vertically, and measure in minims: _____ minims ☐ ☐ ☐

   b. Change the angle of the dropper and dispense 5 more gtt. Measure in minims: _____ minims ☐ ☐ ☐

   c. Dispense 5 more gtt. Do the 15 to 16 gtt equal 15 to 16 minims? _____ ☐ ☐ ☐

   Why or why not? _____ ☐ ☐ ☐

7. How did the oil drops differ from the water drops in final quantity dispensed? _____

   _____ ☐ ☐ ☐

8. Clean up the materials and return the equipment to storage. ☐ ☐ ☐

Equipment: Using the 3.0-ml syringe:

9. Draw up 0.5 ml of water. How many minims are contained in the 0.5 ml? _____ ☐ ☐ ☐

10. The physician orders 0.66 ml. The syringe is marked off in tenths (1/10s). Using Table 1–7 as a reference, draw up the order in minims. How many minims are there in 0.66 ml? _____ ☐ ☐ ☐

Practice Problem Answer Section

ANSWERS P. 5: 1. 16   2. 12   3. 4   4. 9   5. 20   6. 19   7. 40   8. 14   9. 400   10. 1060
11. xi   12. xviii   13. xxiii   14. xxvii   15. xxxiv   16. xxxix   17. Liii   18. Lxxvii   19. Cxxi
20. CCCLxxvi   21. 7   22. 25   23. 209   24. 9   25. 17   26. 90   27. 30   28. 21   29. 15
30. 39

ANSWERS P. 6: 1. 2-1/2 tablets every day   2. One four times a day   3. Two every 4
hours when required   4. One two times a day for 10 days   5. Dispense 50 tablets
6. Dispense 4 ounces   7. Directions on label: 1 drop in the right eye at bedtime
8. Dispense 40 tablets and label: as desired   9. One capsule three times a day before meals
10. 3 drops in enough water to equal two ounces after meals   11. 25 milligrams
immediately then every four hours as needed   12. Ten cubic centimeters in water four
times a day for ten days   13. One-sixth grain intramuscularly every three to four hours as
needed   14. Two drops in both eyes three times a day for three days   15. One tablet
before meals and at bedtime   16. One and one-half teaspoons every 12 hours   17. 50
milligrams intramuscularly as needed for nausea or vomiting   18. Two teaspoons as
needed for fever greater than 101°F   19. 8 milliequivalents two times a day   20. 20 units
subcutaneously before breakfast and at 4 o'clock P.M.   21. 15 cubic centimeters four times
a day   22. Five milligrams two times a day-times 4 doses, then 3 milligrams two times a
day for 4 doses, then 2 milligrams two times a day for 4 doses, then 1 milligram two times
a day   23. One milligram per day times 2 days then discontinue   24. 80 milligrams
immediately   25. Four milligrams per kilogram   26. Two liters intravenously then
discontinue   27. One tablet after meals when required   28. One-one fiftieth of a
grain . . . under the tongue; may repeat every 5 minutes 3 times   29. 0.1 milligram every
12 hours times 10 days   30. 10 drops in water every 6 hours   31. 1 dram in 8 ounces juice
mix and drink quickly

ANSWERS P. 8: 1. 1000 liters (amount)   2. 100 liters (amount)   3. 10 liters (amount)
4. 0.1 liter (amount)   5. 0.01 liter (amount)   6. 0.001 liter (amount)   7. 1000.0 g
(strength)   8. 100.0 g (strength)   9. 10.0 g (strength)   10. 0.1 g (strength)   11. 0.01 g
(strength)   12. 0.001 g (strength)

ANSWERS P. 9: 1. 1   2. 10   3. 30   4. 32   5. 0.5   6. 0.01   7. 500   8. 0.95   9. 750
10. 1.5

ANSWERS P. 10: 1. 1000   2. 1   3. 25   4. 1   5. 500   6. 15   7. 200   8. 500   9. 0.125
10. 0.75   11. 2700   12. 10,000   13. 0.005   14. 0.25   15. 2000

ANSWERS P. 15: 1. 10   2. 15   3. 3   4. 2   5. 2   6. 101.2   7. 3   8. 1.5   9. 2   10. 0.5

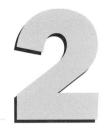

The Controlled Substances Act and Prescriptions

OBJECTIVES

WRITTEN COMPETENCY 2–1: Complete a calendar of federal responsibilities.

WRITTEN COMPETENCY 2–2: Complete the writing of three prescriptions

TERMINAL PERFORMANCE OBJECTIVE (PROCEDURE 2–1): Complete a federal triplicate order form.

TERMINAL PERFORMANCE OBJECTIVE (PROCEDURE 2–2): Transmit a prescription order to the pharmacist.

CONVERSION DRILL FOR SKILL: Convert measurements to their most frequently used approximate equivalents.

The Evaluation of Drugs

Through archeologic and anthropologic discoveries, there is ample evidence that the practice of pharmacology, using animal and plant extracts and minerals, was used extensively by primitive societies since the dawn of time. By medieval times, pharmacology had far advanced from the oral tradition, passed down from generation to generation, to exotic formulas for the relief of symptoms formally recorded in great volumes known as pharmacopeia, or books of drug preparations. Dr. Oliver Wendell Holmes once said of one of these volumes: "if the whole materia medica . . . were sunk to the bottom of the sea, it would be all the better for mankind and all the worse for the fishes." Although the majority of oral traditions and recorded remedies are worthless, many of the same preparations used by the ancient Egyptians, Hebrews, Greeks, Arabs, and Native Americans, such as digitalis, ipecac, and quinine, are still used in medicine today.

In the 19th century, pharmacology became a science and, for the first time, drug properties were studied for their safety and true value. Now, with the advancements in biochemistry, molecular biology, and enzyme chemistry, newly discovered chemicals must be submitted to a long and difficult series of development through biologic tests, animal studies, clinical evaluation studies, safety-in-human studies, efficacy (usefulness) studies, and postrelease evaluations. Only a small number of chemicals, therefore, ever make it to the market as drugs.

DRUG DEVELOPMENT

Once a compound is discovered, *screening tests* are used first to determine whether or not the compound has the activity of the particular kind that is being sought. Once the presence of a particular action is established, *biologic assays* are conducted on animals and microorganisms to determine the relative amounts of that compound necessary to bring about desired activities. Eventually, biologic assays determine the strength of a compound necessary to bring about a desired activity in future human testing.

After a drug is determined to have a specific therapeutic activity *in theory*, *preclinical trials* are conducted on groups of animals to determine that the drug activity is in fact therapeutic and that it is safe. Most drugs have too low a safety margin for use in human tissues, however. Of the thousands of compounds tested to this point, most fail to pass the trials of effectiveness and toxicity, or pass preclinical trials but development is discontinued because further research would be too expensive. These discontinued drugs, called *orphan drugs*, could be used to treat disease, but will never become available for use by patients because of the cost involved. In 1983, the government passed the Orphan Drug Act to encourage further work on these drugs in the form of grants to researchers.

Drugs that are shown to be reasonably safe in preclinical toxicity tests may be cleared for limited *clinical studies* in controlled settings. Clinical studies are performed on human subjects who have volunteered for the testing. During this phase a drug must prove to be as effective as expected, not produce unacceptable side effects or toxic effects, have a high benefit-to-risk ratio, and be as effective as other drugs already on the market.

After long years of successful testing, a drug may be approved for marketing to the general public. But even after approval, manufacturers must continue to furnish additional information concerning the drug's safety and usefulness. Should a drug prove to be unsafe or have unreasonable side effects at any time, its approval can be reversed or altered. One example is hexachlorophene (pHisoHex), a hospital antiseptic that had been used by hospital personnel for handwashing and to bathe newborn infants. After it was discovered that hexachlorophene could cause central nervous system toxicity and death in infants, its approval for use in soaps, cosmetics, and toiletries was reversed by the federal Food and Drug Administration (FDA).

LEGAL REGULATION

Since the turn of this century, the United States government has passed important legislation and subsequent amendments to protect the public's health (Table 2–1). This body of

TABLE 2–1. **History of Federal Legislation
Regulating the Clinical Use of Drugs and Preventing Drug Abuse**

Year	Affecting Clinical Use	Drug Abuse Prevention
1906	Pure Food and Drug Act	
1914		Harrison Narcotic Act
1938	Federal Food, Drug, and Cosmetic Act of 1938	
1951		Durham Humphrey Amendment
1962	Kefauver-Harris Act	
1965		Drug Abuse Control Amendments of 1965
1970		Comprehensive Drug Abuse Prevention and Control Act of 1970 (Controlled Substances Act)
1974		Narcotic Addict Treatment Act
1978		Psychotropic Substances Act
1980		Coast Guard—Importation of Controlled Substances Enforcement Act
1980		Infant Formula Act (marijuana penalties)
1983	Orphan Drug Act	
1984		Comprehensive Crime Control Act
1986		Anti-Drug Abuse Act and Criminal Law and Procedure Act

legislation empowers the government to control and restrict the sale of worthless or dangerous drugs, prevent the marketing of impure drugs, and eliminate the use of false labels and misleading claims of therapeutic usefulness.

The FDA, an agency of the Department of Health and Human Services (HHS), was established in 1936 and is responsible for the regulation of the manufacture and sale of all prescription and over-the-counter (OTC) drugs. The FDA approves the investigational use of all drugs in humans, ensures that drugs are effective as well as safe, and sets standards for the purity, strength, and composition of all drug products during the manufacturing process, so that the composition of all trade brands and generic brands of a particular drug are equally therapeutic and safe. When the drug is approved, the company is given exclusive patent rights for 17 years before other companies can manufacture the drug generically. This is to recover the costs of research and development.

In 1973, the government established the Drug Enforcement Administration (DEA) in the Department of Justice to coordinate all activities directly related to the enforcement of laws respecting narcotics and dangerous drugs. The establishment of the DEA was in response to an alarming increase in drug abuse and the need to control drug traffic, by regulating all persons in the process of drug production and distribution.

Other federal agencies include the Federal Trade Commission (FTC) and the Division of Biological Standards of the National Institutes of Health. The FTC controls the advertising of nonprescription drugs and is charged with protecting the public from false advertising and the deceptive practices of OTC manufacturers. The Division of Biological Standards sets the quality requirement for biologic products such as vaccines, antitoxins, immune sera, and blood derivatives. These agencies work together to enforce all federal legislation affecting the clinical and nonclinical use of drugs.

THE FEDERAL CONTROLLED SUBSTANCES ACT (CSA)

The DEA is the federal law enforcement agency responsible for the control of narcotic and dangerous drug abuse* and for combating drug diversion.† As a branch of the Department

---

* CSA, 1970.
† 1984 Drug Diversion Control Amendments and Controlled Substance Registrant Protection Act of 1984.

TABLE 2–2. **Classification of Controlled Substances**

Schedule I

Characteristics
- High potential for abuse
- No currently accepted medical use in treatment in the United States
- Lack of accepted safety for use under medical supervision

Examples
- Narcotics—heroin
- Depressants—methaqualone (Quaalude)
- Hallucinogens—LSD, mescaline, peyote, amphetamine variants (e.g., MDA), phencyclidine (PCP)
- Cannabis—marijuana, tetrahydrocannabinol (TCH)

Schedule II

Characteristics
- High potential for abuse
- Currently accepted for medical use in treatment in the United States with severe restrictions
- Abuse may lead to severe psychologic or physical dependence

Examples
- Narcotics—opium, morphine, codeine, hydromorphine (Dilaudid), meperidine (Demerol), methadone, oxycodone (Percodan)
- Depressants—barbiturates (amobarbital, pentobarbital, secobarbital)
- Stimulants—cocaine, amphetamine, phenmetrazine (Preludin), methylphenidate (Ritalin)
- Cannabis—tetrahydrocannabinol (Marinol)*

Schedule III

Characteristics
- Potential for abuse is less than drugs in schedules I and II
- Currently accepted for medical use in treatment in the United States
- Abuse may lead to moderate or low physical dependence or high psychologic dependence

Examples
- Narcotics—-Paregoric (opium derivative), certain codeine combinations (e.g., Tylenol or Empirin with codeine)
- Depressants—certain derivatives of barbituric acid, glutethimide (Doriden), methyprylon (Noludar), any suppository dosage form containing amobarbital, secobarbital, or pentobarbital
- Stimulants—benzphetamine

Schedule IV

Characteristics
- Low potential for abuse relative to the drugs in schedule III
- Currently accepted for medical use in treatment in the United States
- Abuse may lead to limited physical dependence or psychologic dependence relative to the drugs in schedule III

Examples
- Narcotics—propoxyphene (Darvon), pentazocine (Talwin)
- Depressants—chloral hydrate, barbital, phenobarbital, methylphenobarbital, benzodiazepines (Ativan, Dalmane, diazepam [Valium], Librium, Xanax, Serax, Tranxene, Verstran, Halcion, Paxipam, Restoril), meprobamate (Equanil, Miltown), ethchlorvynol (Placidyl), ethinamate (Valmid), paraldehyde
- Stimulants—diethylpropion (Tenuate), phentermine

Schedule V

Characteristics
- Low potential for abuse relative to the drugs in schedule IV
- Currently accepted for medical use in treatment in the United States
- Abuse may lead to limited physical dependence or psychologic dependence relative to the drugs in schedule IV

Examples
- Narcotics—preparations containing limited quantities of narcotics, generally for antitussive and antidiarrheal purposes

*Has been used effectively to control nausea in cancer patients, when all other antinausea treatments have failed.

of Justice, it was established in 1973 to investigate drug smuggling, trafficking, and diversion; to enforce federal laws; and to prevent drug abuse and drug diversion through public education.

Under these federal laws, the physician, the pharmacist, and all medical office personnel share the responsibility for controlling and monitoring the following:

- The drug use of patients
- Illegal "script" writing
- Theft of controlled substances from physicians' offices
- Theft of prescription blanks
- Willful and intentional drug diversion by medical personnel
- Records required by law
- The duty to public reporting

Controlled substances, which include narcotics, stimulants and depressants, opium, and cocaine, have legitimate clinical use in the treatment of patients when they are prescribed for patient comfort and well-being. Because these drugs all have the potential to alter consciousness or mental functioning, prescribing controlled substances requires special precautions because of their potential for abuse, addiction, and dependence.

SCHEDULES OF CONTROLLED SUBSTANCES

The drugs that fall under the jurisdiction of the CSA are divided into five categories, known as schedules C-I, C-II, C-III, C-IV, and C-V. Schedule C-I has the highest potential for abuse, and schedule C-V the lowest. Table 2–2 provides schedule descriptions and examples of drugs in each schedule. Drugs may move within the categories because of their potential for abuse. For a complete listing of drugs included and exempted from these schedules, obtain the Code of Federal Regulations mentioned earlier. Table 2–3 lists addresses of the DEA Domestic Field Offices throughout the United States.

The law also provides the mechanism for adding new substances to be controlled, the reclassification of substances to lesser or greater control, and decontrolling substances (removal from the schedule). Proceedings can be initiated by the HHS, the DEA, or any other interested person or group. When a petition is received to add or delete a drug from a certain schedule or to change the schedule of a drug, the DEA begins investigating the drug. A scientific study is then conducted by the HHS, and additional information is solicited from the FDA and the National Institute on Drug Abuse.

If it is determined that a drug or other substance should be controlled, decontrolled, or rescheduled, the DEA publishes a proposal in the Federal Register, inviting all interested parties to respond to the proposal or request a hearing. The DEA will evaluate all the comments and arrange for a public hearing (if called for), then publish a final order in the Federal Register. Unless challenged in the United States Court of Appeals within 30 days, the final order will be enacted into law on a specified date.

The central issue for investigation is whether or not a drug has the potential for abuse. If a potential for abuse cannot be established, the drug cannot be placed on the controlled substance list. Each of the following items is used as an indicator that a substance has the potential for abuse:

1. There is evidence that the substance is being used in amounts sufficient to create a hazard to the individuals using the drug or to the safety of the community.
2. There is significant diversion of the substance from legitimate drug channels.
3. Individuals are taking the substance on their own initiative, rather than by the advice of the medical community.
4. The substance contains a new drug related in action to a drug already on the controlled substance list.

TABLE 2–3. **Drug Enforcement Administration Field Offices
With Assigned Diversion Investigator Personnel**

Location	*Jurisdiction*
Albuquerque District Office Suite 100 4775 Indian School Road, N.E. Albuquerque, New Mexico 87110 (505) 262-6283	New Mexico
Atlanta Division 75 Spring Street, S.W. Room 740 Atlanta, Georgia 30303 (404) 331-7328	Georgia South Carolina
Baltimore District Office 200 St. Paul Plaza, Suite 2222 Baltimore, Maryland 21202 (410) 962-4800	Maryland
Boston Division 50 Staniford Street Suite 200 Boston, Massachusetts 02114 (617) 565-2800	Maine Massachusetts New Hampshire Rhode Island Vermont
Buffalo Resident Office 28 Church Street Suite 300 Buffalo, New York 14202 (716) 846-4421	Western and Central New York
Camden Resident Office 1000 Crawford Place Suite 200 Mt. Laurel, New Jersey 08054 (609) 757-5006	Southern New Jersey
Charleston Resident Office 2 Monongalia Street Suite 202 Charleston, West Virginia 25302 (304) 347-5209	West Virginia
Chicago Division 500 Dirksen Federal Bldg. 219 South Dearborn Street Suite 500 Chicago, Illinois 60604 (312) 353-7875	Central and Northern Illinois
Cleveland Resident Office Courthouse Square 310 Lakeside Avenue, Suite 395 Cleveland, Ohio 44113 (216) 522-3705	Northern Ohio
Columbus Resident Office 78 East Chestnut St. Room 409 Columbus, Ohio 43215 (614) 469-2595	Central and Southern Ohio
Dallas Division Northern Texas 1880 Regal Row Dallas, Texas 75235 (214) 767-7250	Northern Texas

Table continued on following page

TABLE 2–3. **Drug Enforcement Administration Field Offices
With Assigned Diversion Investigator Personnel** (*Continued*)

Location	Jurisdiction
Denver Division 115 Inverness Drive East Englewood, Colorado 80112 (303) 784-6381	Colorado
Des Moines Resident Office Room 937, Federal Building 210 Walnut Street Des Moines, Iowa 50309 (515) 284-4700	Iowa
Detroit Division 357 Federal Building 231 W. Lafayette Detroit, Michigan 48226 (313) 226-7290	Michigan
Ft. Lauderdale Resident Office 1475 W. Cypress Creek Blvd. Suite 301 Ft. Lauderdale, Florida 33309 (305) 527-7094	Southern Florida
Fresno Resident Office 1260 M Street, Room 200 Fresno, California 93721 (209) 487-5402	Central California
Greensboro Resident Office 2300 W. Meadowview Road Suite 218 Greensboro, North Carolina 27407 (919) 333-5052	North Carolina
Harrisburg Resident Office P.O. Box 557 Harrisburg, Pennsylvania 17108-0557 (717) 782-2270	Central Pennsylvania
Hartford Resident Office 450 Main Street Room 628 Hartford, Connecticut 06103 (203) 240-3230	Connecticut
Honolulu Resident Office Room 3129 300 Ala Moana Boulevard P.O. Box 50163 Honolulu, Hawaii 96850 (808) 541-1930	Hawaii Trust Territories
Houston Division 333 West Loop North Suite 300 Houston, Texas 77024-7707 (713) 681-1771	Eastern and Southern Texas
Indianapolis Resident Office 575 N. Pennsylvania Room 290 Indianapolis, Indiana 46204 (317) 269-7977	Indiana
Kansas City Resident Office 8600 Farley, Suite 200 Overland Park, Kansas 66212 (913) 236-3176	Kansas Western Missouri

Table continued on following page

TABLE 2–3. **Drug Enforcement Administration Field Offices
With Assigned Diversion Investigator Personnel** (*Continued*)

Location	*Jurisdiction*
Little Rock Resident Office 10825 Financial Parkway Suite 317 Little Rock, Arkansas 72211-3557 (501) 378-5981	Arkansas
Long Island District Office 1 Huntington Quadrangle Suite 1C-02 Melville, New York 11747 (516) 420-4532	Long Island, New York
Los Angeles Division World Trade Center Edward Roybal Federal Building 255 East Temple Street, 20th Floor Los Angeles, California 90012 (213) 894-4016	South Central California Nevada
Louisville Resident Office 1006 Federal Building 600 Martin Luther King, Jr. Place Louisville, Kentucky 40202 (502) 582-5908	Kentucky
Miami Division 8400 N.W. 53rd St. Miami, Florida 33166 (305) 591-4980	Southern Florida and Eastern Coast of Florida
Milwaukee Resident Office 1000 Water Street, Suite 1010 Milwaukee, Wisconsin 53202 (414) 297-3395	Wisconsin
Minneapolis Resident Office 402 Federal Building 110 S. 4th Street Minneapolis, Minnesota 55401 (612) 348-1729	Minnesota North Dakota
Mobile Resident Office 1110 Mountlimar Suite 270 Mobile, Alabama 36609 (205) 441-5831	Alabama
Nashville Resident Office 801 Broadway, Room A929 Nashville, Tennessee 37203 (615) 736-5988	Tennessee
Newark Division Federal Office Building 970 Broad Street Newark, New Jersey 07102 (201) 645-3482	Central and Northern New Jersey
New Orleans Division 3838 N. Causeway Blvd., Suite 1800 Three Lake Center New Orleans, Louisiana 70002 (504) 585-5665	Louisiana Mississippi
New York Division 99 Tenth Avenue New York, New York 10011 (212) 337-1575	Northern and Southern New York

Table continued on following page

TABLE 2–3. **Drug Enforcement Administration Field Offices With Assigned Diversion Investigator Personnel** (*Continued*)

Location	*Jurisdiction*
Oklahoma City Resident Office Federal Building 200 N.W. Fifth Street Suite 960 Oklahoma City, Oklahoma 73102 (405) 231-4141	Oklahoma
Omaha Resident Office 106 South 15th Street Room 1003 Omaha, Nebraska 68102 (402) 221-4222	Nebraska South Dakota
Philadelphia Division William J. Green Federal Building 600 Arch Street Room 10224 Philadelphia, Pennsylvania 19106 (215) 597-9540	Delaware Eastern Pennsylvania
Phoenix Division 3010 N. 2nd Street Suite 301 Phoenix, Arizona 85012 (602) 640-5700	Arizona
Pittsburgh Resident Office Federal Building 1000 Liberty Avenue Room 2306 Pittsburgh, Pennsylvania 15222 (412) 644-3390	Western Pennsylvania
Portland Resident Office 1220 S.W. 3rd Avenue Room 1525 Portland, Oregon 97204 (503) 326-3371	Oregon
Richmond Resident Office 8600 Staples Mill Road Suite B Richmond, Virginia 23240 (804) 771-8163	Central, Southeastern and Southwestern Virginia
Sacramento Resident Office 1860 Howe Avenue Suite 250 Sacramento, California 95825 (916) 978-4225	North Central and Northeastern California
Salt Lake City Resident Office American Towers III 47 West 200 South, Room 401 Salt Lake City, Utah 84101 (801) 524-4156	Utah
San Antonio District Office 10127 Morocco Suite 200 San Antonio, Texas 78216 (512) 525-2900	Central and Western Texas
San Diego Division 402 W. 35th Street National City, California 90250 (619) 585-4200	Southern California

Table continued on following page

TABLE 2–3. **Drug Enforcement Administration Field Offices
With Assigned Diversion Investigator Personnel** (*Continued*)

Location	*Jurisdiction*
St. Louis Division United Missouri Bank Building 7911 Forsythe Boulevard Suite 500 St. Louis, Missouri 63105 (314) 425-3241	Eastern Missouri Southern Illinois
San Francisco Division 450 Golden Gate Avenue P.O. Box 36035 San Francisco, California 94102 (415) 556-3325	Central and Northern Coast California
San Juan District Office Casa Lee Building 2432 Loiza Street Santurce, Puerto Rico 00913 (809) 253-4234	Puerto Rico Virgin Islands
Seattle Division 220 West Mercer Street Suite 104 Seattle, Washington 98119 (206) 442-5443	Washington State Montana Alaska Idaho
Tampa Resident Office 5426 Bay Center Drive Tampa, Florida 33609 (813) 228-2486	Central, Northcentral and Northwestern Florida
Washington, DC Division 400 Sixth Street, S.W. Room 2558 Washington, DC 20024 (202) 401-7834	District of Columbia Northern Virginia Southern Maryland

Regulation

The provisions of the CSA require that the physician and medical office personnel comply with certain regulations governing recordkeeping, registration, drug distribution, dispensing to patients, and security. Of the many pamphlets published by the Department of Justice, "The Physician's Manual: An Informational Outline of the Controlled Substance Act of 1970," and the "Manual for Mid-Level Providers" are recommended. These booklets summarize the law as it is published by the government in Chapter II of the Code of Federal Regulations, Title 21, Food and Drugs, Chapter 13—Drug Abuse Prevention and Control, Part 1301 to end. They are available from the United States Department of Justice, Drug Enforcement Administration, Washington, DC 20537.

RECORDKEEPING

The CSA requires that complete and accurate records be kept of all quantities of controlled substances purchased, distributed, dispensed, and returned. Records must be:

- Kept separate from other records (including the patient chart)
- Readily retrievable
- Retained for at least 2 years. Check with your state DEA office.
- Available for inspection by DEA at all times. There is a maximum $25,000 fine for each record-keeping infraction.

In medical practice, the three terms *administer*, *dispense*, and *prescribe* are used to describe three separate medication situations. When a drug is administered, a specific dose is taken by the patient during the visit. A drug is dispensed when a quantity of medication is given to the patient for a fee, and the patient continues taking the medication at home. Dispensing also includes manufacturer samples given to patients. A prescribed medication is filled by the pharmacist: only the written order (prescription) is completed at the time of the visit.

A physician who dispenses controlled substances is required to keep a record of each transaction. A physician who regularly administers controlled substances is required to keep records if patients are charged for the drugs, either separately or as a part of the office charge. If a physician both dispenses and administers a controlled substance from the *same inventory*, whether occasionally or regularly, records must be kept of each transaction. A physician who occasionally administers a controlled substance and *does not* dispense the controlled substance from the same inventory is not required to keep separate records. If the occasional administration of controlled substances is recorded only in patients' files, these files must be readily accessible for DEA inspection.

A physician who only prescribes schedule II, III, IV, and V controlled substances need not keep records of these transactions, other than the normal practice of recording the information on each patient's chart or history. Some states may, however, require the physician to keep a separate file of prescription copies. Check your state laws with the field DEA office.

Other situations that require special recordkeeping procedures include narcotic treatment programs and drug research programs. Narcotic treatment programs (e.g., methadone clinics) are carefully regulated by the Narcotic Addict Treatment Act of 1974 (PL 93-281) and require separate and more detailed records for controlled substances that are prescribed, dispensed, or administered for maintenance or detoxification treatment. Physicians are required to register separately as a narcotic treatment program. Separate authorization also is required for any handling of a schedule I substance in any research program.

REGISTRATION

Every physician who prescribes, administers, or dispenses controlled substances must register with the DEA. Exceptions include physicians who are interns, residents, from a foreign country, or on the staff of a Veterans Administration facility, who dispense and prescribe using a special code under the registration of a hospital or other institution. Each registered physician will receive a specific DEA registration number and a Controlled Substance Registration Certificate (Fig. 2–1). Each registration is valid for 3 years.

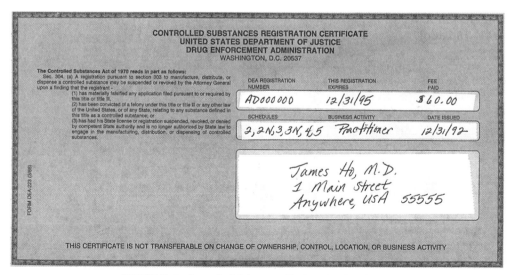

FIGURE 2–1. Controlled Substance Registration Certificate.

To apply for registration, obtain a Form DEA-224 (Fig. 2–2) from any DEA field office. Complete instructions are on the form. The physician completes the appropriate sections and the registration form is returned, with a check, to the Drug Enforcement Administration, Central Station, PO Box 28083, Washington, DC, 20038-8083. The registration fee is $210.00 for a 3-year registration.

FIGURE 2–2. Application for DEA Registration. (*A*) Front. (*B*) Back.

Special attention should be paid to item 2 on Form DEA-224. If the office intends to stock any controlled substances, each applicable block under item 2 should be checked. Once this form is processed, the DEA will issue the office Federal Triplicate Supply Order forms used for purchasing schedule II drugs from drug manufacturers and suppliers.

Renewal applications are handled differently. They are completed and mailed to Atlanta, Georgia, rather than to Washington, DC. Sixty days before the expiration of the physician's current Controlled Substances Registration Certificate, the DEA will send Form 224a, Renewal Application (Fig. 2–3). If the renewal notification is not received by the physician within 45 days of the expiration date, *it is the physician's responsibility to notify the DEA that the renewal application has not been received.* Every practice should develop a reminder mechanism to prevent registration expiration.

A DEA Registration Certificate is always specific to a single site. A separate DEA Registration Certificate must be obtained if the physician dispenses and/or administers controlled substances at another office. If the physician only prescribes at other facilities, however, a separate registration is not required, provided the additional sites are within the same state. If a practice is about to relocate, the physician must provide notice to the DEA and request modification of the Registration Certificate prior to the effective date of the move.

When a physician decides to retire or sell a practice, the DEA should be called for information and guidance. The Registration Certificate and any unused order forms must be returned to the nearest DEA field office. Before mailing, all unused order forms should be voided, for protection from theft in the mail. Unused controlled substances should not be disposed of. The local DEA office will explain how and where to dispose of any controlled substances remaining in the office's inventory (see also section on security).

INVENTORY REQUIREMENTS

The first inventory of all stocks of controlled substances on hand must be conducted on the first date the physician engages in CSA activities. If no drugs are on hand at the time of the initial inventory, a zero (0) inventory should be recorded. Figure 2–4*A* is a sample inventory with each of its required components.

A new inventory is required *every 2 years* following the date of the initial inventory. Labeled as a "Biennial Inventory," the inventory must include the beginning date of business, the end date of business, and the initials of the person taking the inventory. The biennial inventory should contain exactly the same information as the initial inventory. If the biennial inventory cannot be conducted on the required date, written permission for an alternate date may be obtained from the nearest DEA field office, provided advance written notification is given to the DEA field office and the new date is within 6 months of the required date.

Inventories and records of schedule II substances must be maintained *separately* from all other records of the office. Schedule III, IV, and V inventories and records must be maintained separately or otherwise be readily retrievable from the ordinary professional and business records, including computer-generated records.

Although the law requires only periodic review of controlled substances, the medical facility may elect to take inventory and update records more frequently on a voluntary basis. The recommended method is to record the use of each controlled substance at the time it is used. An alternative would be to complete records at the conclusion of each workday. A record of controlled drug use (Fig. 2–4*B*) can be completed each time a controlled substance is administered to a patient. This record of use then can be checked against the inventory, not only at required times but at any time, to account for the inventory on hand and to detect immediately any loss or theft.

ORDER FORMS

Schedule II controlled substances used in the office or in the physician's medical bag may be ordered from suppliers using only the Federal Triplicate Order Form, DEA-222 (Fig. 2–5).

Form DEA-224a (8/90)

RENEWAL
APPLICATION FOR DEA REGISTRATION
UNDER
CONTROLLED SUBSTANCES ACT OF 1970

*Read Instructions Before
Completing Application*

No registration may be issued unless a completed
application form has been received (21 CFR 1301.21)

If Drug Schedule(s) checked under Item 1 differ
from that shown at the right, check this box.
☐

REGISTRANT BUSINESS NAME AND ADDRESS

OMB No. 1117-0014

DEA
REGISTRATION
NUMBER

YOUR CURRENT
REGISTRATION
EXPIRES ON

RETURN *THIS* APPLICATION
with $60 FEE
MAKE *CHECK OR MONEY ORDER* PAYABLE TO:
DRUG ENFORCEMENT ADMINISTRATION
AND
RETURN COMPLETED APPLICATION
IN ATTACHED ENVELOPE.

FOR INFORMATION: Call **(202) 307-7255**
See "Privacy Act" Information on Reverse

1. DRUG SCHEDULES: (Check ☑ all applicable schedules in which you intend to handle controlled substances — see reverse of Instruction sheet.)

SCHEDULE 2	SCHEDULE 2N	SCHEDULE 3	SCHEDULE 3N	SCHEDULE 4	SCHEDULE 5
☐ NARCOTIC	☐ NONNARCOTIC	☐ NARCOTIC	☐ NONNARCOTIC	☐	☐

2. **ALL APPLICANTS MUST ANSWER THE FOLLOWING:**

STATE LICENSE

(a) Are you currently authorized to prescribe, distribute, dispense, conduct research, or otherwise handle the controlled substances in the schedules for which you are applying, under the laws of the **State** or jurisdiction in which you are operating or propose to operate?

☐ YES-**State** License Number(s) _____

State Controlled Substance
License No. (If required) _____

☐ Not Applicable   ☐ Pending

(b) Has the applicant ever been convicted of a crime in connection with controlled substances under State or Federal law, or ever surrendered or had a Federal controlled substance registration revoked, suspended, restricted or denied, or ever had a State professional license or controlled substance registration revoked, suspended, denied, restricted or placed on probation?   ☐ YES   ☐ NO

(c) If the applicant is a corporation (other than a corporation whose stock is owned and traded by the public), association, partnership, or pharmacy, has any officer, partner, stockholder or proprietor been convicted of a crime in connection with controlled substances under State or Federal law, or ever surrendered or had a Federal controlled substance registration revoked, suspended, restricted or denied, or ever had a State professional license or controlled substance registration revoked, suspended, denied, restricted or placed on probation?   ☐ YES   ☐ NO   ☐ NOT APPLICABLE

IF THE ANSWER TO QUESTIONS 2(b) or (c) is YES, include a statement using the space provided on the REVERSE of this part.

Print or Type Name Here - Sign Below   Applicant's Business Phone No.

**SIGN
HERE** ▶ _____
Signature of applicant or authorized individual   Date

A   Title (If the applicant is a corporation, institution, or other entity, enter the TITLE of the person signing on behalf of the applicant. (e.g., President, Dean, Procurement Officer, etc.....))

3. **CERTIFICATION FOR FEE EXEMPTION**

☐ CHECK THIS BLOCK IF INDIVIDUAL NAMED HEREON IS A FEDERAL, STATE, OR LOCAL OFFICIAL.
The Undersigned hereby certifies that the applicant herein is an officer or employee of a Federal, State or local agency who, in the course of such employment, is authorized to obtain, dispense, or prescribe controlled substances or is authorized to conduct research, instructional activity or chemical analysis with controlled substances, and is exempt from the payment of this application fee.

Signature of Certifying Official   Date

Print or Type Name

Print or Type Title

Name of Institution or Agency

WARNING: SECTION 843 (a) (4) OF TITLE 21, UNITED STATES CODE, STATES THAT ANY PERSON WHO KNOWINGLY OR INTENTIONALLY FURNISHES FALSE OR FRAUDULENT INFORMATION IN THIS APPLICATION IS SUBJECT TO IMPRISONMENT FOR NOT MORE THAN FOUR YEARS, A FINE OF NOT MORE THAN $30,000.00 OR BOTH.

All inquiries relating to your DEA registration must be directed to the following:

TELEPHONE INQUIRIES
Call: (202) 307-7255

WRITTEN INQUIRIES
Drug Enforcement Administration - ODRR
Washington, D.C. 20537

• Explanation for answering "Yes", to question(s) 2 (b) or (c):

Applicants who have answered "yes" to questions 2(b) or (c) are required to submit a statement explaining such response(s). The space provided below should be used for this purpose and must be separately signed. If this response involves the revocation, suspension or restriction of a Federal controlled substance registration, provide your previous registration number and the circumstances of its revocation, suspension or restriction. If this response involves the revocation, suspension or restriction of a State professional license or controlled substance registration, provide the license and/or registration number, the names of the issuing state and agency and the circumstances.

PRINT or TYPE Name Here - Sign Below

▶ _____
Signature

▶ _____
Date

PRIVACY ACT INFORMATION

AUTHORITY: Section 302 and 303 of the Controlled Substances Act of 1970 (PL 91-513)

PURPOSE: To obtain information required to register applicants pursuant to the Controlled Substances Act of 1970

ROUTINE USES: The Controlled Substance Act Registration Records produces special reports as required for statistical analytical purposes. Disclosures of information from this system are made to the following categories of users for the purposes stated:

A. Other Federal law enforcement and regulatory agencies for law enforcement and regulatory purposes.

B. State and local law enforcement and regulatory agencies for law enforcement and regulatory purposes.

C. Persons registered under the Controlled Substances Act (Public Law 91-513) for the purpose of verifying the registration of customers and practitioners.

B   EFFECT: Failure to complete form will preclude processing of the application.

FIGURE 2–3. Renewal Application for DEA Registration. (*A*) Front. (*B*) Back.

```
Registrant Name: _John Ho, M.D._    DEA Reg.#: _AD0000000_
Address: __1 Main Street_____
City St Zip: __Anytown, US  00000-0000_____

Inventory of Schedule:  II /X/     III,IV,V /_/

Inventory Date: _1/1/98_____

Inventory Time: Opening of business /X/
                Close of business  /_/
```

Drug/Preparation	#Containers	Contents[+]	CS Content[++]
morphine sulfate tabs	3 pkgs	100 tabs	1/4 gr(16mg)
Demerol HCl ampule	10	1.0 ml	25 mg
Percocet	1 btl	50 tabs	5.0 mg

The above stock controlled substances was inventoried by the person(s) signed below, who attest(s) that the above inventory is maintained at the location appearing at the top of this inventory and has been maintained at the location appearing at the top of this inventory for at least two years.

Jane Smith, CMA
Inventoried by

Sara Joy, CMA
Inventoried by

[+] Number of grams, tablets, ounces, or other units per container.
[++]Controlled substance content of each unit.

A

Drug Name	Patient	Dose	Date	Hour	MD	MA

Reviewed by   Reviewed by
_____, CMA   _____, MD

B

FIGURE 2–4. (*A*) Sample inventory of controlled substances. (*B*) Controlled Substance Patient Use Record.

See Reverse of PURCHASER'S Copy for Instructions	No order form may be issued for Schedule I and II substances unless a completed application form has been received. (21 CFR 1305.04).		OMB APPROVAL No. 1117-0010

TO: (Name of Supplier) ACME WHOLESALE DRUGS   STREET ADDRESS 600 NORTH AVE

CITY and STATE ANYTOWN, USA   DATE TODAY'S DATE

LINE No.	No. of Packages	Size of Package	Name of Item	NATIONAL DRUG CODE	No. of Packages Received	Date Received
1	3	100	Sodium pentothal Capsules, 100 mg	| | | | | | | | | | | |	3	0/0/9-
2	2	100	Secobarbital Capsules, 100 mg	| | | | | | | | | | | |	2	0/0/9-
3	3	100	Desoxyn Tablets, 5 mg	| | | | | | | | | | | |	3	0/0/9-
4	1	30 ml	Demerol, 50 mg/ml	| | | | | | | | | | | |	1	0/0/9-
5	2	PINT	Robitussin A-C, 2 mg/ml	| | | | | | | | | | | |	2	0/0/9-
6				| | | | | | | | | | | |		
7				| | | | | | | | | | | |		
8				| | | | | | | | | | | |		
9				| | | | | | | | | | | |		
10				| | | | | | | | | | | |		

5 ◄ NO. OF LINES COMPLETED   SIGNATURE OF PURCHASER OR HIS ATTORNEY OR AGENT

Date Issued 12/31/97   DEA Registration No. AD.000000   Name and Address of Registrant

Schedules 2,2N,3,3N,4,5

Registered as a Practitioner   No. of this Order Form PO 123456

JAMES HO, M.D.
1 MAIN STREET
ANYWHERE, USA 55555-0000

DEA Form -222 (Aug. 1990)

U.S. OFFICIAL ORDER FORMS - SCHEDULES I & II
DRUG ENFORCEMENT ADMINISTRATION
PURCHASER'S Copy 3

FIGURE 2–5. The Federal Triplicate Order Form is used to order schedule C-II controlled substances.

Initial order forms are requested by checking block 3 of the Application Form, DEA-224 (see Fig. 2–2). Checking block 3 ensures that the DEA will mail a first book of Federal Triplicate Order Forms and a separate Requisition Form DEA-222a (see Fig. 2–3) is used to order more Federal Triplicate Order Form books. There is no charge for additional books.

Physicians purchasing schedules III through V controlled substances do not have to use the Federal Triplicate Order Form; however, records of suppliers' invoices or a log book must be maintained for a 2-year period, preferably using the same information as on the federal form DEA-222. It is advisable to include the date of receipt and quantity received on the invoice or in the log book. For schedule III through V substances, the supplier is still under obligation to verify that the physician has a current, valid registration.

SECURITY

DEA registrants are required by regulation to maintain security for the storage and distribution of controlled substances. Controlled substances must be kept separate from other drugs and placed in a securely locked, substantially constructed cabinet, and the stock of controlled substances should be kept to a minimum. If larger amounts are necessary, the office should at least have an alarm system and a highly rated safe. At all times, access to controlled substances should be restricted to an absolute minimum number of employees.

In the case of theft or loss of office inventory, the DEA field office must be notified immediately. The field office will provide information on what reports will need to be filed. The physician will need to complete Form DEA-106, Report of Theft or Loss of Controlled Substances (Fig. 2–6). In cases of theft, the facility is required to notify also the local police department. It is important to note that *any* theft or loss is significant and, under public reporting regulations, must be reported, even if the loss is a single tablet or a single unit dose.

In cases of damaged or contaminated controlled substances, the local DEA office should be contacted for disposal instructions and to request the disposal Form DEA-41. The local office will guide you through the procedures.

U.S. DEPARTMENT OF JUSTICE / DRUG ENFORCEMENT ADMINISTRATION
REPORT OF THEFT OR LOSS OF CONTROLLED SUBSTANCES

OMB APPROVAL
No. 1117-0001

DEA MANUAL AUTHORITY:
Diversion Investigators 5124
FFS: 630-02

Federal Regulations require registrants to submit a detailed report of any theft or loss of Controlled Substances to the Drug Enforcement Administration.
Complete the front and back of this form in triplicate. Forward the original and duplicate copies to the nearest DEA Office. Retain the triplicate copy for your records. Some states may also require a copy of this report.

1. NAME AND ADDRESS OF REGISTRANT (Include ZIP Code)

ZIP CODE

2. PHONE NO. (Include Area Code)

3. DEA REGISTRATION NUMBER

2 ltr. prefix   7 digit suffix

4. DATE OF THEFT OR LOSS

5. PRINCIPAL BUSINESS OF REGISTRANT (Check one)

1 ☐ Pharmacy   5 ☐ Distributor
2 ☐ Practitioner   6 ☐ Methadone Program
3 ☐ Manufacturer   7 ☐ Other (specify)
4 ☐ Hospital/Clinic

6. COUNTY IN WHICH REGISTRANT IS LOCATED

7. WAS THEFT REPORTED TO POLICE?

☐ YES   ☐ NO

8. NAME AND TELEPHONE NUMBER OF POLICE DEPARTMENT (Include Area Code)

9. NUMBER OF THEFTS OR LOSSES REGISTRANT HAS EXPERIENCED IN THE PAST 24 MONTHS ?

10. TYPE OF THEFT OR LOSS (Check one and complete items below as appropriate)

1 ☐ Night break-in   3 ☐ Employee pilferage   5 ☐ Other (Explain)
2 ☐ Armed robbery   4 ☐ Customer theft   6 ☐ Lost in transit (Complete Item 14)

11. IF ARMED ROBBERY, WAS ANYONE:

KILLED ?   ☐ No   ☐ Yes (How many) _____
INJURED ? ☐ No   ☐ Yes (How many) _____

12. PURCHASE VALUE TO REGISTRANT OF CONTROLLED SUBSTANCES TAKEN ?

$

13. WERE ANY PHARMACEUTICALS OR MERCHANDISE TAKEN ?

☐ No   ☐ Yes (Est. Value)

$

14. IF LOST IN TRANSIT, COMPLETE THE FOLLOWING:

A. Name of Common Carrier

B. Name of Consignee

C. Consignee's DEA Registration Number

D. Was the carton received by the customer ?

☐ Yes   ☐ No

E. If received, did it appear to be tampered with ?

☐ Yes   ☐ No

F. Have you experienced losses in transit from this same carrier in the past ?

☐ No   ☐ Yes (How Many) _____

15. WHAT IDENTIFYING MARKS, SYMBOLS, OR PRICE CODES WERE ON THE LABELS OF THESE CONTAINERS THAT WOULD ASSIST IN IDENTIFYING THE PRODUCTS ?

16. IF OFFICIAL CONTROLLED SUBSTANCE ORDER FORMS (DEA-222) WERE STOLEN, GIVE NUMBERS

17. WHAT SECURITY MEASURES HAVE BEEN TAKEN TO PREVENT FUTURE THEFTS OR LOSSES ?

DEA Form (Dec. 1985) — **106**   Previous edition dated 3/83 is OBSOLETE.   CONTINUE ON REVERSE

A

FIGURE 2–6. Report of Theft or Loss of Controlled Substances Form. (*A*) Front.

LIST OF CONTROLLED SUBSTANCES LOST

Trade Name of Substance or Preparation	Name of Controlled Substance in Preparation	Dosage Strength and Form	Quantity
Examples: Desoxyn	Methamphetamine Hydrochloride	5 Mg Tablets	3 x 100
Demerol	Meperidine Hydrochloride	50 Mg/ml Vial	5 x 30 ml
Robitussin A-C	Codeine Phosphate	2 Mg/cc Liquid	12 Pints
1.			
2.			
3.			
4.			
5.			
6.			
7.			
8.			
9.			
10.			
11.			
12.			
13.			
14.			
15.			
16.			
17.			
18.			
19.			
20.			
21.			
22.			
23.			
24.			
25.			
26.			
27.			
28.			
29.			
30.			
31.			
32.			
33.			
34.			
35.			
36.			
37.			
38.			
39.			
40.			
41.			
42.			
43.			
44.			
45.			
46.			
47.			
48.			
49.			
50.			

I certify that the foregoing information is correct to the best of my knowledge and belief.

Signature   Title   Date

☆U.S. GOVERNMENT PRINTING OFFICE: 1988 - 241-707/9555

B

FIGURE 2–6 (*Continued*). (*B*) Back.

Prescription Orders

Regardless of a drug's classification or whether or not it is a controlled substance, the way in which a physician prescribes or orders that drug is regulated. The physician and everyone who approves or interacts with a drug order must follow certain protocols. It is the physician, physician assistant, or nurse practitioner who initiates the order for a prescription medication. In the office, the physician may write the order on a prescription form and give it to the patient to have filled at a local pharmacy, or may actually dispense the medication from the office supply. For legal documentation, the physician or the medical assistant will note on the patient's record the medication order and, if applicable, that the medication was dispensed to the patient. The usual rules for charting apply. Each medication entry must document the date (and time, if necessary), the name of the medication, the strength, the amount, directions to the patient, route, technique (if applicable), and signature. Chart the entries without skipping lines. Blank spaces can be filled inadvertently with misinformation. For example:

1/1/90 T:100.4 P:80 R:16 BP:130/68

CC: Patient complains of fever, chills, sore throat, cough, and muscular pain. Dx: Viral URI with secondary bronchitis. Tx: Bed rest, fluids, ASA. Rx: Amoxil 250 mg; Disp: #28; Sig: qid; refill 1×. 1/1/90 Med disp to pt per Dr's order. Sara Ivy (signature of health professional)

Except for schedule II drugs, the physician may hand an order to the medical assistant to transmit by telephone order to the pharmacist. In these cases, the patient may have been seen in the office or at home, or may have consulted with the physician by telephone, and may not be able to take a written prescription to the pharmacy.

The authority for prescribing cannot be delegated to anyone else. However, the medical assistant making calls to or receiving calls from pharmacists regarding a new prescription may act as the physician's agent and transmit the physician's order.

For verbal prescription orders, first the physician writes the prescription order in the patient's medical record, then the medical assistant uses the record to relay the order to the pharmacist. If the physician writes the order on a notepad, the medical assistant may call in the order, then enter the order on the patient's record and place the record on the physician's desk for initialing or signature. The patient's record must include every prescription ordered, including refills, whether or not the patient was seen in the office.

Some physicians prefer to call the pharmacies directly. The medical assistant obtains the name and phone number of the pharmacy from the patient and either the medical assistant or the physician calls in the order. Other physicians prefer that the pharmacists call their offices. In this case, the medical assistant instructs the patient to call the pharmacy and give the pharmacist the doctor's name and phone number.

Either way, it is the medical assistant's responsibility to see that the order is relayed to the pharmacist within a reasonable time. Written orders should not be filed until one is sure the pharmacist has been called and has received the information.

The same rules apply for patients requesting refills. Each refill must be treated as a new prescription. The medical assistant is not authorized to approve a refill request, by either a patient or a pharmacist, no matter what the drug may be. If the physician intends for a patient to be able to refill a prescription at will, the physician will designate a refill "prn" on the original prescription. All refill requests must be (1) approved by the physician and (2) entered on the patient's record. There may be standing orders or protocols in a practice to cover specific situations.

The pharmacist is the physician's partner in the patient treatment plan. Medical assistants must always respond to pharmacist telephone calls immediately. If the pharmacist telephones to verify information about a prescription order, the call should be transferred or the information relayed immediately to the physician.

THE PRESCRIPTION FORM

The prescription is written in a very traditional manner, and it contains eight parts (Fig. 2–7):

1. Date. Federal drug laws limit the length of time that a prescription may be filled—usually to 6 months.
2. Full name and address of the patient. This section may also include the patient's age, which may alert the pharmacist to potential age-related needs of the patient, and which also makes it more difficult for someone to use another person's prescription.
3. Superscription. This is the symbol "Rx," which is the abbreviation for the Latin word *recipe* and means "take."
4. Inscription. This is the main body of the order. It includes the name of the drug, the dosage form, and the amount of the dose (strength).
5. Subscription. This section includes the amount to be dispensed and any special directions to the pharmacist for preparing the drug.
6. Signature. This is written on the form as "Sig," which is the abbreviation for the Latin *signetur* and means "write on label." This section is labeling information for the patient and includes instructions such as the time and frequency of the dose, storage information, food precautions, and so on.
7. Refill information. Federal law regulates the number and frequency of refills allowed for certain controlled substances. If refills are not authorized, this should be specified on the form. Refills are authorized by writing in the number of times a prescription may be refilled or "prn" for prescriptions that may be refilled whenever the patient needs more medication.
8. Physician's signature. The physician's manual signature must be followed by the licensed title of the physician, and DEA number, when applicable to controlled substances.

All prescription orders are dated as of, and signed by the physician on, the day of issue and should include the full name and address of the patient, and the name, address, and registration number (when applicable) of the physician. The physician signs a prescription order in the same manner as a legal document. Where a verbal order is not permitted by law, the prescription must be written in ink or typewritten and must be manually signed by the physician.

James Ho, MD
1 Main Street
Anywhere, US 00000–00

DEA# AD000000 Phone: 555-1212

Patient: Adam Miller Age: 38
Address: 29 Elmcrest 00506 Date: 1/1/98

Rx Amoxil 250 mg
Disp: #28
Sig: i b.i.d.

Generic OK No
Refill: None, (1) 2, 3, 4, 5

James Ho, M.D.

Copy 1 of 2

FIGURE 2–7. Sample prescription form.

The prescription may be prepared by the medical assistant for the signature of the physician, but the prescribing physician is ultimately responsible in case the prescription order is not medically correct or does not conform to all the essential aspects of the law and regulations.

PRESCRIPTIONS FOR CONTROLLED SUBSTANCES

The guidelines listed here should be followed for all prescription orders for controlled substances. The prescription must be:

1. Dated as of and signed on the date of issue.
2. Completed with the full name and address of the patient.
3. Completed with the name, address, and registration number of the physician.
4. Written in ink or typewritten.
5. Safeguarded by writing out the actual amount prescribed in addition to giving the arabic number or roman numeral (to discourage alterations).
6. Written to avoid orders for large quantities, unless it is absolutely determined by the physician that such quantities are necessary.
7. Manually signed by the physician. The medical assistant may prepare the prescription for signature, however. (Some pharmacists maintain a reference file of physician's signatures as a control against forgery.)
8. Filled with the following patient label: "CAUTION: Federal law prohibits the transfer of this drug to any person other than the patient for whom it was prescribed."

In addition, schedule II prescriptions:

1. Must be written and presented to the pharmacist, except in an emergency (see below).
2. May not be refilled.
3. May require the use of multiple-copy prescriptions. (Although the CSA does not require the physician to maintain copies of prescriptions, certain states require the use of multiple-copy prescriptions) (Fig. 2–8).

Emergency telephone prescription orders for schedule II drugs may be filled under the following conditions:

1. The case is a bona fide emergency; that is, the immediate administration of the drug is necessary, no alternative treatment is available, and it is not possible for the physician to provide a signed, written order for the drug at that time.

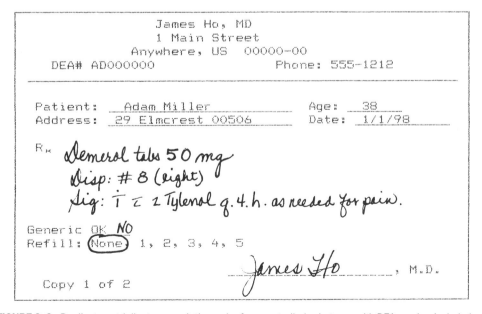

FIGURE 2–8. Duplicate or triplicate prescription order for a controlled substance with DEA number included and "no refill" noted.

2. The drug must be limited to the amount needed only during the emergency period.
3. The physician must furnish a signed, written order to the pharmacy within 72 hours; otherwise, the pharmacist is required to notify the DEA.

Schedules III and IV prescriptions:

1. May be issued orally, by telephone, or in writing to the pharmacist.
2. May include authorized refills up to five times, or within 6 months, whichever occurs first.

Schedule V prescriptions:

1. May be issued orally, by telephone, or in writing to the pharmacist.
2. May include authorized refills up to five times, or within 6 months, whichever occurs first.
3. Some schedule V drugs, such as Robitussin A-C, may be purchased OTC, but must be signed for by the customer.

SAFE CHARTING OF PRESCRIPTIONS

1. Place a space between a number and its unit of measurement.
   correct: 2 mg   incorrect: 2mg
2. Omit periods after abbreviations.
   correct: mg   incorrect: mg.
3. Never place a decimal after a whole number. If the decimal is not seen, the patient would mistakenly receive 10 times the correct dose.
   correct: 2 mg   incorrect: 2.0 mg
4. Always place a decimal and zero before a fraction of a whole number.
   correct: 0.2 ml   incorrect: .2 ml
5. Do not abbreviate the Unit measurement. It could be mistaken for a zero or the abbreviation for micron.
   correct: Unit   incorrect: U
6. Use mcg rather than μg
   correct: mcg   incorrect: μg
7. QD (once daily) can be mistaken for QID (four times a day), 4 times the intended dose or for OD (right eye).
   correct: once daily   incorrect: QD, OD
8. Do not use chemical names. The numbers contained in them can be mistaken for the number of doses to give.
9. Do not abbreviate drug names, as abbreviations can be unrecognizable to others.

WRITING PRESCRIPTIONS

1. Do not abbreviate. Fully written prescriptions prevent tampering with information by others, prevent the pharmacist or patient from making a mistake, and eliminate the need for further clarification.
2. Write out the patient's full name: first, initial, last, and address.
3. Include the age and weight, if possible, for children and the elderly.
4. Write the full name of the drug, dosage form, and strength.
5. Print the full name of the drug, if it is rarely used or a new drug.
6. Always include the number or amount to be dispensed.
7. Include complete patient instructions, including why the medication is being taken.
8. Indicate recognized contraindications for a prescribed drug to eliminate the need for further clarification.

Over-The-Counter Drugs

A medication that may be purchased without a prescription is an OTC drug. These drugs are available to the public for the purposes of self-treating various mild or chronic symptoms.

Just as with prescription drugs, the FDA controls the quality and safety of nonprescription medications. The safety of these drugs is usually not in question: they are considered safe because their dosages are low. Among the considered safe and useful OTC drugs are Tylenol, aspirin, Motrin, and Actifed. These drugs are used to treat pain, fever, or cold symptoms. Motrin and Actifed are two examples of OTC drugs that were previously available by prescription only. Medications frequently ordered and not considered dangerous are becoming available in lower dosage form OTC in increasing numbers. This does not minimize the side effects and dangers of taking medications without the knowledge of the physician. FDA postrelease studies may yet reverse some approvals for drugs sold OTC.

Some OTC drugs have such low dosages, however, that their *effectiveness* is often questioned. Low dosage means that a drug is minimally therapeutic or not therapeutic at all, and most drugs probably exert more of a placebo effect rather than a therapeutic effect. On the other hand, OTC drugs may be overused or manufactured in combination with other chemicals and may be dangerous. Examples of combination drugs are cold remedies that contain several chemicals, each intended for the treatment of different cold symptoms. Although OTC dosages are low, patients may overmedicate themselves, or the combination of chemicals may be undesirable for particular patients or even unsafe. Most people take OTC drugs without reading what is in them or their contraindications for usage. Any drug not used as directed may be potentially life-threatening.

OTC drugs also are used to treat gastrointestinal (GI) disturbances, infections, allergies, constipation, undesired weight gain, and sleep disorders. The public also has access to a great variety of vitamins, minerals, and nutritional supplements for self-diagnosed deficiencies. The main danger with people treating themselves is that self-medicating often delays appropriate and needed medical attention. Likewise, the use of OTC drugs may hide serious underlying conditions.

General patient teaching about OTC medicines should include the following safety measures. Teach patients to:

1. Read package inserts and labels.
2. Use only the recommended dosages for age and weight.
3. Avoid doubling or halving doses.
4. Avoid medicines when directions or indications are unclear.
5. Discard expired or unlabeled medicines.
6. Avoid using tobacco and alcohol with medicines.
7. Avoid combining prescription and OTC medicines, unless advised to do so by the physician.
8. Know all family drug allergies and intolerances before taking or giving a medicine.
9. Be aware that many OTC drugs are contraindicated in pregnant or nursing mothers, small children, and the elderly.
10. Know their pharmacists and to check with their pharmacists if they have any questions.

Another danger is the misuse of OTC drugs. Too often, patients forget that OTC preparations are really drugs. Even the most seemingly harmless drug can result in dependence or interact with other prescribed medications, leading to toxic or other harmful effects.

It is therefore important when collecting a medical history from the patient to ask the patient specifically to report the use of any OTC drug and to take every opportunity to include information about OTC drugs in patient education plans. Here are a few specific teaching points to keep in mind when instructing patients about OTC drugs:

1. Cough and cold remedies often contain caffeine, for no medical reason.
2. Cough and cold remedies often contain combinations that are unessential. For ex-

ample, some combinations contain both an antihistamine and a decongestant. Antihistamines are useful in allergy conditions, but not in conditions that are caused by viral or bacterial infections.

3. Cough and cold remedies cause drowsiness and can impair judgment.

4. Antihistamine cough and cold medicines may cause excitability in children.

5. Nasal spray decongestants can cause rebound (swelling) of nasal tissue and increase rather than relieve nasal congestion, especially after continuous use.

6. Patients receiving long-term antacid therapy should be advised by a physician as to the types of antacids to use. Antacids with magnesium have a laxative effect. Antacids that contain aluminum or calcium have a constipating effect.

7. Sodium bicarbonate is rarely prescribed anymore because of its high sodium content and because it may cause "acid rebound," which is an increase in stomach acid secretions.

8. Bismuth subsalicylates (Pepto-Bismol) contains aspirinlike components, and should not be taken with aspirin or used by patients with aspirin allergy, chickenpox, or flu.

9. Laxatives may cause chronic constipation or may lead to patient psychologic and physical dependency, or both.

10. Laxatives should not be used in the presence of abdominal pain.

11. Vitamin and mineral overdose may produce serious toxic and possible lethal effects, especially in children, pregnant or lactating women, and the elderly.

12. Sleep medications are usually antihistamines and should be used with caution by patients with certain types of glaucoma, with peptic ulcers, and with urinary tract conditions.

13. Ophthalmic preparations should be kept sterile and not used by anyone other than the purchaser.

14. Vaginal douching may mask actual infections or cause a serious imbalance of the delicate normal flora of the vagina, or both.

15. Antiaging skin products have not yet been proved effective, and may cause side effects.

16. Weight-reducing products are ineffective without appropriate and concurrent lifestyle changes.

17. Asthma medicines should be used only in cases of confirmed history of asthma.

Guidelines for the Prevention of Drug Abuse or Misuse

Patients usually comply with the physician's directions for the proper use of medications dispensed to them. However, the physician often must issue to the patient drugs that may be abused or misused, without having any real control of the patient's intended or unintended future actions. Because of this abuse potential, everyone involved in patient care should practice the precautions to prevent the various activities that may be used by patients to obtain prescription drugs illegally or to obtain prescription drugs legally for misuse.

1. Be cautious of patients who self-diagnose and self-prescribe. Patients may falsify illnesses to obtain prescription medications.

2. Carefully monitor patients who habitually telephone for controlled substance refills yet refuse to make appointments to come into the office.

3. Be cautious of a series of new patients all complaining of the same illness.

4. Be cautious of patients who say that other physicians have been prescribing controlled substances for them. Request patient medical records from previous physicians for verification.

5. Inform patients of the effects of prescription drugs and how and why to use them.

6. Keep prescription blanks in a safe and inaccessible place.

7. Minimize the number of prescription pads in use, and keep pads in an assigned place, out of the patient's sight.
8. Do not use prescription blanks as notepads. A drug user could erase the note and forge a prescription order.
9. Never sign prescription orders in advance.
10. Maintain only a minimum stock of controlled substances in the office and in the physician's medical bag.
11. Keep the physician's medical bag safe from public access.
12. Keep careful records of all controlled substances administered, prescribed, or dispensed and of all telephone requests and approvals for refills. After completing a telephone refill, pull the patient's medical record and record the refill on the patient's chart.

In addition to these general office policies, physicians practice careful medicine when they refrain from prescribing excessive quantities of controlled substances or issuing orders for longer periods than needed. These two practices may prevent drug abuse or dependency or keep a patient from diverting the medication to other persons.

Our duty to the patient and to good medical practice, when working with prescriptions and controlled substances in the office, requires a constant interest in and concern about patient health; good judgment and watchfulness of proper drug use; careful documentation, both medically and when required by law; and attention to security.

Written Competency 2–1

Performance Competence: Complete a calendar of federal responsibilities with at least six of the seven duties correct, within 15 minutes. Do not award partial credit for incomplete or incorrect answers.

Complete the following controlled substances calendar of duties and responsibilities by stating what procedures have to be completed on each date.

1. Day 1:

2. Receipt of controlled substances from supplier:

3. Daily:

4. Biennially:

5. Triennially:

6. Moving a practice:

7. Selling a practice:

Score: _____

See Appendix B for answers.

Written Competency 2–2

Performance Competence: Complete the writing of three prescriptions, on the blanks provided, with 100 percent accuracy within 10 minutes. Do not award partial credit for incomplete or incorrect transcription.

1. Patient: John Doe, 115 Main St. Anywhere, USA, age 22. Original prescription: Demerol tablets, 50 mg, 12 tablets. Directions: Take one tablet with two Tylenol every 4 to 6 hours as needed for pain. Use your knowledge of the Controlled Substances Act requirements (Table 2–2) to respond to the patient's request for a refill.

James Ho, MD
1 Main Street
Anywhere, US 00000-00
DEA# AD000000   Phone: 555–1212

_____

Patient: _____ Age: _____
Address: _____ Date: _____

R$_\text{X}$

Generic OK _____
Refill: None, 1, 2, 3, 4, 5

_____, M.D.
Copy 1 of 2   DEA #: _____

---

2. Patient: Mary Jones, 495 West Elm St, Anywhere, USA, age 45. Dispense Darvocet-N 50 mg, 60 tablets. Directions: Take two tablets every 4 hours, not to exceed 600 mg per day. Include the maximum number of refills that would be allowed for this drug under the Controlled Substances Act. No generic substitutes are allowed.

James Ho, MD
1 Main Street
Anywhere, US 00000-00
DEA# AD000000   Phone: 555–1212

_____

Patient: _____ Age: _____
Address: _____ Date: _____

R$_\text{X}$

Generic OK _____
Refill: None, 1, 2, 3, 4, 5

_____, M.D.
Copy 1 of 2   DEA #: _____

---

3. Patient: Jerry Miller, 10 E 29th St, Anywhere, USA, age 65. Dispense Naprosyn 250 mg, 100 tablets. Directions: Take three tablets to start, then one tablet every 8 hours until the pain has subsided. Refill prn.

James Ho, MD
1 Main Street
Anywhere, US 00000-00
DEA# AD000000   Phone: 555–1212

_____

Patient: _____   Age: _____
Address: _____   Date: _____

R$_x$

Generic OK _____
Refill: None, 1, 2, 3, 4, 5

                               _____, M.D.
Copy 1 of 2   DEA #: _____

4. Patient: Jane Wiggs, 123 Main St., age 35 is to receive Amoxil 250 mg by mouth q8h × 10 days; no refills; may use generic. Dispense 30 capsules.

James Ho, MD
1 Main Street
Anywhere, US 00000-00
DEA# AD000000   Phone: 555–1212

_____

Patient: _____   Age: _____
Address: _____   Date: _____

R$_x$

Generic OK _____
Refill: None, 1, 2, 3, 4, 5

                               _____, M.D.
Copy 1 of 2   DEA #: _____

5. Patient: Mary Smith, 1 West St., age 75 is to take Premarin 0.625 by mouth daily. Dispense 60 and refill 6 times and dispense as written.

```
┌─────────────────────────────────────────┐
│             James Ho, MD                 │
│             1 Main Street                │
│           Anywhere, US 00000-00          │
│      DEA# AD000000     Phone: 555–1212   │
│   _____  │
│                                          │
│   Patient: _____  Age: _____ │
│   Address: _____   Date: _____ │
│                                          │
│   Rx                                     │
│                                          │
│                                          │
│   Generic OK _____                    │
│   Refill: None,  1,  2,  3,  4,  5       │
│                                          │
│                         _____, M.D.│
│   Copy 1 of 2          DEA #: _____    │
└─────────────────────────────────────────┘
```

6. Patient: Joe Baker, 1512 North Ave., age 21 to receive Tylenol #3. Take 1 or 2 by mouth as needed for pain, dispense 30; no refills; may substitute.

```
┌─────────────────────────────────────────┐
│             James Ho, MD                 │
│             1 Main Street                │
│           Anywhere, US 00000-00          │
│      DEA# AD000000      Phone: 555–1212  │
│   _____  │
│                                          │
│   Patient: _____  Age: _____ │
│   Address: _____   Date: _____ │
│                                          │
│   Rx                                     │
│                                          │
│                                          │
│   Generic OK _____                    │
│   Refill: None,  1,  2,  3,  4,  5       │
│                                          │
│                         _____, M.D.│
│   Copy 1 of 2          DEA #: _____    │
└─────────────────────────────────────────┘
```

7. Patient: Nancy Jones, 550 Atlantic Ave., age 67 to receive Lanoxin 125 mcg by mouth every morning. Dispense 30, check pulse before taking; withhold if pulse below 50 and call doctor; refill 12 times; dispense as written.

```
┌─────────────────────────────────────────────┐
│              James Ho, MD                     │
│              1 Main Street                    │
│           Anywhere, US 00000-00               │
│     DEA# AD000000     Phone: 555–1212         │
│   ─────────────────────────────────────       │
│                                               │
│   Patient: _____   Age: _____   │
│   Address: _____    Date: _____    │
│                                               │
│   Rₓ                                          │
│                                               │
│                                               │
│   Generic OK _____                         │
│   Refill: None,  1,  2,  3,  4,  5            │
│                                               │
│                            _____, M.D.  │
│   Copy 1 of 2          DEA #: _____         │
└─────────────────────────────────────────────┘
```

8. Patient: Jack Smith, 1531 South St., age 48, to take Coumadin 3 mg by mouth every evening, dispense 300–1 mg tabs to take 3 tabs each day; refill 3 times; dispense as written.

```
┌─────────────────────────────────────────────┐
│              James Ho, MD                     │
│              1 Main Street                    │
│           Anywhere, US 00000-00               │
│     DEA# AD000000     Phone: 555–1212         │
│   ─────────────────────────────────────       │
│                                               │
│   Patient: _____   Age: _____   │
│   Address: _____    Date: _____    │
│                                               │
│   Rₓ                                          │
│                                               │
│                                               │
│   Generic OK _____                         │
│   Refill: None,  1,  2,  3,  4,  5            │
│                                               │
│                            _____, M.D.  │
│   Copy 1 of 2          DEA #: _____         │
└─────────────────────────────────────────────┘
```

9. Patient: John Max, 324 Main St., age 23, to receive Biaxin 500 mg by mouth bid for 14 days; may refill one time. Dispense 28.

```
              James Ho, MD
              1 Main Street
           Anywhere, US 00000-00
      DEA# AD000000    Phone: 555–1212
      _____


      Patient: _____   Age: _____
      Address: _____    Date: _____

      Rx



      Generic OK _____
      Refill: None,  1,  2,  3,  4,  5


                           _____, M.D.
      Copy 1 of 2          DEA #: _____
```

10. Patient: Pat Reed, 475 West St., age 58, to take Furosemide 40mg each am; dispense 30; may substitute, refill 12 times.

```
              James Ho, MD
              1 Main Street
           Anywhere, US 00000-00
      DEA# AD000000    Phone: 555–1212
      _____


      Patient: _____   Age: _____
      Address: _____    Date: _____

      Rx



      Generic OK _____
      Refill: None,  1,  2,  3,  4,  5


                           _____, M.D.
      Copy 1 of 2          DEA #: _____
```

11. Patient: Denise Jones, 980 Atlantic Ave., age 19, take Ortho Novum 7/7/7-28; take 1 each am; dispense 12 months.

```
┌─────────────────────────────────────────────┐
│                                             │
│                 James Ho, MD                │
│                 1 Main Street               │
│              Anywhere, US 00000-00          │
│        DEA# AD000000     Phone: 555–1212    │
│        ─────────────────────────────────    │
│                                             │
│                                             │
│     Patient: _____   Age: _____ │
│     Address: _____    Date: _____  │
│                                             │
│     Rₓ                                      │
│                                             │
│                                             │
│                                             │
│     Generic OK _____                     │
│     Refill: None, 1, 2, 3, 4, 5             │
│                                             │
│                         _____, M.D.   │
│     Copy 1 of 2         DEA #: _____      │
│                                             │
└─────────────────────────────────────────────┘
```

12. Patient: Jack Jones, 5934 Main St., age 35, take Prozac 20 mg by mouth bid; dispense 60; refill 2 times; may substitute.

```
┌─────────────────────────────────────────────┐
│                                             │
│                 James Ho, MD                │
│                 1 Main Street               │
│              Anywhere, US 00000-00          │
│        DEA# AD000000     Phone: 555–1212    │
│        ─────────────────────────────────    │
│                                             │
│                                             │
│     Patient: _____   Age: _____ │
│     Address: _____    Date: _____  │
│                                             │
│     Rₓ                                      │
│                                             │
│                                             │
│                                             │
│     Generic OK _____                     │
│     Refill: None, 1, 2, 3, 4, 5             │
│                                             │
│                         _____, M.D.   │
│     Copy 1 of 2         DEA #: _____      │
│                                             │
└─────────────────────────────────────────────┘
```

See Appendix B for answers.

Score: _____

Terminal Performance Objective/Competency

Procedure 2–1: Complete a Federal Triplicate Order Form (DEA-222) for Schedule II Controlled Substances

EQUIPMENT	Form DEA-222 Physician's Registration Certificate (see Fig. 2–1)

ORDER

(See form on page 62)

Three packages of sodium pentobarbital capsules, 100 mg, 100 capsules; 2 packages of secobarbital capsules, 100 mg, 100 capsules; three bottles of Desoxyn tablets, 5 mg, 100 tablets; one 30-ml vial Demerol, 50 mg per ml; 2 pt Robitussin A-C, 2 mg per ml liquid.

Part I Performance Competence: Complete the Federal Triplicate Order Form (DEA-222) for schedule II controlled substances in mailable quality (so that the form will not be returned by the supplier) and within reasonable job production time, as stated by your evaluator.

Part II Performance Competence: Complete the Federal Triplicate Order Form representing receipt of the entire order accurately and within reasonable job production time, as stated by your evaluator.

	V	**S**	**U** *
PROCEDURAL STEPS 1. Use ink or typewriter.	☐	☐	☐
2. Copies 1 and 2 must not be separated nor the carbon removed, or suppliers will refuse to fill the order.	☐	☐	☐
3. The triplicate copy is to be retained by the office, at the registered address, and be available for inspection by the DEA for at least 2 years after the date of the order.	☐	☐	☐
4. Do not erase errors or make alterations. If you make an error, void and keep on file.	☐	☐	☐
5. If more than 10 items are ordered, additional order forms must be used.	☐	☐	☐
6. The order must be dated as the day it is submitted for filing and signed by the physician exactly as the registration is signed.	☐	☐	☐
7. Only one item may be entered on a single line. A line item is any number of units with the same description—that is, the same drug and same size of container.	☐	☐	☐
8. Enter the number of items ordered or the supplier will refuse to fill the order.	☐	☐	☐

---

*V = Value, to be filled in if assigning points or other specific values to each step.
 S = Satisfactory completion of the step.
 U = Unsatisfactory completion of the step or step incomplete; needs more practice.

9. Fill in the remaining blocks using the information on the Registration Certificate (see Fig. 2–1).   ☐ ☐ ☐

10. Assume receipt of all schedule II items. Date the receipt and enter the number of items received in the spaces provided on the right hand side of the triplicate copy.   ☐ ☐ ☐

11. Initial by date received.   ☐ ☐ ☐

See Reverse of PURCHASER'S **Copy for Instructions**	No order form may be issued for Schedule I and II substances unless a completed application form has been received, (21 CFR 1305.04).	**OMB APPROVAL** **No. 1117-0010**
TO: *(Name of Supplier)*	STREET ADDRESS	

CITY and STATE			DATE		NATIONAL DRUG CODE	TO BE FILLED IN BY PURCHASER	
L I N E No	____ **TO BE FILLED IN BY PURCHASER** ____					No. of Packages Received	Date Received
	No. of Packages	Size of Package	Name of Item				
1							
2							
3							
4							
5							
6							
7							
8							
9							
10							

◀ **NO. OF LINES COMPLETED**   SIGNATURE OF PURCHASER OR HIS ATTORNEY OR AGENT

Date Issued	DEA Registration No.	Name and Address of Registrant
Schedules **2 , 2N, 3 , 3N , 4 , 5**		
Registered as a	No. of this Order Form	

DEA Form -222
(Aug 1990)

U.S. OFFICIAL ORDER FORMS - SCHEDULES I & II
DRUG ENFORCEMENT ADMINISTRATION
PURCHASER'S Copy 3

Date: _____ Competency achieved: Y _____ N _____

Designated reasonable time standard: _____

Actual completion time: _____

Terminal Performance Objective/Competency

Procedure 2–2: Transmit a Prescription Order to the Pharmacist

EQUIPMENT

Patient chart with order
Pharmacy telephone number
Audio tape cassette and tape recorder

ORDER

For: Andrew Smith, age 2 years, 800 Eastern Avenue, New York, NY 10011
Rx: Spectra suspension
300 ml
Sig: 1 tsp q12h × 10 days for otitis media.
Shake well, refrigerate, drink lots of water.
Ref: None. Substitution: None.

Performance Competence: Using an audio cassette tape, simulate a telephone call to a pharmacist and transmit the foregoing order with complete accuracy and within a reasonable time so that the pharmacist is not delayed in his or her duties.

	V	S	U*
PROCEDURAL STEPS			
1. Have the written order in front of you.	☐	☐	☐
2. Check to be sure you understand the order.	☐	☐	☐
3. Confirm any unusual order with the physician.	☐	☐	☐
4. Place your call and ask to speak to the pharmacist.	☐	☐	☐
5. State the name of the physician and that you are calling in a prescription for a certain patient.	☐	☐	☐
6. State the name of the drug.	☐	☐	☐
7. State the drug strength (such as mg or gr).	☐	☐	☐
8. State the amount to be dispensed (number of tablets, oz, and so on).	☐	☐	☐
9. State the directions to the patient.	☐	☐	☐
10. State the refill authorization.	☐	☐	☐
11. State whether or not a generic substitution is permissible.	☐	☐	☐
12. Wait for the pharmacist to read back the order and confirm.	☐	☐	☐
13. If it has not already been done, record the order on the patient's chart.	☐	☐	☐
14. Place the chart on the physician's desk for initialing or signature.	☐	☐	☐

*V = Value, to be filled in if assigning points or other specific values to each step.
S = Satisfactory completion of the step.
U = Unsatisfactory completion of the step or step incomplete; needs more practice.

Date: _____ Competency achieved: Y _____ N _____

Designated reasonable time standard: _____

Actual completion time: _____

Conversion Drill for Skill

Using Table 1–7 and the conversion formula, convert the following within 10 minutes. Do not give yourself credit for partial or incorrect answers. Strive for a score of 100 percent. If you score less than 100 percent, return to Chapter 1, and reread the section on conversions.

1. 1/60 gr   = _____ mg

2. 1/300 mg = _____ g

3. 5 mcg   = _____ mg

4. 10 kg   = _____ lb

5. 2 tsp   = _____ ml

6. 30 minims = _____ ml

7. 256 oz   = _____ gal

8. 88 lb   = _____ kg

9. 300 mg   = _____ gr

10. 0.5 ml   = _____ minims

11. 132 lbs   = _____ Kg

12. gr 1/6   = _____ mg

13. 250 mcg   = _____ mg

14. 1500 cc   = _____ L

15. 600 ml   = _____ oz

16. gtt xx   = _____ cc

17. 300 mg   = _____ gr

18. 0.75 g   = _____ mg

19. gr xv   = _____ g

20. dram vii = _____ cc

21. 12 oz   = _____ ml

22. 12.5 cc   = _____ ml

23. 30 mg   = _____ gr

24. 44 Kg   = _____ lb

25. 1/150 gr = _____ mcg

Score: _____

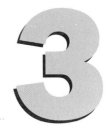

Forms of Medication and Patient Care Applications

OBJECTIVES

WRITTEN COMPETENCY 3–1: Identify the various forms of medication and the general rules for their use.

TERMINAL PERFORMANCE OBJECTIVE (PROCEDURE 3–1): Divide or crush tablets for preparing fractions of a dose.

CONVERSION DRILL FOR SKILL: Convert measurements to their most frequently used approximate equivalents.

History of Drug Forms

From the beginning of recorded time, humans have used plants, minerals, and animal sources for medicinal purposes, for religious ceremonies, and for their mystical and magic powers. Eventually, a great deal of healing knowledge was learned and passed down from generation to generation through medicine lore. Over time, primitive humankind gradually learned those plants, fruits, and barks that were good food to eat, those that caused discomfort or poisoning, those that could be used for healing effects, and even those that could be used to create psychologic changes such as euphoria and hallucination.

Early in the 19th century, chemical science began to flourish. Chemists were able to extract pure substances from plants and animals, and these purer forms began to replace the more natural but crude drug forms. In 1805, the first pure drug extracted from a plant was that of morphine refined from opium. Later in the same century, pharmacology was further advanced through discoveries in organic synthetic chemistry, and laboratory techniques were developed to manufacture artificial substances once found only in nature. One of the first synthesized drugs was salicylate. Synthesized salicylate was combined with natural acetic acid to form acetylsalicylic acid, or aspirin.

In the 20th century, both pure chemicals, isolated and extracted from natural substances, and synthetic substitutes, resembling organic chemicals in nature, are used separately and in combination in drug therapy. Although we no longer think of our medications as being locally gathered from the floors of rain forests, it is estimated that less than 1 percent of the plants inhabiting this earth have been discovered. The continued search for new medicinal cures from natural substances is as equally important as developing new synthetic substances in the laboratory.

From primitive humanity to modern medicine, certain forms for dispensing pharmaceutic products have evolved. Some forms, like the mineral oils, are used today just as they were 1500 years ago, yet other forms, such as dermal patches, have been introduced only within the last few years. Today drugs are manufactured, prepared, and used in a large variety of solid and liquid dosage forms.

Solid Preparations

Solid preparations are the most commonly used medication forms in most medical settings. Solid preparations include tablets, capsules, powders, and crystals, usually for oral dosages. Tablets and capsules are most often available in the dosage ordered, but occasionally instructions must be given to patients who must self-administer fractions of tablets at home.

The physician usually orders tablets and capsules by the number of tablets or capsules to be given. Tablets and capsules are available in dosages of grams, milligrams, micrograms, or grains. Certain drugs are available in one dosage size only. In this case the physician may order simply by the number of tablets (e.g., one tablet four times a day). However, tetracycline (Achromycin) dosage is available in both 250-mg capsules and 500-mg capsules. In this case, the physician must state both the number *and* the capsule strength (e.g., 250 mg, one tablet four times a day).

Powders and crystals are measured and added to liquids before use. If a drug is not available in a pediatric liquid or tablet form, children's doses may also be prepared by grinding tablets into a powder and dissolving the powder in a specific amount of water. Fractions of a dose can then be measured in a syringe or medicine cup. Specific instructions for this will be discussed in Chapter 7.

The types of solid preparations are described here in alphabetic order. In addition, examples of each type and special patient education sections are included.

1. *Buccal tablet*—tablet that is placed in the buccal cavity (the area between the gum and cheek). These tablets are designed to dissolve rapidly for absorption by the venous capillaries in the mouth.

   Example: Nitroglycerin (vasodilator, used for angina pectoris)

   PATIENT EDUCATION: Instruct the patient not to swallow or chew the tablet and not to take the tablet with water. Water would dissolve the tablet and prevent capillary absorption.

2. *Buffered tablet*—solid preparation combined with buffering agents such as aluminum glycinate and magnesium carbonate. Buffering agents may be used to decrease the amount of acid (pH) in a drug, which can reduce the frequency and severity of stomach irritation. Whether or not buffering tablets are actually effective is controversial, however.

   Example: Bufferin (a drug used to reduce fever, inflammation, and pain)

3. *Caplet*—solid, compressed powder or granules in the shape of a capsule, sometimes coated for easy swallowing (Fig. 3–1*A*).

   Example: Motrin, Advil, Aleve, Naprosyn, Daypro, or Medipren caplets (used to reduce inflammation and pain)

4. *Capsule*—gelatin-coated powder or granules that dissolve in stomach acids or occasionally in the intestine (Fig. 3–1*B*). They are often sealed for protection from altering the use or content of the drug.

   Example: Benadryl capsules (used primarily to reduce allergic reactions)

5. *Compact*—medication-dispensing container designed as a daily reminder (Fig. 3–1*C*). It holds medication for 1 month and is usually used for dispensing birth control pills over a 21-day or 28-day period.

   Example: Ortho-Novum 7/7/7 (used for birth control)

6. *Enteric-coated tablet*—tablets covered with a substance that delays the dissolution of drugs that may cause nausea or vomiting if they come into contact with the stomach lining. Enteric-coated medications are dissolved not by gastric acids but by the alkaline secretions in the upper part of the intestine.

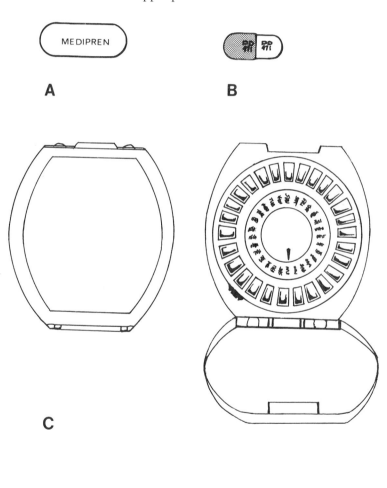

A

B

C

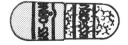

D

FIGURE 3–1. Examples of the various drug forms. (*A*) Caplet. (*B*) Capsule. (*C*) Compact containing 1 month's supply medication (usually 21 or 28 tablets). (*D*) Spansule (time-release capsule).

Example: Ecotrin (enteric-coated aspirin, used to reduce fever, inflammation, and pain)

7. *Gelcap*—soft gelatin shell manufactured in one piece with drug in a liquid form inside the shell.

   Example: Vitamin supplements, such as Vitamin A or Vitamin E; Procardia

8. *Lozenge*—a medication contained in a candy or fruit base, dissolved in the mouth (see also Troche).

   Example: Cēpacol cough drops (used to reduce cough)

9. *Powder*—fine particles made from grinding a solid, not in much use today. Some effervescent antacids and laxative powders are used for relief of gastrointestinal (GI) distress, such as indigestion and constipation.

   Example: Metamucil (produces bulk in the bowel and used as a laxative)

10. *Spansule*—time-release capsules. Spansules are usually clear capsules, with visible multicolored granules inside (Fig. 3–1*D*) (see also Time-release capsule or tablet).

    Example: Tuss-Ornade spansules (used to reduce cough and congestion)

    PATIENT EDUCATION: **Time-release products should never be opened or broken up, as this could result in rapid absorption and overdose.**

11. *Sublingual tablet*—tablet designed to dissolve rapidly for absorption by the venous capillaries under the tongue.

    Example: Nitroglycerin (used to relieve pain caused by angina and to dilate the coronary vessels)

    PATIENT EDUCATION: **Instruct the patient not to swallow or chew the tablet and not to take the tablet with water.**

12. *Tablet*—compressed powder or granules, of different shapes and sizes. Some tablets are scored for breaking in half or in quarters. Tablets break up quickly into a powder in the stomach. Many are covered with sugar to disguise the taste of the drugs.

    Example: Aspirin (used to reduce fever, inflammation, and pain)

    PATIENT EDUCATION: **Tablets that are scored in halves or quarters may be assumed to be manufactured with an equal distribution of medication. You may break or cut these tablets into half- or quarter-doses. Tablets that are not scored cannot be assumed to have equally distributed medication and should not be divided. Tablets should not be divided by crushing. The amounts are too small to be accurately measured. You can, however, crush a tablet and administer the entire tablet in a small amount of semisolid food.**

    The term *pill* is passe, as it does not apply to any solid preparation in common use today. A pill is a small globular (beadlike) mass, usually but rarely compounded by the pharmacist.

13. *Time-release capsule or tablet*—capsule or spansule containing granules that are released slowly for prolonged action.

    Example: Inderal (used to manage high blood pressure)

    PATIENT EDUCATION: **These products should never be opened or broken up, as this could result in rapid absorption and overdose.**

14. *Troche*—a medication contained in a candy or fruit base, dissolved in the mouth (see also Lozenge).

Liquid Preparations

Most liquid preparations are available in one strength only. The physician orders the exact amount to give—for instance, 1 teaspoonful (tsp) or 1 ounce (oz). The types of liquid preparations are described here in alphabetic order. In addition, examples and special patient education sections are included.

1. *Aromatic water*—aqueous solution usually saturated with a volatile (easily evaporated) spicy substance; usually used to disguise salty substances dissolved in water.

   Example: Cinnamon oil, spearmint oil, or peppermint (aromatic waters may be used as digestive stimulants)

2. *Douche solution*—diluted aqueous solutions for irrigating the vagina.

   Example: Betadine douche (used as a cleaning solution and an anti-infective; also used to cleanse wounds in the topical treatment of acne)

3. *Elixir*—aqueous solutions with alcohol, sweetened and flavored. Adults often prefer this form to syrups. Alcohol is able to dissolve volatile oils and other substances not soluble in aqueous solutions.

   Example: Elixir of terpin hydrate and codeine (a C-V controlled substance used to suppress the coughing reflex)

   PATIENT EDUCATION: **Children often find elixirs too strong-tasting. For children, the physician may suggest diluting the dose of an elixir with water. Dilute only the dose to be given; adding water to the bottle may cause precipitation of the drug.**

   Elixirs must be used with caution with diabetics and alcoholics. Because of the sugar and alcohol content, patients receiving disulfiram (Antabuse), a drug used to help the alcoholic abstain from alcohol, should not use elixirs. Alcohol mixed with Antabuse causes severe nausea and vomiting.

4. *Emulsion*—water and oil mixtures, similar to homogenized milk. These preparations may be diluted with water just prior to administration.

   Example: Cod liver oil (sometimes used as a laxative)

5. *Extract and fluidextract*—highly concentrated preparations made by evaporating the alcoholic solvents of plants until a syrupy mass, plastic mass, or dry powder is left.

   Example: Fluidextract of belladonna or belladonna extract (used to reduce intestinal spasm and diarrhea)

6. *Gel (magma)*—viscous suspensions of minerals in liquid, usually in gelatinous or pastelike form.

   Example: Milk of magnesia (an antacid used to treat indigestion by neutralizing stomach acid)

   PATIENT EDUCATION: **Shake well before use. Because of inaccurate measurement due to residue, disposable cups are preferred.**

7. *Suspension*—finely divided, undissolved substances dispersed in a liquid vehicle when the medication is dispensed.

   Example: Amoxicillin suspension (used to treat bacterial infections)

   PATIENT EDUCATION: **After reconstitution, suspensions have a shelf life usually limited to 7 days at room temperature or 14 days under refrigeration. Shake well before use.**

   To prepare oral suspensions, shake container to loosen powder, measure water as indicated, add half the water and shake vigorously to avoid lumps, add the remaining water, then shake vigorously again. Discard after 14 days.

   Shake well before each use. Because of inaccurate measurement due to residue, disposable cups are preferred.

8. *Syrup*—aqueous solutions of sugar to which flavors are added, mostly used for children. The use of syrups is preferred to putting drugs in milk or fruit juice, as the latter may cause children to remember the off-taste and later refuse to drink milk or juice, or to not drink the entire amount necessary for the total dosage.

Example: Ipecac syrup (used to induce vomiting when certain poisonous substances have been ingested)

PATIENT EDUCATION: **Do not emphasize the flavor or call the medicine "candy" to fool the child; this could result in an overdose.**

Syrups must be used with caution in patients with diabetes. Always question an order for a drug in syrup form for the diabetic patient.

9. *Tincture*—an alcoholic or hydroalcoholic solution, usually using prepared plants with solvents containing alcohol. Tinctures are very potent therapeutic drugs.

Example: Tincture of opium, tincture of belladonna, and paregoric (camphorated tincture of opium) (mainly used to reduce intestinal motility and spasm and to treat severe forms of diarrhea)

Liquid Topical and Local Preparations

Most liquid topical and local preparations are applied to the skin and mucous membranes. They are available from stock supplies or are prepared by the pharmacist in the strength ordered by the physician. Occasionally solutions will be prepared for patient use or patients will need instructions for preparing solutions for topical use in the home.

Drugs are usually applied to the skin or mucous membranes for their local effect; that is, to treat one area only. However, the skin or mucous membranes may be the route by which a drug is introduced into the body so that it may enter the bloodstream and create a systemic (general) effect. The types of liquid topical and local preparations are described here in alphabetic order. In addition, examples and special patient education sections are included.

1. *Aerosol*—a liquid spray containing measured amounts of medication delivered by bulb nebulizers or oral inhalers and rapidly absorbed into the bloodstream (See also metered dose inhaler and nebulizer inhaler).

Example: Epinephrine inhalant (local effect: to treat bronchial asthma and bronchospasm; systemic effect: a cardiac stimulant)

2. *Colloid suspension*—a suspension in which the undissolved particles are very small. Water is added for use.

Example: Aveeno (oatmeal) bath (used locally to relieve itchy, sore, sensitive skin)

3. *Dermal cream*—a skin cream allowing a slow, sustained release of medication. It can be absorbed through the skin of others if touched.

Example: Nitro Cream (used systemically to relieve pain caused by angina and to dilate the coronary vessels)

PATIENT EDUCATION: **After administration, wash hands as quickly as possible. Wear gloves when applying to another person.**

4. *Dermal patch*—a skin patch permitting a slow, sustained release of medication, absorbed through the skin over a period of hours or days (Fig. 3–2).

Example: Estrogen, testosterone, nicotine, fetanyl, clonidine, nitroglycerin, or scopolamine (nitroglycerin used systemically to relieve pain caused by angina and to dilate the coronary vessels; scopolamine used systemically to relieve motion sickness)

PATIENT EDUCATION: **If administering, keep hands away from the mouth and eyes, and wash hands after application. Dispose of carefully, and keep out of the reach of children and animals. Rotate site to avoid skin irritation.**

5. *Liniment*—drug combined with oil, soap, alcohol, or water applied locally to produce a feeling of heat.

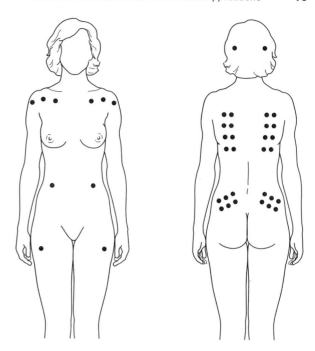

FIGURE 3–2. Recommended areas for transdermal patches. Behind the ear: scopolamine. Upper chest and upper arms: nicotine and nitroglycerin. Buttocks: estrogen patches.

Example: Camphor liniment (used to relieve local musculoskeletal pain and aches)

6. *Lotion*—aqueous solution of suspended ingredients, used to treat skin conditions.

    Example: Calamine lotion (used to relieve local skin irritation)

7. *Metered dose inhaler (MDI)*—A handheld aerosol that delivers a fine mist of medication to the respiratory tract, including the lungs.

    Example: albuterol, a bronchodilator used in airway obstruction due to asthma or chronic obstructive pulmonary disease (COPD) (Fig. 3–3).

8. *Nasal spray*—A solution prepared as a nasal spray.

    Example: beclomethasone, a corticosteroid used to treat bronchial asthma or seasonal rhinitis; calcitonin, a hormone used to treat postmenopausal osteoporosis.

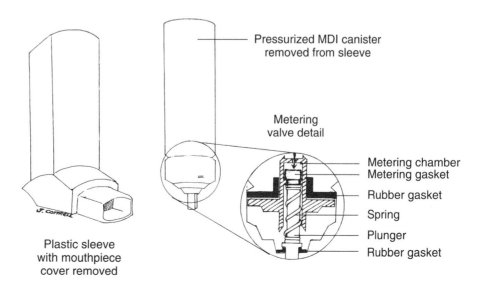

Pressurized MDI canister removed from sleeve

Metering valve detail

Metering chamber
Metering gasket

Rubber gasket

Spring

Plunger

Rubber gasket

Plastic sleeve with mouthpiece cover removed

FIGURE 3–3. Metered dose inhaler system.

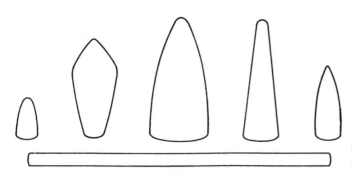

FIGURE 3–4. Suppository shapes (not actual size).

9. *Nebulization inhaler*—An aerosol or spray device (nebulizer) used for producing a fine spray or mist. Medications are prepared for nebulization from concentrates or solutions.

   Example: albuterol (see metered dose inhaler), isoproterenol, used in airway obstruction due to asthma or chronic obstructive pulmonary disease (COPD).

10. *Spirit*—a solution of volatile (easily evaporating) material in alcohol; may be diluted with water or inhaled.

    Example: Aromatic spirit of ammonia

    PATIENT EDUCATION: **In cases of simple fainting, the use of aromatic spirits of ammonia (smelling salts) or any other chemical substance is no longer recommended.**

11. *Suppository*—a medicated mass designed to melt at body temperature and used for introduction into the rectum, urethra, or vagina (Fig. 3–4). Materials used include cocoa butter and glycerin.

    Example: glycerin suppository (used locally to moisten stool and relieve constipation)

    PATIENT EDUCATION: **Rectal suppositories must be in contact with the intestinal mucosa. Suppositories inserted into stool will not be effectively absorbed.**

12. *Tampon*—a pack, pad, or plug made from cotton or sponge and impregnated with medication.

13. *Tincture*—an alcoholic or hydroalcoholic solution, prepared from nonvegetable chemicals.

    Example: Tincture of iodine, for use on the skin or mucous membranes, as an antiseptic.

14. *Translingual spray:* A fine mist delivered in metered doses, sprayed into the mouth under the tongue.

    Example: nitroglycerin, used for the treatment of angina pectoris.

Liquid Preparations for Injection

Liquid preparations for injection are sterile solutions sealed in vials or ampules (Fig. 3–5); these will be discussed in greater detail in Chapter 6. All injectable solutions are measured in milliliters (ml) or minims because syringes are measured this way. The types of liquid local preparations for injection are described here in alphabetic order. In addition, examples and specific techniques of injection are included that will be explained in detail in Chapter 6.

1. *Colloid suspension*—a gelatinous suspension in which the undissolved particles are very small. This is a repository form of drug, which means the consistency is designed for slow intramuscular absorption.

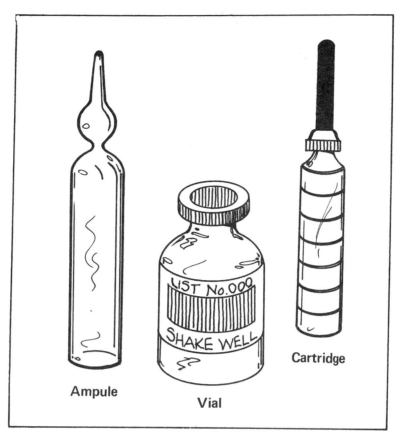

FIGURE 3–5. Containers for injectable medications. (From Frew, MA, and Frew, DR: Clinical Procedures for Medical Assisting. FA Davis, Philadelphia, 1990, p 303, with permission.)

Example: Novolin R (used to treat diabetes mellitus)

2. *Insoluble ester solution*—compound formed from an alcohol and an acid by removing water. Repository form for slow IM release and absorption.

   Example: Testosterone dissolved in vegetable oil (used to treat hormonal imbalances and breast cancer)

   SPECIFIC TECHNIQUES: These are given deep IM and often using Z-tract injection method. (See also Chapter 5.)

3. *Insoluble salt solution*—Repository form for slow intramuscular (IM) release and absorption.

   Example: Penicillin G, Procaine aqueous (used to treat bacterial infections)

   SPECIFIC TECHNIQUES: Shake until no sediment is visible. Larger-gauge needles are required. When applicable, Z-tract injection method avoids irritation to the tissues. (See also Chapter 5.)

4. *Oil solution or suspension*—drug suspended in a fatty substance to slow (repository form) intramuscular absorption.

   Example: Poison ivy serum (used to desensitize the patient to poison ivy skin reactions, in case of future exposure)

5. *Powders and crystals*—dry forms of a medication that need reconstituting (adding liquid) with sterile water labeled "for injection" or sterile normal (isotonic) saline.

   Example: M-M-R vaccine (measles, mumps, and rubella live virus vaccine)

6. *Sterile normal (isotonic) saline*—an aqueous solution of salt in sterile water that is the same osmotic pressure as blood serum and used to dilute drugs for injection and for

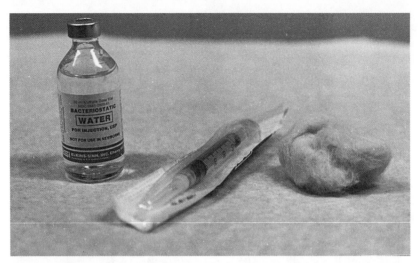

FIGURE 3–6. Sterile water is used to dilute drugs for injections. (From Frew, MA, and Frew, DR: Clinical Procedures for Medical Assisting. FA Davis, Philadelphia, 1990, p 308, with permission.)

wound care and irrigation. Normal saline is considered less irritating to the tissues than sterile water.

Example: Bacteriostatic sterile sodium chloride

SPECIFIC TECHNIQUES: Multidose vials of sterile isotonic saline contain a bacteriostatic preservative that has been found to cause seizures in infants up to 1 month of age or older when used to reconstitute drugs for IM injection. Diluents in single-dose vials that do not contain preservatives should be used for infants.

7. *Sterile water*—a solution (aqueous) of sterile water, purified first by distillation, used to dilute drugs for injection and for wound care and irrigation (Fig. 3–6).

Example: Sterile water, *USP.*

SPECIFIC TECHNIQUES: Multidose vials of sterile isotonic saline contain a bacteriostatic preservative that has been found to cause seizures in infants up to 1 month of age or older when used to reconstitute drugs for IM injection. Diluents in single-dose vials that do not contain preservatives should be used for infants.

Oral Dosage Forms That Should Not Be Crushed

In general, it is not advisable to crush or alter in any other way certain medications. Yet there are many situations in which crushing or dividing a tablet may be necessary. For example, an adult patient may have a physical disability or a psychological barrier, making swallowing a tablet difficult. Small children, critically ill patients, and patients with nasogastric tubes also are not able to swallow solid forms of medication.

There are specific reasons why certain drugs should not be crushed or altered in any way. Consult with a pharmacist or the package insert if there is any doubt. The pharmacist may be able to recommend whether a liquid form exists or if the solid form can be compounded. In general, the following medication forms should not be altered.

1. *Extended-release products*—This type of product is designed to release medication over a long time period. This can be accomplished by centering the drug within multiple layers. As the layers melt, medication is released, all at once or in stages. Slow-K is

an example of a slow-release tablet. Some capsules contain beads that are dissolved by the body at differing rates. Inderal is an example.

2. *Irritating medications*—Tablets that irritate the stomach are "enteric-coated" to protect the mucous membranes of the mouth and stomach until the drug passes on to the intestine. Ecotrin (enteric-coated aspirin) is an example.

3. *Offensive-tasting medications*—Unpleasant-tasting medications are usually coated with sugar by the manufacturer. Crushing the tablet releases the underlying medication, which then leaves an unpleasant taste in the mouth. Motrin is an example.

4. *Sublingual medications*—Medications intended to dissolve under the tongue should be left intact, otherwise the absorption rate could be too fast or even ineffective. Nitroglycerin is an example.

5. *Effervescent tablets*—These tablets are dropped into a liquid to create a solution. Some effervescent tablets lose their ability to dissolve quickly when crushed.

Written Competency 3–1

Performance Competence: Select the one answer or completion that is *best* in each of the 10 questions, with at least 90 percent accuracy and within 15 minutes. Do not give yourself credit for questions left unanswered.

1. Acceptable methods for dividing medications into fractions of a dose include:
   (a) Opening capsules, then adding a premeasured amount of water.
   (b) Crushing tablets into a powder, then dividing the powder into fractions with a blade.
   (c) Opening spansules, then adding a premeasured amount of water.
   (d) Cutting scored tablets and administering a portion of the tablet followed by water.
   (e) All of the above.

2. Medication forms that are swallowed include:
   (a) Buccal tablets.
   (b) Troches.
   (c) Sublingual tablets.
   (d) Caplets.
   (e) All of the above.

3. Each of the following is a true statement about an oral suspension medication EXCEPT:
   (a) Most have to be reconstituted.
   (b) Underdosage may occur due to medication residue.
   (c) They are shaken before each use.
   (d) After reconstitution, they have a usual shelf life of 7 to 14 days.
   (e) Oral syringes are preferred for drug delivery.

4. Drug preparations that must be used with caution with the diabetic patient include:
   (a) Extracts.
   (b) Time-release capsules.
   (c) Fluidextracts.
   (d) Syrups.
   (e) Enteric-coated tablets.

5. Each of the following is an injectable drug preparation that slows drug absorption in the body EXCEPT:
   (a) Aqueous solutions.
   (b) Colloid suspensions.
   (c) Insoluble salt solutions.
   (d) Insoluble ester solutions.

6. Alcohol-free preparations include:
   (a) Aromatic waters.
   (b) Elixirs.
   (c) Tinctures.
   (d) Emulsions.
   (e) Liniments.

7. The injectable drug solution that is most like the fluids bathing the human tissues is:
   (a) Sterile water.
   (b) Isotonic saline.
   (c) Insoluble salt solution.
   (d) Oil suspension.
   (e) Colloid suspension.

8. Of the following medications, which will be totally absorbed into the bloodstream first?
   (a) Sublingual tablet.
   (b) Enteric-coated tablet.

(c) Buffered tablet.

(d) Time-release capsule.

(e) Dermal patch.

9. Of the following medications, which will be totally absorbed into the bloodstream first?

(a) Suppository.

(b) Aerosol.

(c) Colloid suspension injection.

(d) Oil suspension injection.

(e) Insoluble salt solution injection.

10. Children find which of the following drug forms particularly strong-tasting?

(a) Elixirs.

(b) Syrups.

(c) Emulsions.

(d) Tinctures.

(e) Suspensions.

Score: _____

See Appendix B for answers.

Terminal Performance Objective/Competency

Procedure 3–1: Divide or Crush Tablets for Preparing Fractions of a Dose

EQUIPMENT   Tablets that are scored
Small scoring knife
Two metal teaspoons

Performance Competence: Complete each step of this procedure with exact accuracy and within reasonable job production time, as stated by your evaluator.

| | V | S | U* |

PROCEDURAL STEPS

1. Break scored tablets in half by grasping each half between your thumbs and index fingers until you can break a tablet exactly in two.

   □ □ □

2. Break quarter-scored tablets into quarters by placing the knife blade in the wedge of the score and bearing down with even pressure, until you can cut a tablet exactly into four quarters.

   □ □ □

3. Place a tablet on one spoon, then nestle the second spoon on top of the tablet.

   □ □ □

   or

   Place the tablet in a medicine cup, then place another medicine cup on top and crush the tablet.

   □ □ □

---

*V = Value, to be filled in if assigning points or other specific values to each step, of if step is to be delineated as a critical step.

S = Satisfactory completion of the step.

U = Unsatisfactory completion of the step or step incomplete; needs more practice.

4. Crush the tablet between the two spoons and mix the tablet with a small amount of semisolid food.

□ □ □

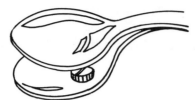

Date: _____ Competency achieved: Y _____ N _____

Designated reasonable time standard: _____

Actual completion time: _____

Conversion Drill for Skill

Using Table 1–7 and the conversion formula, convert the following within 10 minutes. Do not give yourself credit for partial or incorrect answers. Strive for a score of 100 percent. If you score less than 100 percent, return to Chapter 1, and reread the section on conversions.

1. 0.5 ml   = _____ minims (choose the *one best* conversion)

2. 0.66 ml   = _____ minims (choose the *one best* conversion)

3. 2.5 oz   = _____ ml

4. 64 ml   = _____ tbs

5. 0.5 gal   = _____ oz

6. 250 mg   = _____ g

7. 250 lb   = _____ kg

8. 114 lb   = _____ kg

9. 92 lb   = _____ kg

10. 168 lb   = _____ kg

11. 2 tsp   = _____ cc

12. 3 Tbls   = _____ cc

13. dr. iv   = _____ cc

14. gtt xx   = _____ cc

15. oz iv   = _____ cc

16. 150 mcg   = _____ mg

17. 0.25 g   = _____ mg

18. gr v   = _____ mg

19. gr 1/6   = _____ mg

20. gr 1/4   = _____ mg

21. gr 1/2   = _____ mcg

22. 0.175 mg   = _____ mcg

23. 600 mg   = _____ gr

24. gr xv   = _____ g

25. 1500 cc   = _____ L

Score: _____

See Appendix B for answers.

Drug Classifications and Interactions

OBJECTIVES **WRITTEN COMPETENCY 4–1:** Classify drugs according to their therapeutic effects.

WRITTEN COMPETENCY 4–2: Match drugs to their classifications.

WRITTEN COMPETENCY 4–3: Answer true–false statements about drug names and classifications.

WRITTEN COMPETENCY 4–4: Apply concepts of drug–patient interactions and drug–drug interactions to patient care situations.

WRITTEN COMPETENCY 4–5: Apply concepts of drug–patient and drug–drug interactions to patient care situations.

TERMINAL PERFORMANCE OBJECTIVE (PROCEDURE 4–1): Use drug references for proper drug identification and classification.

ASSIGNMENT 4–1: Use drug references to create drug information guides.

CONVERSION DRILL FOR SKILL: Convert body weight measurements to their most frequently used approximate equivalents and calculate dosages based on body weight.

Before administering medications and providing patient care, it is important to understand what specific actions drugs have on the body and, more importantly, how the body responds to those effects and what adverse effects and conditions might alter, favorably or unfavorably, a patient's response to a drug's intended action. Understanding the concepts of drug interactions with and effects on the body is made easier by classifying drugs according to distinguishing groups.

Drugs are grouped and named by various subjects according to their natural relationships to one another within each grouping. The nomenclature (names) and classifications of drugs form the basic discipline for understanding how drugs are alike as well as how they differ from one another. Use Table 4–1 as a guide as this chapter discusses the various ways of classifying drugs.

Drug Nomenclature

Drugs are first distinguished by their names. Each drug may have as many as four different names—an organic name, a chemical name, a generic name, and a brand (trade) name. A drug's name may be different in each of the four categories, or one name may be used for more than one category. Table 4–2 compares the brand, generic, and organic names of some commonly prescribed drugs.

The *brand (trade) name* of a drug is each manufacturer's trademark designation. Many companies manufacture the same generic drug, but with different brand names. Each brand name is owned by a company and begins with a capital letter. Brand names for digitoxin include Crystodigin and Purodigin; those for digoxin include Lanoxin and Lanoxicaps.

To reduce the proliferation of confusing names, the Food and Drug Administration (FDA) now requires that each drug have an *official name*. An official name may be selected from among a drug's chemical, generic, and brand names, but the generic name is usually chosen. Official names contain the initials *USP* after it; for example, digoxin, *USP* or digitoxin, *USP*. Generic names are not capitalized.

Drug Classifications

Body System. Drug classifications can be confusing, as there are so many ways to group drugs. Drugs may be classified by *body systems*. For instance, drugs that act on the heart and blood vessels may be classified under cardiovascular drugs. Digoxin (Lanoxin) is an example. Drugs that are used to treat muscle or joint disorders may be classified as musculoskeletal drugs. Cyclobenzaprine (Flexeril) is a musculoskeletal drug used to treat muscle spasm.

General Use. Drugs may be classified according to *general use*. Nitrogen mustard (Mustargen) is used to treat cancer (CA) and may be classified under chemotherapeutic* agents. Tetanus toxoid is used to immunize against the disease tetany (lockjaw) and is classified as an immunologic agent. Dexamethasone (Decadron), used to decrease inflammation, may be classified under general use as an adrenocorticosteroid.

---

* "Chemotherapy" was originally used to describe the use of chemicals to treat infections but is now used to describe the action of drugs used specifically to destroy cancer cells.

TABLE 4–1. Examples of How Drugs Can Be Classified

Name	System	General Use	Family	Therapeutic	Primary Action	Indication	Pharmacologic
Lanoxin	Cardiovascular	Cardiac arrhythmia	Cardiac glycosides	Antiarrhythmic	Promotes calcium movement	Congestive heart failure	Digitalis glycoside
Tetanus Toxoid, *USP*	Immune	Immunologic	Biologics	Prophylaxis	Active immunity	Vaccination	Tetanus toxoid
Mustargen	Varies	Chemotherapy	Nitrogen mustards	Antineoplastic	Causes cellular death	CA (cancer)	Alkylating agent
Decadron	Respiratory	Adrenocorticosteroid	Corticosteroids	Anti-inflammatory	Suppresses immune response	Edema and allergies	glucocorticoid
Bicillin L-A	Varies	Antibacterial	Penicillins	Antimicrobial	Kills bacteria	Bacterial infections	Natural penicillin
Insulin	Endocrine	Insulin replacement	Antidiabetic agents	Hypoglycemic	Increases glucose movement	Diabetes mellitus	Pancreatic hormone
Duricef	Varies	Antibacterial	Cephalosporins	Antimicrobial	Kills bacteria	Bacterial infections	First-generation cephalosporin
Riopan	Digestive	Ulcer medications	Antacids	Antiulcer	Neutralizes stomach acid	Peptic ulcer	Magnesium compound
Monistat	Integument	Yeastlike fungal prophylaxis	Synthetic antifungals	Antifungal	Kills fungus	*Candida* infections	Imidazole derivative
Valium	CNS	Nonbarbiturate sedative	Benzodiazepines	Antianxiety	Acts as CNS depressant	Tension, anxiety	benzodiazepine
Lasix	Urinary	Diuresis	Loop diuretics	Diuretic	Increases urine output	Edema	Loop diuretic
HydroDIURIL	Urinary, cardiovascular	Diuresis	Thiazide diuretics	Antihypertensive diuretic	Increases urine output, lowers blood pressure	Edema, hypertension	benzothiadiazine
Aspirin	Immune	Analgesia	Non-narcotic analgesics	Analgesic, antipyretic, anti-inflammatory	Inhibits prostaglandin production	Mild to moderate pain and inflammation, fever	salicylate

TABLE 4–2. **Examples of Drug Names**

Brand	Generic	Organic
Lanoxin	digoxin, *USP*	*Digitalis lanata*
Crystodigin	digitoxin, *USP*	*Digitalis purpurea*
Bayer	aspirin, *USP*	acetylsalicylic acid
Tylenol	acetaminophen, *USP*	para-aminophenol (coal tar and aniline)
Riopan	magaldrate, *USP*	aluminum and magnesium
Bicillin L-A	penicillin G potassium, *USP*	benzylpenicillin
Adrenalin	epinephrine HCl, *USP*	epinephrine

Family. Drugs also may be categorized according to *family*. These names are usually subdivisions of other classifications. For example, all antibiotics that are derived from the natural mold *Penicillium notatum* may be classified under penicillins. Newer antibiotics of the cephalosporin family were introduced in the 1960s. Although similar in chemical structure and action to the penicillins, these newer antibiotics may be classified as cephalosporins, and further subclassified as first-generation cephalosporins, second-generation cephalosporins, or third-generation cephalosporins. Even though both groups may be classified under the same general purpose (prophylaxis [prevention] of bacterial infections), they can be separately classified by family.

Therapeutic Effect. Two other common methods of classifying drugs include grouping drugs by their *therapeutic effects* or their *action* on certain organs or tissues. Magaldrate (Riopan) is a magnesium compound that is classified therapeutically as an antiulcer agent. Classified by action, Riopan is an antacid, neutralizing hydrochloric acid in the stomach. As another example, diazepam (Valium) is classified therapeutically as an antianxiety/anticonvulsant agent; by action it is classified as a central nervous system (CNS) depressant and seizure suppressant.

Indication. Some drugs may have more than one therapeutic effect or action and, therefore, are used for more than one condition, or indication, (e.g., Valium). Although furosemide (Lasix) is classified strictly as a diuretic (an agent that promotes urine secretion), another diuretic, hydrochlorothiazide (HydroDIURIL), may be used to treat hypertension as well. Thus, HydroDIURIL may be classified as a diuretic *and* as an antihypertensive. Epinephrine (Adrenalin) constricts the blood vessels and, as such, is classified as a vasoconstrictor; yet it can also dilate the respiratory passages and therefore is additionally classified as a bronchodilator used for the treatment of asthma. Aspirin is another example: aspirin is classified as an analgesic (relieves pain), antipyretic (reduces fever), and anti-inflammatory agent, all in one.

Whether a drug has one primary use or many primary uses, it can be classified in a variety of ways. Grouping drugs is confusing, and classifications are often mixed and matched or overlap with other classifications. Table 4–1 lists a few of the ways in which drugs can be classified.

Terminology Used in Describing Drugs

When giving information about a drug, a particular sequence is used in pharmacology references, drug guides, and package inserts. This sequence is usually detailed as follows:

1. **Action.** Action is the physiological effect a drug has on the body cells. It defines how the drug works and is not necessarily the reason why the drug is used.
2. **Therapeutic classification.** This defines the type of drug according to its use in treating a disease or disorder. This differs from a drug's pharmacologic classifica-

tion, which defines a drug according to its pharmacologic family. For example, the therapeutic classification of aspirin is "non-narcotic analgesic, anti-inflammatory, and antipyretic," whereas its pharmacologic classification is "salicylates."

3. **Pregnancy risk category.** This refers to the five categories (A, B, C, D, and X), established by the FDA to indicate the level of risk for birth defects (see Chapter 5, Table 5–1).

4. **Indication(s).** This is the primary condition(s) treated by a particular drug.

5. **Contraindications.** Conditions that make the administration of the drug undesirable or improper are given here. For example, aspirin appears to impede blood clotting and its administration is contraindicated in patients with gastrointestinal (GI) bleeding (ulcers) and bleeding disorders. Aspirin may increase the risk of Reye's syndrome when taken by children and teenagers with fever and certain viral infections. Because of the risk of Reye's syndrome, aspirin is contraindicated for children or teenagers with chickenpox or influenzalike symptoms.

6. **Adverse reactions or side effects.** This includes commonly observed undesirable secondary effects; that is, effects other than the primary effect being sought by the administration of the drug. Adverse reactions usually result in patient discomfort. "Untoward reactions" and "side effects" are also used to describe adverse reactions. Not all side effects, however, are adverse—they are simply unintended.

7. **Hypersensitivity.** Drug allergies, which occur in some patients and not in others, come under this category. Allergic reactions occur when the body has been previously exposed (and sensitized) to a particular drug and then is re-exposed to the same drug. Hypersensitivity is always a contraindication to the administration of the drug in question.

8. **Idiosyncrasies.** Patients who are abnormally sensitive to small doses of a drug the *first* time a drug is administered are said to have idiosyncrasies. Idiosyncrasies are usually due to hereditary defects that result in an abnormal or unusual response to a drug.

9. **Dependence.** The need to use a drug to relieve tension or discomfort or to achieve pleasure and euphoria is called *psychologic dependence. Habituation* refers to a mild form of psychologic dependence (e.g., as on the caffeine in coffee). *Physical dependence* is the need to use a drug continuously to produce a certain "normal" function. Discontinuation of a drug on which a patient is physically dependent may lead to withdrawal symptoms. Withdrawal symptoms differ from person to person, depending on the type of addiction and the amount of drug being used. Withdrawal symptoms may be mild or potentially severe and dangerous if characterized by convulsions and death.

10. **Dosage.** Unless otherwise noted, dosage refers to the usual adult dosage (amount of the drug to take), method of administration (route), and timing.

11. **Administration.** This is the drug's storage and specific pointers on how to administer particular drugs.

12. **Patient education.** Included here is general patient information about the drugs they are taking such as the condition(s) for which their drug is administered, the drug's common side effects, and when to call the physician to report any unusual conditions or adverse reactions. Compliance and safe use should be the primary goals of each patient education situation. Other patient guidelines may include specific information, such as expressing the importance of taking all the drug prescribed or explaining what the "prn" order means.

13. **Precautions.** These are risks due to special conditions of the patient, drug, or environment that need to be considered for the safe use of the drug. For example, aspirin should be used *with caution* in children with fever and dehydration because aspirin toxicity could develop quickly. Another precaution may be to stop the use of aspirin 1 week prior to surgery.

14. **Toxic effects.** These are the poisonous effects of drug overdose. Toxic effects may result from life-threatening adverse reactions or idiosyncrasies, a single overdose of the medication, or the accumulation of a medication in blood levels over time.

Uses of Drugs

Drug therapy is defined as the correct and accurate administration of prescribed drugs as part of the patient care plan. There are actually five types of uses for administering drugs as part of the patient care plan.

Therapeutic Uses. Drug therapy is most often thought of in the context of a cure—for example, antibiotics cure bacterial infections. Drugs used for curative, or healing, purposes are often termed *therapeutic*.

Palliative Uses. Drugs may be used for *palliative* reasons, meaning to make the patient comfortable and to relieve pain or other symptoms; in other words, drugs may be used not to cure but to provide relief from a disease or condition. The use of nonsteroidal anti-inflammatory drugs (NSAIDs) for the relief of pain in arthritis is an example of a palliative drug.

Prophylactic Uses. Prophylaxis means "to prevent from occurring." In these instances, drugs are used to prevent the occurrence of a disease or a condition. Vaccines and toxoids are examples of prophylactic drugs; birth control pills are another.

Diagnostic Uses. Drugs also may be used *diagnostically*, as when dyes are injected for radiographic studies and antigen sera are used to test for skin allergy.

Replacement Uses. Replacement drugs include vitamins, minerals, and supplementary food products; insulin for patients with diabetes; and other hormones used to treat illnesses such as thyroid extract for hypothyroidism and estrogens for menopause.

Factors Altering the Usual Effects of Drugs

The experienced health care provider soon learns that the response of one person to a drug is not always the same as that of another to the same drug. In fact, the same dose of a particular medication may affect patients in many different ways. Whereas some patients may be extremely sensitive to a medication, others may be entirely resistant to its effect. When treating a patient, the physician follows the usual protocol of starting with the average recommended dose, and then he or she assesses the patient's response for any necessary alterations in dosage. Many different factors may alter a patient's response to a medication. These factors are listed as follows:

1. *Weight.* Given the same dose, it can generally be said that the greater the patient's weight, the less powerful a drug's effect; and the less the patient's weight, the more powerful the effect. For this reason, many drug dosages are calculated and administered on the basis of the ratio of milligrams of the drug to kilograms of patient body weight.

2. *Age.* Age has its greatest significance in drug therapy when treating the very young and the very old. The underdeveloped body systems in newborns and the deteriorating body systems of the elderly may change the rate at which these age groups transform and metabolize drugs in their bodies.

3. *Sex.* Gender sometimes affects the patient's response to a drug. Because women's muscles usually have a higher fat content and therefore a poorer blood supply than do men's, women tend to absorb intramuscularly injected medications more slowly than men do. The menstrual cycle and birth control pill (BCP) use may alter hormone levels in women, sometimes decreasing the body's immune response. For example, antibiotic levels may not be as effective when treating infections in women during certain times of the menstrual cycle.

4. *Normal physiologic state.* Each person has his or her own pattern of adrenal steroid production and secretion, acid–base balance, and water or electrolyte balance. This pattern is the *diurnal rhythm*, defined as increased cellular activity during the daytime. Usually diurnal rhythms make the CNS more resistant to certain depressant

drugs and steroids during the daylight hours. For this reason, sleep-inducing drugs are much less effective during the day and steroid therapy is much safer when given in the morning.

5. *Pathology.* Diseases of the organs and tissues that assist the body in drug transformation and elimination can affect a patient's ability to respond to the intended use of a drug, especially diseases of the liver and kidneys. Patients who are being treated for multiple disorders may be excessively resistant or sensitive to a particular drug when it is used in combination with others.

6. *Genetic.* Some patients inherit the ability to break down certain drugs rapidly and require higher daily doses of drugs, whereas others, lacking certain drug-metabolizing enzymes, metabolize drugs so slowly that even the administration of ordinary doses at usual intervals results in drug accumulation at toxic levels. These patients require dosage decreased below usual levels.

7. *Allergy.* In some patients, the presence of a drug stimulates the patient's immune system to produce antibodies. When the same medication is given again, an immune reaction occurs, causing one or many of the types of allergic response.

8. *Psychologic.* A patient's response to a drug is often influenced by beliefs, hopes, fears, previous experiences, and mental attitudes. For this reason, a *placebo* may be administered to satisfy a patient's psychologic need for treatment. Placebos may take the form of a sugar pill or an injection of sterile water, or of a lesser or greater dose of medication being prescribed.

9. *Environmental.* Factors such as temperature alter a patient's physiology and thus affect the patient's response to a drug. Heat dilates the vessels and increases blood flow. Therefore, drugs that dilate blood vessels (e.g., antihypertensives) may have to be decreased during the summer months or during vacations in the tropics.

10. *Tolerance.* Tolerance is a phenomenon of reduced responsiveness to a drug. Tolerance may be inherited or acquired when a patient takes a drug for a long time.

11. *Cumulative action.* The accumulation of a drug in the body results in drug toxicity. This usually happens when a drug is taken at intervals too short to allow for the elimination of previous drug levels. This increased concentration results in a much greater drug effect on the body and toxic side effects.

12. *Other medications.* Many patients, especially the elderly, are treated with more than one drug at a time. In addition, many patients combine prescription drugs with over-the-counter medications. Multiple drugs can interact to produce effects that are often undesirable and sometimes dangerous. Harmful drug interactions can decrease efficacy or increase toxicity.

13. *Route of administration.* The same drug administered by different routes can exert different effects on the body. For example, a drug taken orally may be therapeutic, but given intravenously, it may be fatal in the same patient.

Drug–Drug Interactions

Perhaps the single most common factor altering the usual response to drugs is the combined effects of drugs on the body. When one drug is given with another, its effects may differ from when the drug is administered alone. One drug may increase or decrease the effects of another, by either physical or chemical means.

When combining drugs, *synergism* occurs when the presence of one drug *increases* the intensity or prolongs the duration of the effects of another drug. Synergism may result when two drugs produce the same type of effect, even though they may act on different sites or by different mechanisms. Synergism can have harmful effects. For example, combining two drugs that can lower blood pressure in different ways may cause a much more dangerous drop in blood pressure than when either drug is given alone. Synergistic combinations also can be intended for their medical advantages. An example is the combining of codeine and aspirin. Although codeine and aspirin reduce pain at different sites and by different mechanisms (codeine acts on the CNS, aspirin in the tissues where the pain is centered), the combination may relieve pain more effectively than when each is used alone.

Potentiation is a term that describes a synergistic action, but in a much different way. Potentiation occurs when only one of the two drugs exerts the action that is made greater by the presence of the other drug. One drug, although inactive, intensifies the effects of a second, active drug. For example, the effects of anticoagulants may be potentiated by the use of some anti-inflammatory agents such as phenylbutazone (Butazolidin). A patient whose condition has been stabilized by anticoagulants may face the potential of unexpected bleeding should he or she begin concurrent Butazolidin therapy.

Antagonism is the opposite of synergism. When combining drugs, antagonism occurs when the presence of one drug *decreases* the intensity or shortens the duration of the effects of another drug. Antagonism may occur when two drugs affect the body's physiology in opposing ways, so that the effects of one drug cancel out those of another. Use of tetracycline and other antibiotics have been associated with BCP failure. Although the exact cause is not known, it is thought that antibiotics decrease the normal intestinal flora, which in turn is responsible for a decreased absorption of the hormones contained in the BCPs. A drop in drug-induced hormone levels could permit pregnancy to occur. Antagonism also occurs when two drugs combine chemically to neutralize one another. This is the principle behind deliberately giving an antidote in a case of poisoning.

A drug may be synergistic with some drugs and antagonistic with others. For example, antacids may prematurely release enteric-coated drugs in the stomach and either increase or cancel out their effects. Some antacids are antagonistic to the effects of anticoagulants and tetracycline-type antibiotics. Their presence in the stomach can reduce the body's ability to absorb anticoagulants or tetracyline, resulting in an increased risk to blood clotting or a delayed recovery from an infection.

More than 7000 drugs are available for clinical use, with more than 55 million different drug–drug interactions possible. Although there are relatively few serious interactions, the health care provider has the responsibility to help prevent drug–drug interactions that might delay a patient's recovery or even endanger the patient. Health care providers are charged with ensuring that patients are knowledgeable about dose scheduling and aware of the most common side effects of drugs that may occur from drug–drug interactions. Patients are urged to disclose all medications being taken at home and to understand or question the precise directions given for taking medications. The use of over-the-counter (OTC) drugs should be kept to a minimum, especially products containing aspirin and antacids, unless approved of by the physician. The best way to prevent adverse drug reactions is to understand the basic relationship of the commonly used drugs to one another. As a part of every medication education plan, it is important to ask the patient about any over-the-counter drugs taken within the last 30 days.

Drug Reference Materials

It is not possible to learn everything written about clinical pharmacology, even concerning a single drug. To research everything written about a single drug or keep up-to-date on the studies being conducted on a single drug would represent a full-time, ongoing process. It is important, however, to be as knowledgeable as possible about the specific drugs encountered on a regular basis for administration or patient teaching.

The pharmacist is the best source of information. Pharmacists are available by telephone to give advice about drug–drug or drug–food interactions. As most pharmacies now keep patient records on computer, a patient's prescription drug history can be retrieved easily. One should also read pertinent product information that is made available by the manufacturer, then use expanded reference sources such as those listed here. Each drug's role in patient care should be discussed with the physician or pharmacist before it is administered for the first time. Information to be used in patient education discussions or handouts should be reviewed with the physician. One should ensure through questioning that dosage requirements, primary actions on the body, secondary actions (adverse effects), contraindications, drug interactions, and the possible toxic effects are understood for each drug administered or discussed with patients in the teaching situation. A thorough knowledge of a drug makes it possible to predict the likely signs and symptoms of a toxic reaction or overdose, and the measures that would be necessary to treat a life-threatening situation.

Keeping current about drug therapy requires concentration and perseverance and the special discipline of paying attention to detail. As a new drug is encountered, its classification should be learned and its similarities to and differences from a known drug in the same classification should be compared. When in doubt, one should ask the physician or look up information in one of the many drug references available. The 50 most commonly prescribed drugs are included as Appendix A in this text. References used to learn about drugs follow.

1. *Package inserts.* This is the most up-to-date and important source for drug product information. Each drug package includes an information sheet describing all the significant aspects of administration, including indications for use, dosage recommendations, contraindications of use, warnings and precautions, adverse reactions, drug interactions, chemical formulation of the drug, clinical studies, altered laboratory values, and special directions for usage in special age groups and in pregnancy.

    For each drug commonly prescribed and administered, its package insert should be preserved alphabetically in a notebook for instant reference and made available to all staff. To ensure that product information is current, the notebook should be periodically reviewed with the local pharmaceutical sales representatives or the pharmacist. Inserts could then be routinely updated by replacing old inserts with new ones.

2. *Physician's Desk Reference (PDR).* This reference is published annually by the Medical Economics Company. It is complimentary to physicians and pharmacists who subscribe to *Medical Economics Magazine.* It also can be purchased from the company or in most retail book stores. The information contained in the *Reference* is taken from the literature printed as package inserts of more than 2800 prescribed drugs. The material is listed alphabetically, first by manufacturer and then by brand name, and contains cross-referencing sections for quick and easy use according to usage, therapeutic classification, generic name, manufacturer's name, brand name, and photographic color reproduction.

3. *Family Physician's Compendium of Drug Therapy.* This reference is published annually by the McGraw-Hill Book Company and is available directly from the company or in retail book stores. The drugs in the *Compendium* include nearly all the medications routinely prescribed or recommended by family physicians. Drug information is arranged by therapeutic category, then in alphabetic sequence by brand name. It also includes photographic color plates for visual identification of products. One can locate any product, by brand name or generic name, in the general index at the back of the book. There is also a special section on significant new drugs, a glossary of medical and pharmaceutic terms, and a directory with emergency telephone numbers of the following: pharmaceutical manufacturers, drug information centers, poison control centers, pain clinics, voluntary health organizations, and other counseling and referral services. McGraw-Hill Book Company also publishes the *Compendium* for various specialty practices.

Other references that may occasionally be used by the physician include the following:

- *Drug Handbooks,* published by medical publishers, such as F. A. Davis. These handbooks are easy to use and contain only the information pertinent to drug administration and patient teaching.
- *Drug Cards.* Drug cards may be purchased from medical publishers or created on computer to suit the needs of an individual medical practice. Some drug cards are designed for the health care practitioner; others, for patient use. Figure 4–1 is an example of a drug card designed for practitioner use. A less technical card should be designed for patient use.

Generic: **conjugated estrogen**
Trade: Premarin
Category: Hormone

Dose/Route: oral 0.3 mg to 2.5 mg
Injectable 25 mg/5 mL (give deep IM in large muscle)
Vaginal cream 0.625 mg/g
Dose depends on the condition being treated

Action: replaces or increases the level of estrogen in the body

Use: treatment of the following conditions—abnormal uterine bleeding, menopausal symptoms, postmenopausal replacement therapy, atrophic vaginitis, postpartum breast engorgement, breast cancer, prostrate cancer

Side effects:
CNS: headache, dizziness, and depression
CV: hypertension, edema, and thrombophlebitis
GI: nausea and vomiting, weight changes
GU: breakthrough bleeding, altered menstrual flow
in men—testicular atrophy, impotence
Skin: urticaria, acne, flushing
Other: breast changes, leg cramps, elevated blood sugar,
and changes in libido

Interactions: physicians should be notified if patient is taking any of the following drugs—steroids, oral anticoagulants, cyclosporin, bromocriptine, and tamoxifen

Contraindications: patients with thromboletic disorders, use caution with patients having the following conditions—hypertension, gallbladder disease, seizures, heart failure, hepatic and renal failure, bone and blood disorders

Patient education:
Teach self breast exam
Instruct on the need for yearly exam and pap
Inform of possible side effects
Used to promote cardiac and skeletal health
The need to take as ordered to get therapeutic effect in relieving menopausal symptoms
Report any suspected pregnancy immediately
If having nausea, take at bedtime or with food
Warn of possible breast tenderness
Instruct diabetic patients to closely monitor blood sugars

FIGURE 4–1. Sample drug card for practitioner's use.

TABLE 4–3. Therapeutic Classification of Drugs

Therapeutic Classification	Action	Use	Examples
Analgesic/anti-inflammatory (non-narcotic, NSAID)	Produces anti-inflammatory, analgesic, and antipyretic effects by inhibiting prostaglandin synthesis	Mild to moderate pain arising from the integumental structures; gout; rheumatoid diseases; arthritis	Relafen, Advil, Medipren, Nuprin, Ultram
Analgesic/anti-inflammatory/antipyretic (non-narcotic)	Relieves pain; dilates peripheral vascular system and increases heat loss, thus reducing body temperature; blocks pain impulse generation	Fever; mild to moderate pain arising from the integumental structures; gout; arthritis; rheumatoid diseases	Aspirin, Tylenol, OTC aspirin products
Analgesic/antitussive (narcotic)	Controlled substance that depresses the cough reflex and GI motility; alters both perception of and emotional response to pain by a means still unknown	Severe pain, especially originating from coronary, pulmonary, or peripheral organs; preoperative medication; diarrhea and dysentery; cough suppression	Hydrocodone, Demerol, MSO_4, MS Contin, Roxanol, Percocet, Percodan, Darvon, Tylenol with Codeine, Propacet 100, Darvocet-N, Paveral, Nubain
Anesthetic, local	Blocks initiation and transmission of nerve impulses to the brain	Local anesthesia during minor surgery; topical application for relief of skin and mucous membrane irritation	Americaine Otic, Xylocaine
Antacid/antiflatulent	Neutralizes hydrochloric acid in the stomach; disperses intestinal gas	Treatment of indigestion and peptic ulcers; abdominal distention	Maalox, Mylanta, Riopan, Pepcid
Antianemic/hematinic	Provides elemental iron or vitamin B_{12} vitamin for the formation of hemoglobin	Treatment of iron-deficiency anemias	$Vitamin_{12}$, Folvite, Feosol, Imferon
Antianginal agent	Dilates peripheral blood vessels of the heart and reduces cardiac oxygen demand	Angina pectoris	Nitrostat, Procardia, Cardizem
Antianxiety agent (antihistaminic)	CNS depressant, working similarly to the effects of histamine (see Antihistamine)	Emotional upset; nervous tension; muscle relaxation; neuroses; management of drug withdrawal; vomiting	Atarax, Vistaril
Antianxiety agent	CNS depressant and smooth muscle relaxant	Emotional upset; nervous tension; muscle relaxation; neuroses; management of drug withdrawal	Xanax, Valium
Antiarthritic/antigout agent	Diminishes inflammation of the musculoskeletal system	Arthritis, gout, and other inflammatory conditions	Feldene, Benemid
Antiarrhythmic	Regulates the rate of the heart beat	Cardiac arrhythmias	Lanoxin (digitalis glycoside), Calan (calcium channel blocker)

Table continued on following page

TABLE 4–3. **Therapeutic Classification of Drugs** (*Continued*)

Therapeutic Classification	Action	Use	Examples
Anticoagulant	Inhibits vitamin K–dependent activation of blood coagulation factors II, VII, IX, and X in the liver	Thrombophlebitis, post-myocardial infarction prophylaxis	Coumadin, Heparin
Anticonvulsant	Depresses the brain's motor center or stimulates the seizure threshold of the CNS	Treatment of epilepsy and other neurologic disorders	Phenobarbital, Valium, Dilantin, Fosphenytoin
Antidepressant	Inhibits the CNS neuronal uptake of serotonin	Short-term management of depressive illnesses	Prozac, Elavil, Zoloft, Paxil
Antidiarrheal/antispasmodic	Decreases the motility of the GI tract; antispasmodic	Diarrhea, dysentery, flatulence, and GI disorders	Imodium, Donnatal, Antispas (parenteral), Bentyl, belladonna
Antifungal agent	Kills or prevents the growth of fungi and yeast	Vaginal candidiasis, thrush, athlete's foot, and other mycoses	Monistat, Nitroral
Antihistamine/ antinauseant/ antiemetic	Competes with histamine at cell receptor sites; prevents abnormal amounts of histamine produced in the body, but does not reverse histamine-mediated responses	Treatment of allergic reactions; severe nausea and vomiting	Benadryl, Benylin, Phenergan injection, Seldane, Claritin
Antihyperlipidemic	Lowers cholesterol levels	Adjunct to diet therapy to reduce cholesterol	Zocor, Pravachol
Antihypertensive	Reduces blood pressure by lessening resistance to blood flow, through relaxation of vasoconstricted peripheral vessels	Hypertension, migraine headache, arteriosclerosis, and angina pectoris	Beta-adrenergic blockers (Inderal, Lopressor, Tenormin); calcium-channel blockers (Procardia XL, Norvase, Cardizem, Calan); angiotensin-converting enzyme (ACE) inhibitors (Capoten, Vasotec, Zestril, Prinivil)
Antihypoglycemic	Raises serum glucose levels	Coma of insulin shock therapy; insulin-induced hypoglycemia	Glucagon
Anti-infective, topical	Adjunctive antibiotic therapy to prevent secondary infections	Wounds; second- and third-degree burns	Silvdene Cream
Anti-inflammatory agent (corticosteroid)	Group of natural hormones that have a marked anti-inflammatory effect; suppresses the immune response	Allergic states; eye conditions; hematologic and neoplastic conditions; acute emergencies; acute and chronic skin conditions	Decadron L-A Suspension, Cortef, Hydrocortone, Solu-Cortef, Depo-Medrol, Solu-Medrol, Kenalog-10, Kenalog-40
Anti-inflammatory, NSAID (non-narcotic, nonsteroidal)	Produces anti-inflammatory effects by inhibiting prostaglandin synthesis	Mild to moderate pain arising from the integumental structures; gout; arthritis; rheumatoid diseases	Naprosyn, Motrin, Voltaren

Classification	Action	Use	Examples
Antimicrobial agent (antibiotics)	Kills micro-organisms, inhibits the growth of microorganisms, or prevents the reproduction of microorganisms	Treatment of diseases caused by bacteria, spirochetes, or rickettsiae; not effective for viruses	Trimox, Biaxin, Veetids, Zithromax Z-Pak, Duricef, Ancef, Kefzol, Mefoxin, Ceftin, Claforan, Rocephen, Keflex, Keftab, E-Mycin, Eryped, Erythrocin, Ilosone, Pediamycin, Blephamide, Amcill, Omnipen, Principen, Bicillin L-A, Amoxil, Pen-Vee K, Doryx, Vibramycin, Achromycin, Sumycin, Cipro, Ceclor, Augmentin
Antinauseant/antiemetic	Acts on the medulla of the brain and the vestibular mechanisms of the ear	Nausea, vomiting, vertigo, and motion sickness	Tigan, Compazine
Antipruritic	Reduces the reaction of the skin to irritation; see also anti-inflammatory agents (corticosteroid)	Acute contact dermatitis	Calamine, cocoa butter, collodion, zinc oxide
Antiseptic agent	Prevents growth of surface microorganisms	Skin irritations and cleansing	Hydrogen peroxide, Mercurochrome
Antiulcer agent	Competitively inhibits histamine thereby decreasing gastric secretion or forming a barrier at the ulcer site	Duodenal and gastric ulcers	Tagamet, Zantac, Carafate, antacids, Prilosec
Bronchodilator/antiasthmatic	Dilates the muscular walls of the bronchi; breaks up mucous secretions	Asthma, chronic obstructive pulmonary disease	Albuterol, Alupent, Metaprel, Brethine, Adrenalin 1:1000, Broncaid Mist, Theo-Dur, Ventolin, Proventil
Bronchodilator/vasopressor (anticholinergic, adrenergic)	Dilates the muscular walls of the bronchi; increases vasoconstriction	Bronchitis, asthma, allergic conditions; used in shock to increase blood pressure and open bronchial passages	Aminophyllin, Adrenalin 1:1000, Atrovent
Bronchodilator/vasopressor/decongestant	Dilates the muscular walls of the bronchi; vasoconstricts; dries mucous secretions	Bronchitis, asthma, allergic conditions, nasal congestion	Sus-Phrine, Broncaid Mist
Cardiotonic	Increases strength of myocardial contraction; pulse strengthens and slows	Congestive heart failure	Lanoxin (digoxin), Crystodigin (digitoxin)
Cauterizing agent	Germicidal activity created by metal ions; denatures protein by producing a corrosive effect	Prevention of gonorrheal ophthalmia neonatorum, wound cauterization, local antiseptic	Silver nitrate

Table continued on following page

TABLE 4–3. **Therapeutic Classification of Drugs** (*Continued*)

Therapeutic Classification	Action	Use	Examples
Contraceptive	Suppresses ovulation	Prevention of conception	Lo/Ovral, Ortho-Novum, Triphasil, Ortho-Novum 7/7/7-28
Cough suppressant (antitussive)	Depresses the cough reflex in the medulla of the brain	Allergies, upper respiratory infections, colds	Narcotic (Actifed with Codeine, Ambenyl, Dimetane-DC Syrup, Hycodan Tablets and Syrup), Ambenyl-D, Benadryl, Tuss-Ornade
Cough expectorant	Liquifies mucus and promotes the ejection of mucus from the respiratory tract	Bronchitis, upper respiratory infections, colds	Benylin Syrup, Organidin, Robitussin, Triaminic Expectorant
Diuretic	Increases the production of urine by acting on the renal tubules in the kidney	Control of edema in cardiac disease, such as hypertension; sometimes used to control premenstrual fluid retention	Lasix, Maxzide, Dyazide, Triamterene/HCTZ
Emetic	Stimulates vomiting by irritating the gastic mucosa	To induce vomiting when poisonous substances have been ingested; drug overdose	Ipecac Syrup
Hormone replacement (androgen, estrogen, progestin, corticosteroid, thyroid, testosterone)	Replaces hormonal deficiencies in the body; artificially regulates hormone production	Treatment of functional and dysfunctional uterine bleeding; diabetes; major constituent of birth control pills	Depo-Provera, Provera, Humulin N, Insulin, Premarin, Synthroid, Prempro, Levoxyl
Hypoglycemic	Lowers serum glucose levels	Diabetes mellitus that cannot be controlled by diet alone	Glucophage (oral), Regular (Humulin BR, Humulin R); Prompt Insulin Zinc Suspension (Semilente Iletin I, Semilente); Isophane and Regular (Novolin 70/30); Isophane NPH (Humulin N, Insulatard NPH Human, Novolin N); Insulin Zinc Suspension (Humulin L, Novolin L); Protamine Zinc (PZI); sulfonylureas (Diabinese Micronase, Orinase, Tolinase)
Hypolipidemic	Inhibits early enzyme synthesis of cholesterol	Reduction of low-density lipoprotein and total cholesterol levels in primary hypercholesterolemia	Mevacor

Muscle relaxant	Reduces transmission of impulses from the spinal cord to skeletal muscle	Muscle spasm	Flexeril, Robaxin
Potassium supplement	Replaces and maintains potassium levels	Hypokalemia	Micro-K, Slow-K, K-Dur
Sedative/hypnotic	Acts on the limbic system, thalamus, and hypothalamus of the CNS to produce hypnotic effects	Insomnia	Halcion, Dalmane, Restoril, Ambien
Urinary analgesic	Exerts local anesthetic action on urinary mucosa by an unknown mechanism	Pain due to urinary tract irritation and infection	Pyridium
Urinary antimicrobial	Decreases bacteria folic acid synthesis	Urinary tract infections	Noroxin, Septra, Septra DS
Vaccine, active immunity	Composed of certain antigens that are usually live disease–causing agents; for innoculation, they are weakened or partially detoxified and cause the body to manufacture its own antibodies	Prevention of communicable disease	DTP, influenza virus vaccine, Heptavax-B, Recombivax HB, Pneumovax 23, M.M.R. II, Orimune
Vasodilator	Dilates the arterioles	Relieves pressure on the urethra in benign prostatic hypertrophy; also used to treat hypertension	Hytrin

Source: Adapted from Frew, MA and Frew, DR: Comprehensive Medical Assisting: Administrative and Clinical Procedures. FA Davis, Philadelphia, 1988, with permission.

- *AMA Drug Evaluations*, published by the American Medical Association
- *The American Hospital Formulary*, published by the American Society of Hospital Pharmacists
- *The United States Pharmacopeia/National Formulary (USP/NF)*, published by the United States government. If a drug name is the same as the official name in this reference, the drug name will contain the initials *USP* after it (e.g., influenza virus vaccine, *USP*). The USP/NF lists all the legal drugs in the United States.

There are many databases available as well as large quantities of material available on the Internet. Care should be taken to use and pass on information only backed by scientific research and legitimate internet sites.

Internet Sites for Pharmacology

- http://omni.cc.purdue.edu/~wrunning/cicnet (HealthWeb)
- http://pharminfo.com (commercial organization)
- http://www.cpb.uokhsc.edu/pharmacy/pharmint.html (geographic locations)
- http://www.rxlist.com (searchable database of more than 4,000 drugs)

Therapeutic Classifications of Drugs

The application of drug therapy to patient care involves knowing as many of the factual details of pharmacology as possible. All the details can never be learned or memorized, but the health care provider can learn the general concepts involving the interaction of drugs with one another and with the body's tissue. This knowledge comes by understanding (1) the basic groupings of drug classifications and (2) the basic drug–patient and drug–drug interactions.

Learning about drugs by first understanding the therapeutic classifications of drugs is the easiest way to build a firm knowledge of pharmacology. Drugs in the same classification will possess many similar properties, usually relating to either the action or the use of the drug. Drugs in the same classification often have similar side effects, contraindications, routes, dosage, and important patient education basics. When a new drug arrives on the market, it will be easy to relate it to the others in the same classification you already know. Differences will be more apparent as well.

Table 4–3 lists the therapeutic classifications of the drugs most commonly encountered in the medical office, either in discussions with patients concerning their prescriptions or when administering drugs. The table does not include all classifications of drugs or all possible indications for which any particular drug may be used.

Written Competency 4–1

Performance Competence: Using Table 4–3, classify drugs according to their therapeutic effects, within 30 minutes and with 100 percent accuracy. Do not give yourself credit for partial or incorrect answers. Do not proceed to Written Competency 4–2 until you have corrected all incomplete or incorrect answers.

1. The therapeutic classification for a drug that liquifies mucus and promotes the ejection of mucus from the respiratory tract is:
   (a) Emetic.
   (b) Antiemetic.
   (c) Antitussive.
   (d) Antihistamine.
   (e) Expectorant.

2. The therapeutic classification for Orimune is:
   (a) Vaccine.
   (b) Antifungal agent.
   (c) Anti-infective agent.
   (d) Antimicrobial agent.
   (e) Anti-inflammatory agent.

3. The therapeutic classification for a drug that slows the heart rate and increases the strength of heart contractions is:
   (a) Antihypertensive.
   (b) Vasopressor.
   (c) Cardiotonic.
   (d) Antianginal agent.
   (e) Antiarrhythmic agent.

4. The therapeutic classification for a drug used to prevent blood clots is:
   (a) Antianginal agent.
   (b) Anticoagulant.
   (c) Antihypertensive.
   (d) Potassium supplement.
   (e) Cardiotonic.

5. The therapeutic classification for OTC drugs that treat pain, arthritis, and fever is:
   (a) Analgesic.
   (b) Anti-inflammatory.
   (c) Antipyretic.
   (d) All of the above.
   (e) None of the above.

6. The therapeutic classification for a drug used to treat insomnia is:
   (a) Anesthetic.
   (b) Antianxiety agent.
   (c) Antidepressant.
   (d) Muscle relaxant.
   (e) Sedative.

7. The therapeutic classification for a drug used to treat diabetes is:
   (a) Hypoglycemic.
   (b) Antihypoglycemic.
   (c) Hypolipodemic.
   (d) Hormone replacement.
   (e) Emetic.

8. The therapeutic classification for a drug used to induce vomiting is:
   (a) Antiemetic.
   (b) Antianemic.
   (c) Antinauseant.
   (d) Emetic.
   (e) Expectorant.

9. One therapeutic classification for Lanoxin is:
   (a) Antihypertensive.
   (b) Diuretic.
   (c) Hypolipodemic.
   (d) Antiarrhythmic.
   (e) Muscle relaxant.

10. An example of a drug classified as an NSAID is:
    (a) Motrin.
    (b) Hydrocortone.
    (c) Flexeril.
    (d) Aspirin.
    (e) Tylenol.

Score: _____

See Appendix B for answers.

Written Competency 4–2

Performance Competence: Using the information in Chapter 4, match the following drugs to their classifications, within 30 minutes and with 80 percent accuracy. Do not give yourself credit for partial or incorrect answers.

(a) Hormone	1. Premarin
(b) Antimicrobial	2. Capoten
(c) Contraceptive	3. Amoxil
(d) Diuretic	4. Lasix
(e) Antihypertensive	5. Triphasil
	6. Inderal
	7. Dyazide
	8. Augmentin
	9. Ortho Novum 7/7/7
	10. Synthroid

Score: _____

See Appendix B for answers.

Written Competency 4–3

Performance Competence: For the following 10 questions, circle True or False, within 30 minutes and with 80 percent accuracy. Correct any FALSE statements, making each statement TRUE. Do not give yourself credit for partial or incorrect answers.

1. Once a drug is available in the generic form, any drug company can produce the drug and use the same trade name.   T   F

2. The most reliable source of information about drug–drug interactions is the drug company's sales representative.   T   F

3. Cephalosporin is a drug classification indicating its general effect.   T   F

4. Each drug can be classified only one way.   T   F

5. A palliative drug is used for its curative effect.   T   F

6. Maalox given with tetracycline is an example of a synergistic effect.   T   F

7. The *USP/NF* lists all the legal drugs in the United States.   T   F

8. Drugs organized in particular categories make drug information more uniform.   T   F

9. The *PDR* is organized into one large index.   T   F

10. Information about one drug in a particular classification provides general information about other drugs in the same classification.   T   F

Score: _____

See Appendix B for answers.

Written Competency 4–4

Performance Competence: Using the information in Chapter 4 and Appendix A or a drug reference such as the *PDR*, apply concepts of drug–patient interactions and drug–drug interactions to a patient care situation. Select and circle the one answer or completion that is *best*, within 30 minutes and with 80 percent accuracy. Do not give yourself credit for partial or incorrect answers.

A patient receiving Coumadin (a coumarin-type anticoagulant) calls and reports that she has had a fever and has been taking aspirin (salicylates) for 5 days.

1. Advise this patient to discontinue the (aspirin) (anticoagulant).

2. This drug–drug combination may result in a(n) (decreased) (increased) prothrombin time.

3. This drug–drug interaction is an example of (synergism) (potentiation).

4. A drug–drug interaction resulting in an unexpected change in the patient's prothrombin time would be an example of an (adverse reaction) (idiosyncrasy).

5. The Coumadin is prescribed for (prophylactic) (palliative) reasons.

6. The underlying factor that altered this patient's usual response to either drug is (cumulation) (pathology).

7. The risk of combining aspirin and Coumadin is an example of a (patient precaution) (contraindication).

8. The patient teaching opportunity here is to warn the patient about (OTC drugs) (anticoagulant dose reduction during illness).

9. As a coumarin derivative, Coumadin is a (generic name) (brand name).

10. The physician will advise the patient to (come into the office for laboratory tests and examination) (reduce the dosage of Coumadin).

Score: _____

See Appendix B for answers.

Written Competency 4–5

Performance Competence: Using the information in Chapter 4, Appendix A, and the *PDR,* apply concepts of drug–patient interactions and drug–drug interactions to a patient care situation. Select and circle the one answer or completion that is *best,* within 30 minutes and with 80 percent accuracy. Do not give yourself credit for partial or incorrect answers.

Ms. Smith is an 80-year-old patient with a history of diabetes mellitis (DM), congestive heart failure (CHF), and hypertension (HTN). She is currently taking Lanoxin, Lasix, Insulin, Premarin, Slow K, and prn aspirin. She calls and complains of vaginal bleeding and frequent urination, especially at night (nocturia). An appointment is made for the same day. On review of her systems, she additionally reports visual problems, ringing in her ears (tinnitis), loss of appetite (anorexia), black stools, a general feeling of tiredness (malaise), muscle cramps, and overall weakness. She also experiences excessive sweating (diaphoresis) in the early morning with confusion and lethargy.

1. Ms. Smith's drug(s) reported to cause black stools include _____.

2. Ms. Smith's drug(s) reported to cause tinnitis as a side effect include _____ _____.

3. Ms. Smith's drug(s) reported to cause increased urination and nocturia include _____ _____.

4. Ms. Smith's drug(s) reported to cause visual problems, anorexia, malaise, muscle cramps, and weakness as side effects include _____.

5. Ms. Smith's drug(s) reported to cause diaphoresis, confusion, and lethargy as side effects include _____.

Score: _____

Terminal Performance Objective/Competency

Procedure 4–1: Use Appendix A, the *PDR,* or Other Reference for Proper Drug Identification or Classification

EQUIPMENT   Appendix A
PDR
Other drug reference

Performance Competence: Complete the following 10 assignments within 30 minutes with 100 percent accuracy:

1. The manufacturer of Capoten. _____

2. The generic names for Dyazide. _____

3. The trade name for furosemide. _____

4. The pregnancy safety level for Premarin. _____

5. The normal adult dose for Amoxil. _____

6. The routes that may be used for administering Lasix. _____

7. A drug classified as a thyroid (hormone replacement) agent. _____

8. The generic name for Inderal. _____

9. The color(s) and shape(s) of Triphasil. _____

10. The color and shape(s) of Ortho Novum 7/7/7. _____

Date: _____ Competency achieved: Y _____ N _____

Designated reasonable time standard: _____

Actual completion time: _____

Assignment 4–1: Use Appendix A, the *PDR*, or Other Reference to Create Drug Information Guides

EQUIPMENT   Appendix A; *PDR;* or other drug reference
Line notepaper or index cards
Drugs: 1st 10 drugs from the 50 Most Commonly Prescribed Drugs List, Appendix A

Performance Competence: Complete a drug guide for each of the drugs listed under Equipment. The ten guides should be completed with 100 percent accuracy and must include the following:

Generic name _____

Brand name (trade name) _____

Classification _____

Controlled substance classification _____

Pregnancy risk category _____

Action _____

Indications use _____

Contraindications _____

Adverse reactions/side effects _____

Dosage/Route _____

Patient education (in terms the patient will understand)

    Compliance issues _____

    Report to the physician when _____

Special alert _____

Date: _____ Competency achieved: Y _____ N _____

Conversion Drill for Skill

Using Table 1–7 and the conversion formula, convert the following weights within 10 minutes. Do not give yourself credit for partial or incorrect answers. Strive for a score of 100 percent. If you score less than 100 percent, return to Chapter 1 and reread the section on conversions.

1. 24 lb = _____ kg

2. 62 lb = _____ kg

3. 86 lb = _____ kg

4. 105 lb = _____ kg

5. 143 lb = _____ kg

6. 6 kg   = _____ lb

7. 10 kg = _____ lb

8. 22 kg = _____ lb

9. 40 kg = _____ lb

10. 100 kg = _____ lb

Using the conversions 1–5 just completed above, calculate the dose for each "patient," using a drug that has the directions to administer 5 mg/kg/day bid. (Ex: A patient weighs 10 Kg. 5 mg × 10 = 50 mg. Divided into two doses per day, 50 mg ÷ 2 = 25 mg per dose.)

11. _____ Kg × 5 mg = _____ mg/day and _____ mg in each dose.

12. _____ Kg × 5 mg = _____ mg/day and _____ mg in each dose.

13. _____ Kg × 5 mg = _____ mg/day and _____ mg in each dose.

14. _____ Kg × 5 mg = _____ mg/day and _____ mg in each dose.

15. _____ Kg × 5 mg = _____ mg/day and _____ mg in each dose.

Convert the following:

16. 0.6 g   = _____ gr

17. 500 mg = _____ G

18. 175 mcg = _____ mg

19. 20 ml   = _____ tsp

20. 240 cc = _____ oz

21. 16 oz   = _____ Tbls

22. dr iii = _____ ml

23. 10 mg   = _____ gr

24. gr xv   = _____ mg

25. 30 cc   = _____ oz

Score: _____

See Appendix B for answers.

5

Safety in Drug Therapy and Patient Care

Universal Blood and Body Fluid Precautions
  Protective skin care and skin barriers
  Handling and disposal of needles and syringes
Safety Precautions for Preparing Medications
  Medication storage
Assessment of the Patient
Medication Allergies (Hypersensitivities)
Patient Education in Drug Therapy
Pediatric Dosage Forms
Pediatric Rules of Safety
The Use of Drugs in Pregnant and Lactating Women
Geriatric Rules of Safety

WRITTEN COMPETENCY 5–1: Apply Rules of Safety for Assessment of the Environment and Patient Assessment to the Clinical Situation

TERMINAL PERFORMANCE OBJECTIVE/COMPETENCY (PROCEDURE 5–1): Prepare a Medication

TERMINAL PERFORMANCE OBJECTIVE/COMPETENCY (PROCEDURE 5–2): Administer a Medication to a Patient

TERMINAL PERFORMANCE OBJECTIVE/COMPETENCY (PROCEDURE 5–3): Prepare a Patient Teaching Guide

TERMINAL PERFORMANCE OBJECTIVE/COMPETENCY (PROCEDURE 5–4): Teach a Patient to Take a Medication

TERMINAL PERFORMANCE OBJECTIVE/COMPETENCY (PROCEDURE 5–5): Create a Bulletin Board That Instructs Patients About Drug Therapy

ASSIGNMENT 5–1: Use Appendix A, the *PDR,* or Other Reference to Create Drug Information Guides

CONVERSION DRILL FOR SKILL

OBJECTIVES **WRITTEN COMPETENCY 5–1:** Apply rules of safety for assessment of the environment and patient assessment to the clinical situation.

TERMINAL PERFORMANCE OBJECTIVE (PROCEDURE 5–1): Prepare a medication.

TERMINAL PERFORMANCE OBJECTIVE (PROCEDURE 5–2): Administer a medication to a patient.

TERMINAL PERFORMANCE OBJECTIVE (PROCEDURE 5–3): Prepare a patient teaching guide.

ASSIGNMENT 5–1: Use drug references to create drug information guides.

CONVERSION DRILL FOR SKILL: Convert measurements to their most frequently used approximate equivalents.

117

Although drugs must successfully pass through a long series of studies before becoming commercial products (see Chapter 2), most have the potential to cause side effects in a small percentage of patients, especially the elderly, pregnant women, and children. Because drugs can never be considered 100 percent safe, drug assessment for every patient never ends nor is it the responsibility of just the manufacturer or any one person.

Each health team member involved in preparing and administering a drug to a patient must be informed about the drug, the illness, and the patient, and constantly be alert to environmental safety and any changes or new information that could make the administration of a drug improper or undesirable. Assessment first involves ensuring that the environment is safe during the preparation of the medication and for the patient at the time of its administration.

Universal Blood and Body Fluid Precautions

Safety begins with aseptic practices. In addition to sterile procedures, the routine use of appropriate barrier precautions (e.g., gloves, masks, gowns, and goggles) may be necessary when *contact* with blood or other body fluids is anticipated. Because administering medications at times may result in contact with blood and other body fluids, a review of barrier protections and the handling of sharp instruments is necessary. Although barriers will not necessarily provide protection from skin puncture, they will provide protection from the other three potential ways of transmitting bloodborne organisms: *splash*, *spill*, and *splatter*.

PROTECTIVE SKIN CARE AND SKIN BARRIERS

Handwashing is necessary before and after each drug preparation and administration using tepid water with a quality grade of surgical soap and followed with an application of hand lotion, to keep the skin moist and intact. *Patient contact of any sort must be avoided if open lesions or broken skin is present on the hands, face, or other exposed body surfaces of the health care worker.* Medical assistants and other health workers should be excused from direct patient care until their skin conditions are healed.

In minor cases of chapped hands, it is important to wear single-use, disposable, nonsterile gloves for personal protection, whether the patient contact is invasive (involving puncture or incision) or noninvasive. If exposure to patient blood or body fluids is expected, gloves must be worn. Every injection is a procedure that invades the underlying tissues, and every needle is exposed to blood and body fluids. Therefore, every injection is a high-risk source of spill, splash, and splatter and gloves should be worn when administering injections.

HANDLING AND DISPOSAL OF NEEDLES AND SYRINGES

"Sharps" (needles and sharp instruments) must be handled with care and concentration. Organized and concise movements for handling a syringe and needle unit are necessary to prevent injury and contamination. After injecting a medication into the patient, every precaution must be taken not to touch the needle. To keep movement around a contaminated needle to a minimum, *do not* recap the needle and *do not* bend, break, or in any other way tamper with a needle after use. At the treatment site, dispose of the intact needle–syringe unit into a closed-system, rigid, puncture-resistant disposal container (Fig. 5–1), and dispose of the container before it becomes three-quarters full.

If a used needle–syringe unit must be transferred to another area for disposal, recap the needle. The procedure for this, however, is very specific. First, recap the needle using *one hand* against a medication tray. *Do not* touch the cap or any part of the needle. Then, carry the syringe unit to the disposal area on the medication tray, held directly in front and above waist level. *Do not* carry needle–syringe units in clothing pockets.

Work surfaces should be cleaned with standard household bleach (5.25 percent sodium

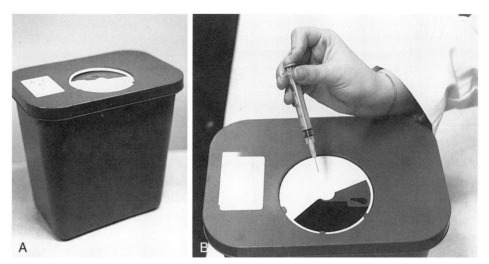

FIGURE 5–1. *A,* A closed-system, rigid, puncture-resistant disposal container. *B,* Disposing of syringe and needle. (From Frew, MA and Frew, DR: Clinical Procedures for Medical Assisting. F. A. Davis, Philadelphia, 1990, p 310 with permission.)

hypochlorite) prepared as a 1:10 (1 part bleach to 10 parts water) dilution fresh each day. Other acceptable cleaning solutions include ethyl alcohol, glutaraldehyde, and stabilized hydrogen peroxide. (For preparation of these stock solutions, see Chapter 8.) Cleaning materials should be placed in hazardous waste bags according to Occupational Safety and Health Administration (OSHA) regulations

Safety Precautions for Preparing Medications

Good habits involving concentration and competence in hand–eye coordination must be developed. Conscientious and deliberate body movements, intelligently applied, are necessary for preserving sterile medication products and preventing the contamination of sterile materials.

In addition to a "sterility conscience," preparing the appropriate drug for treatment requires a commitment to honesty and straightforwardness: be reliable in understanding the language of each drug order written; responsibly recognize and immediately correct an error or break in sterile technique; and honestly report an error made, or the lack of understanding of a drug order.

Safeguarding the patient begins with the "seven rights." Assess each order by asking, "Is this . . . ?"

- The right patient
- The right drug (name and strength)
- The right dose
- The right route
- The right time (e.g., hour, date, time of day, etc.)
- The right technique
- The right documentation

For each drug routinely administered, know its use (indication), adverse reactions, usual dosage, route, storage requirements, and any special directions for the patient. Create medication index cards or a medication notebook for a quick reference (see Chapter 4). Package inserts may be glued to cards or notebook paper and filed or bound in alphabetic order. Other sources include reference books, journals, and textbooks (see Chapter 4).

In the medication room, the steps of safety begin with the *three medication checks.* Compare every medication order with the label the following *three times:*

1. When taking the medication from storage
2. While preparing the medication
3. When replacing the medication in storage (in most circumstances medications are replaced in storage *before* administration to patients; it would not be safe to perform the third check after administering the medication)

Then, these additional steps of safety should be practiced with each drug prepared:

1. Work with adequate lighting and materials.
2. Prepare medications in quiet. Do not converse with others when preparing a drug.
3. Pay attention to the procedure and think through each step. Do not allow the process to become automatic and routine: that is when errors are most likely to occur.
4. Prepare the specific drug ordered. Never substitute without conferring with the physician.
5. Prepare the exact dosage ordered by the physician. If the strength of the medication on hand is not exact, calculate dosage accurately and according to set formulas each time. If the ordered strength is not available by calculation, notify the physician, who may adjust the dosage so that it may be measured exactly.
6. Never hesitate to question an order, for instance, if it is suspected that the dosage ordered is not within normal dosage limits. Consult with the physician.
7. Return drugs to storage immediately *after* use. Drugs should not be left out unattended.
8. If a drug is prepared for the physician to administer, leave the patient's chart, the prepared medication, *and* the drug container together for the physician to perform the "seven rights."
9. Administer only medications you have personally prepared or that have been prepared by the physician.
10. Every medication should be charted by the physician before administration and then initialled or otherwise signed after administration, designating that the order was indeed carried through.
11. Chart every medication with a routine that will prevent duplication or omission.

MEDICATION STORAGE

Medications are manufactured with a variety of storage needs, under sterile and nonsterile conditions. Drugs may require dry storage at room temperature (59° to 86°F), refrigeration (approximately 40°F), or freezing (below 32°F). Directions for the storage of each medication is clearly stated on the label, the package insert, and the shipping container label (Fig. 5–2). When drugs are received into inventory, their labels should be checked for storage requirements.

In addition to temperature requirements, some medications must be stored away from sunlight; however, it is advisable to store *all* medications in cool, clean areas, away from direct sunlight as well as patients and the public. Do not leave medications unattended or unlocked in areas accessible to patients.

Whether medications are stored on the shelf or in the refrigerator, shelve medications in alphabetic order and rotate those medications that will expire first to the front of the shelf. De-

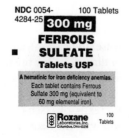

The seal of this package bears our name, Roxane. If the seal is broken or our name does not appear, do not use. **Usual Dose:** Adults, 1 tablet 3 times daily with meals. Children, as directed by physician. **Caution:** As with any drug, if you are pregnant or nursing a baby, seek the advice of a health professional before using this product. **Warning:** Keep this and all drugs out of the reach of children. In case of accidental overdose, seek professional assistance or contact a poison control center immediately. Store at Controlled Room Temperature 15°-30°C (59°-86°F). Protect from Moisture.

NDC 0054-4284-25   100 Tablets
300 mg
FERROUS SULFATE
Tablets USP
A hematinic for iron deficiency anemias. Each tablet contains Ferrous Sulfate 300 mg (equivalent to 60 mg elemental iron).
Roxane Laboratories, Inc. Columbus, Ohio 43216   100 Tablets

4166701 080

FIGURE 5–2. Bottle of ferrous sulfate tablets, USP. (Courtesy of Roxane Laboratories Inc., Columbus, OH.)

velop a system for re-ordering *before* the last amount is used. Know usage rates, and mark or tag the last container with "time to reorder." Record and inventory narcotic medications daily.

The following procedures help to maximize the shelf life and maintain the sterility and safe use of liquid and solid medications (see also Chapter 6, Rules for Stock Drugs):

1. Check expiration dates each time a medication is taken from the shelf. Discard expired drugs.
2. Unless otherwise directed, do not use a drug that has changed color or developed a precipitate.
3. Pour liquids from bottles on the side opposite that of the label. Keep the label against the palm of the hand.
4. Wipe clean the sides of bottles after each use.
5. Do not return unused medications to their containers.
6. Do not relabel medications: discard any medication containers with damaged labels.
7. Do not handle solid medications. Shake solid medications (tablets, and so on) directly from the container into the container lid, then transfer the tablets from the lid into a medication cup.

Assessment of the Patient

As it has been stated, drug therapy requires constant evaluation of the specific drugs being used, the illnesses for which they are used, the environment in which they are used, and, most importantly, the patient. Assessment of the patient in relation to drug therapy includes two main parts: known data about the patient's past medical history and an assessment of the patient's current physical status.

The first aspect of patient data collection is rather simple but important—that of patient identification. In drug therapy it is especially important to ensure that the patient is correctly identified as the one who is to receive a specific medication. When approaching a patient, the only acceptable approach is to *ask the patient to state his or her own name.* Do not call a patient by his or her name and then ask for verification. Too often, patients nod in agreement without really listening. This mistaken compliance is sometimes due to an emotional state or a decreased level of functioning, but, most often, patients trustingly believe that if they are being addressed, the persons addressing them know who they are.

Before the physician writes a medication order, evaluation of the patient's past history is a necessary part of a decision to prescribe a particular medication. The physician's diagnosis and supplemental laboratory results, when available, usually confirm the appropriateness of a medication order, but other factors concerning the patient's past history could alter the desirability of the use of a drug or one drug over another.

Chronic conditions, for example, may contraindicate the use of a drug or require a reduced dosage. The patient may be currently taking other medications, which could cause excess dosage, adverse mixtures of medication, or drug dependencies. The patient may be on a diet that contraindicates the use of a drug—for example, the patient may ingest alcohol, nicotine, or caffeine. Another important factor is allergies—drug reactions, food reactions, and reactions to animal proteins. It is important to know what chemicals and proteins are included in drugs and whether or not the patient already has a known history of allergy to those chemicals or proteins.

In a holistic manner (considering all aspects of the patient as a person), the patient's emotional status is as important as the physical status. Successful drug therapy depends on the patient's level of understanding the disease and how it is to be treated, social support at home, financial ability to continue the treatment, and past patterns of health care compliance.

In carrying out the physician's orders, physical assessment is ongoing. The patient's age, weight, and physical height should be recorded. Patients who are at the extremes of overweight or underweight may need an increase or reduction in the usual adult dosage. Some drugs have such a low margin of safety (see therapeutic index, farther on) that dosage will depend on the exact size of the patient. The patient's age may determine the inappropriateness of a drug or at least an adjusted dosage. Young children and the elderly, for example, have different rates of metabolism and excretion and usually require adjusted rates of dosage.

The physical assessment of the patient includes the evaluation of a particular site or route chosen for the administration. The physician may order a drug to be injected into a particular muscle but, as the site is being prepared, a recent change in pigmentation or a growth is noted, which would make the site ordered inappropriate. The physical condition of the patient can often influence whether the original order should stand or be changed.

Finally, drug assessment includes evaluation of the patient after a medication has been administered. The patient's response to a medication should be closely monitored, especially after a medication has been administered by injection. After injections or the administration of any medication that is known to be capable of bringing on severe adverse reactions, stay with the patient and observe for any unexpected response. With some drugs, patients are asked to wait 20 to 30 minutes, in case of a possibly delayed, unexpected response. Patient education should include undesirable side effects and what to do in case they should occur after the patient has left the facility. When an unexpected response occurs, it is important to add the incident to the patient medical history for future reference.

In summary, every member of the health team participating in drug therapy must scrutinize the appropriateness of every drug ordered and the overall patient situation, specifically:

1. Identify the patient by asking his or her name.
2. Ask the patient about any drug or food allergies.
3. Assess the patient's:
   a. Past history
   b. Age
   c. Weight and height
   d. Medication site contraindications
4. Stay with the patient until all drugs are taken.
5. Observe the patient for untoward reactions.
6. Document the administration and patient education.

Medication Allergies (Hypersensitivities)

It was stated previously that collecting data about patient allergies and reactions to food, drug, and animal products is very important. Medications so closely resemble the same products in food and animals that cause allergic reactions in humans that it is worth going into some detail about how medications cause allergies (hypersensitivities).

Allergens are substances capable of inducing allergy or hypersensitivity. Almost any drug can be or become an allergen to an individual patient. Once a drug to which the patient is allergic (sensitized) comes in contact again with body cells, it will set off a series of reactions that range from drug-induced skin reactions (local inflammation) or generalized body hives to potentially fatal reactions.

For this reason, drug allergy histories are very important. Any allergy should be noted in red on the outside cover of the patient folder and on every page of the medical record. Patients should be asked, before every injection, if they are allergic to products that are similar to any of the drug's components—another reason why safety in drug administration includes a complete knowledge of each drug administered.

In addition to known drug allergies, a patient is always in jeopardy of developing a new drug allergy at any time. The fact that a patient tolerated a medication in the past does not ensure that the patient will not develop a reaction if the drug is given again. Often on first contact with a drug there is no response, but on subsequent contact the body's immune system will react to the drug and cause tissue damage or even fatal systemic failure.

As with any allergy, the presence of an allergic substance releases a very complicated immune response in the body. White blood cells release toxins, antibodies build up and begin to attack the body's own cells, and huge amounts of histamine are released.

Histamine is found in nearly every type of body tissue. Histamine is released in extreme cold, in body injury due to micro-organism invasion or trauma, and in allergic reactions. Histamine produces the following body effects:

1. Histamine dilates blood vessels, thereby decreasing blood pressure. Decreased blood pressure causes fluids to build up in the tissues, producing edema (swelling). One local example of edema is congestion of the nasal passages during colds and allergies. Serious swelling of other structures, such as the larynx and trachea (bronchospasm), however, could pose the life-threatening risk of respiratory failure.
2. Histamine contracts the smooth muscles that control the body's organs. Large amounts of histamine will cause the bronchi (smooth muscle) of the lungs to constrict, causing asthma, for example, or respiratory distress.
3. *Anaphylactic shock* occurs when histamine produces a rapid decrease in blood pressure, edema of the respiratory organs, and bronchospasm. These changes may produce a circulatory shock that is fatal in minutes, if left unattended.
4. Other body reactions to histamine include uterine contractions; increased stomach acid secretion; increased bronchial, intestinal, and salivary secretions; dilation of cerebral blood vessels causing severe headaches; and pain and itching of the sensory nerves of the skin.

Mild histamine-induced reactions may be treated with antihistamines, which block additional effects of histamine, or with corticosteroids, which beneficially alter the histamine response of the patient to asthma-inducing or skin-inflaming agents. The more serious anaphylactic shock and severe asthma attack reactions must be treated with emergency medications ordered by the physician such as epinephrine (Adrenalin), ephedrine, and aminophylline. Cardiopulmonary resuscitation may also be necessary.

Prevention of allergic drug reaction is the responsibility of health care professionals. To protect patients against the harm of allergic response, certain precautions must be taken when giving drugs that are:

- Known to produce an allergic reaction in a large percentage of the population (e.g., antibiotics—especially the penicillins, or contrast media injection during radiographic studies)
- Known to produce histamine reactions such as hives, asthma, and anaphylaxis (e.g., certain vaccines and toxoids)
- Used to desensitize allergic individuals (e.g., pollen-allergen injection therapy [allergy shots])
- Used to treat or reverse an allergic reaction or asthmatic attack in progress

Patients who receive drugs that fall into any of the four aforementioned categories must do the following:

1. Be thoroughly assessed for current health status and history of allergy
2. Remain in the office for *30 minutes* after injections to be observed for local skin reactions, generalized skin or respiratory reactions, or anaphylaxis. If serious, life-threatening allergic reactions occur, they will usually occur within 30 minutes. (This does not preclude the less severe allergic reactions that may occur hours or days later, however.)
3. Be given careful instructions about the way the drug works and specific problems commonly encountered with drug side effects or toxicity. Toxicity is an exaggerated response to a drug. It is usually the result of too large a dose, impaired patient metabolism or excretion abilities, or a particular patient sensitivity to the effects of a drug.

Special procedures are required for drugs known to cause allergy (hypersensitivity) in patients. They include the following:

1. If a patient is asked to wait for a specific time after receiving an injection, the exact time the patient is detained and any other follow-up notes are recorded on the chart as part of the medication documentation; for example:

   1/1/90 3:30 PM Rx: Pollen serum 1:10,000, injection No. 10. Patient asked to wait 30 minutes.

   3:40 PM Small 1 cm local redness and swelling noted at the injection site; 2 tsp Benadryl (per physician order or written protocol) administered for reaction; patient asked to wait another 30 minutes.

   4:10 PM Patient left office; no further local or systemic reactions noted. Allergist called, ordered dosage reduced to 0.1 ml, same schedule. No further instructions given to the patient. Initials.

2. Anytime a patient is asked to wait for observation for allergic reactions following the administration of a medication, the medication and order are not to be put away but should be kept out in a safe place until the patient is discharged to go home. This is done so that, in case of severe reaction, the physician will be able immediately to see the order and the drug administered. Putting away the drug would preclude this double-check and waste valuable time in an emergency.

3. In the drug-sensitive patient or in any situation in which the chance of drug reaction is highly likely, it is recommended that the patient be asked about specific allergies and the full "seven rights" performed a second time immediately before the medication is injected.

If mild reactions, such as local inflammation, occur:

1. The physician may order an antihistamine (e.g., Benadryl liquid or capsules) be given before the patient is discharged to go home.

2. The patient will be asked to stay another 20 to 30 minutes to ensure that the condition improves rather than worsens. When a patient is given any treatment for asthma or allergy, the patient must remain 30 minutes from the time of the treatment, so that the effects of the treatment can be observed and recorded.

3. Should a patient later report developing a mild allergic reaction (anything from diarrhea to rashes or fever) the physician will want to make an immediate decision as to whether or not the patient should continue taking the medication. The incident reaction is reported in the patient's chart, and the patient is considered allergic to that medication from that time on. Thereafter, the patient's medical record is labeled with the allergic substance identified on the outside of the folder and on every page of the medical record.

Patient Education in Drug Therapy

Patient education has been proved to be the first line of support that leads to a patient's compliance (willingness) in following medical treatment and lifestyle change recommendations. Studies have shown that patients who have received well-presented instructions and rationales fare better than patients who have not received information or who do not understand the information given them.

The objectives of patient education are to encourage the patient to:

1. Participate fully in decisions concerning his or her own care; that is, to agree with decisions without being forced to accept the values of the physician and other health care providers

2. Cooperate with the health care team, by communicating honestly positive and negative feelings and expectations of and discouragements regarding treatment, and by keeping appointments and reporting either progress or a lack thereof

3. Follow the treatment recommendations, as directed

4. Integrate the illness and its treatment into his or her own lifestyle; that is, to teach patients how to adjust to diet changes, to changes in habits, and to taking medications that may produce uncomfortable side effects

Drug therapy is a situation in which patients must know and understand certain facts—dosage and timing, for example, because these two factors are essential for correct patient compliance. The following points are important in patient education to ensure drug therapy compliance.

- Make sure the patient has the mental capacity to understand the information by asking certain questions, such as "Do you know what day this is?" or "Do you know what we are about to do?" Choose a time when the patient is mentally alert and not distracted by other conditions. Talk with the patient in an area that is conducive to listening, and present the material at a level the patient can understand.
- Use several senses, such as visual aids with an oral presentation. After information is given, ask the patient to reply with the information. Give simplified direct information; for example, say "Take this medication at 10 AM, 2 PM, and 6 PM," rather than "Take this medication three times each day." Use repetition: Explain, ask the patient to explain back to you, then review the directions once again.

Although the details will vary, always include the following key points of drug therapy:

1. Patient's food or drug allergies
2. Name of the drug
3. Exact dosage
4. Action of the drug
5. Timing of the administration
   a. Exact hour(s) of administration
   b. Food–drug interactions and directions
   c. Drugs to be avoided at bedtime or when driving a car, for example
6. Storage requirements and instructions for preparation
7. Specific over-the-counter (OTC) drug interactions to avoid
8. Comfort measures that would enhance the drug's effect or minimize its side effects
9. Safety tips, such as keeping medications out of the reach of children or notifying other health care providers of the drug being taken
10. Common side effects and signs of toxicity, and how to notify the physician if such signs should occur
11. Problems to expect with sudden cessation of drug therapy

For patients taking multiple drugs, work with the patient to devise systems for therapy reminders:

- Posters or charts
- Calendars or monthly dispensers
- Weekly reminders, such as empty egg cartons or pill boxes

Because pharmaceutic facts are so confusing to the patient, the best teaching plans use patient-teaching handouts. Preprinted teaching plans are available from a variety of sources; it is also easy to design your own. Figure 5–3 is a sample teaching guide that can be used as a master, onto which information can be entered for any teaching situation.

Recording a teaching session is as important as recording the administration of a drug. Methods of recording teaching sessions will vary from place to place. It is important to include the date and time, along with the name of the person who gave the teaching. This provides a legal document that the patient was instructed on the correct use of the medication, understood the directions, and agreed to follow the treatment recommendations. If the patient did not receive instructions, this also should be noted with an explanation of why instructions were not given. The following is an example of teaching documentation.

1/1/90 3:30 PM Rx: Pollen serum 1:10,000 injection No. 10. Patient asked to wait 30 minutes.

PATIENT MEDICATION PLAN

Patient Name _____   Date _____

FOR _____ DRUGS to TREAT _____
                      (classification)   (illness)

- -

(In layman's terms, give here a brief description of how the drug works.)

Instructions: The name of your drug is _____ .
                      The dose ordered for you is _____ .
                      Special storage needs are _____ .

                      The drug should be taken _____ times a day
                      the best times are _____ , _____ , _____ , _____ .

                      This drug should/should not be taken with meals, because food will affect the way the
                      drug is absorbed.

                      Some side-effects that you should be aware of include _____
                      _____ .

                      Activities that should/should not be considered while taking this drug are _____
                      _____ .

                      Tell any _____
                                        (doctor, nurse, dentist, etc.)
                      who takes care of you that you are taking this medication.

                      Keep this and all medications out of the reach of children.

Notify your physician immediately if any of the following occur:

(List specific signs of drug toxicity commonly occurring.)

Avoid abruptly stopping the use of this medication.
Stopping this medication suddenly can cause _____ .

Be sure to complete the full course of this prescription.

Do not use this medication for any other illness, or give this medication to any other person.

FIGURE 5–3. Sample drug therapy teaching guide.

3:40 PM   Small 1 cm local redness and swelling noted at the injection site; 2 tsp Benadryl (per physician order or written protocol) administered for reaction; patient asked to wait another 30 minutes.

4:10 PM   Patient informed that this reaction was minimal and that his allergist would be contacted for further directions. Patient directed to call and set up an appointment with his allergist. Physician recommended Benadryl, 2 tsp q4h for the rest of the day. Patient instructed to call the office if the redness and swelling does not subside by tomorrow or in case of shortness of breath or any difficulty breathing.

4:10 PM   Patient left office; no further local or systemic reactions noted. Allergist called, ordered dosage reduced to 0.1 ml, same schedule. Initials.

Pediatric Dosage Forms

The administration of drugs to children requires a few special precautions. The physiologic processes of children do not fully mature until age 12. A child's body functions and responds differently in drug absorption, distribution, metabolism, and excretion. These factors must be taken into consideration by the physician when prescribing and administering medications to children.

In infants and small children, oral drug absorption may be delayed or enhanced by lower gastric acidity and intramuscular medications may be delayed by underdeveloped muscle mass. Drugs applied to the skin, on the other hand, are usually absorbed faster because the child's body surface area is so much greater in proportion to the internal organs.

The distribution of drugs can occur either more quickly or more slowly than in adults, depending on the drug. Usually distribution is faster, which means that toxicity is more of a concern in children. Occasionally, however, a child's decreased sensitivity to certain compounds requires higher doses per unit of body weight than in adults. Diphtheria immunizations, for example, are administered with higher doses of the diphtheria toxoid for infants than for older children and adults. Until the end of the first year, infant metabolism is lower and drug elimination by the kidneys is decreased.

Some drugs are specially manufactured in reduced-strength pediatric dosage forms, but most pediatric doses are hand-calculated scaled-down adult doses. Adult doses are manufactured for the average adult, usually based on the average weight of 150 pounds. (For this reason care must be taken not to overdose underweight adults and geriatric patients.) Because body weight is the standard by which most drugs are manufactured, lower doses, usually based on body weight, are calculated for children.

Although not particularly accurate, this approach has been successful because most drugs used today in pediatric practice are relatively nontoxic medications with a wide margin of safety (wide therapeutic index). The therapeutic index is a method of assessing the safety of a drug and compares a drug's lethal dose with its effective dose. Drugs that have a low margin of safety (narrow therapeutic index; e.g., digoxin) are drugs in which the levels needed for effective treatment are dangerously close to toxic levels. For this reason, manufacturers now calculate pediatric doses from adult doses by translating dosage into milligrams per kilogram of body weight (see Chapter 8).

> **SPECIFIC TECHNIQUES: Multidose vials of sterile isotonic saline contain a bacteriostatic preservative that has been found to cause seizures in infants up to 1 month of age or older when used to reconstitute drugs for IM injection. Diluents in single-dose vials that do not contain preservatives should be used for infants.**

Pediatric Rules of Safety

Other problems include the child's cooperation and understanding about drug therapy. The child's compliance and education will, of course, depend on the child's level of development and the cooperation of the parents. The following are some general rules for administering medications to the pediatric patient.

DO's

1. Have the attitude that the cooperation of the child is important; otherwise there is a war of the wills.
2. Be empathetic toward a child's negative feelings about receiving a medication. It is natural.
3. Be friendly but firm that the medication must be administered.
4. If you cannot gain the child's cooperation, restrain the child with the help of the mother or other personnel (see farther on).
5. Talk to the child. Use diversion tactics: play, sing, say the alphabet.
6. If the child is old enough, explain that he or she will taste a medication for a minute or, if an injection, that a medication will sting for a minute, but that it is important to hold very still.

7. It is best to keep the knowledge of an injection to the last minute, but do let the child know just before injecting. Keep the needle out of the child's sight.
8. After medicating, offer praise even though the child may not have cooperated. Show support and appreciation.
9. Take opportunities to explain how the treatment will be helpful.
10. Crush tablets for children under age 5.
11. Disguise crushed medication only in nonessential foods. The child may remember the off taste and not eat that food again.
12. A hug with your praise for cooperation works just great!

DON'T's

1. Do not offer bribes for taking a medication. This suggests that medications are bad.
2. Do not allow parents to pretend they are taking the medication first.
3. Do not belittle or make fun of the child's fears.
4. Do not say you want the child to be a "big boy or girl."
5. Do not try to prevent the child from crying. Denying such a physical or emotional reaction to pain or fear is not realistic.
6. Do not offer rewards such as candy, Band-aids, or used medication equipment as toys.
7. Do not force oral medications: they may be accidentally aspirated.
8. Never lie to a child.

To restrain a child, hold the child against your body with one arm around the child supporting the head and neck. Have the child's arm nearest you tucked and secured between your side and the child's. With the other hand, hold the child's free arm and hand. Keep the child's head elevated to prevent aspiration.

The Use of Drugs in Pregnant and Lactating Women

Most drugs pass through the placental barrier and circulate in the blood of the embryo and fetus. The embryo is particularly sensitive to the effects of chemicals during the first trimester. A woman contemplating pregnancy should ideally discontinue all prescription and OTC drugs before becoming pregnant, unless, of course, a drug is specifically prescribed by the physician. During pregnancy, all drugs are theoretically contraindicated unless the potential benefit to the mother outweighs the potential risk to the child.

The Food and Drug Administration (FDA) has established five categories (Table 5–1) for the use of drugs in pregnant and lactating women. When using official package insert information or information from other drug references, pay particular attention to these categories. Learn to look for these special warnings for each drug administered.

TABLE 5–1. **Drug Use in Pregnancy Categories**

Category	Definition
A	Animal and human studies to date have failed to show a risk to the fetus. There appears to be no risk in any of the three trimesters of pregnancy.
B	Animal studies have shown no risk to the fetus, but clinical studies on women are inadequate or incomplete.
C	Animal studies have shown a risk to the fetus, and clinical studies on women are inadequate, incomplete, or unavailable or no animal or human studies are available.
D	There is clinical evidence of risk to the human fetus, but drug use may be acceptable in pregnant women despite its risk.
X	There is clinical evidence that the use of a drug has a high-risk potential to the developing fetus and has resulted in birth defects. These drugs should be contraindicated in pregnancy despite their usefulness in treatment.

These categories are based on animal and human studies, and indicate whether or not a drug systemically absorbed by the fetus can affect reproductive capacity or cause birth defects or both. Some studies also show whether or not a particular drug is excreted in human milk and should be used with caution in lactating mothers.

The categories listed in Table 5–1 are general only, and intended as an alert to read more information before administering a drug or educating patients about a drug. Information about each drug described in the following chapters will include its pregnancy risk category. The categories represent a consensus from drug resource materials. Read package inserts for more detailed information on each specific drug.

Geriatric Rules of Safety

Like the pediatric patient, elderly persons are more sensitive to the effects of drugs and present potential problems unique to this life stage. The metabolism in the geriatric patient is considerably slowed, which alters the rates of drug absorption, distribution, metabolism, and excretion.

Elderly patients have increased fatty tissue and decreased muscle tissue, which results in delayed absorption and the accumulation of drugs in their body tissues. Various other physiologic changes increase and prolong the distribution of drugs in the body system and increase sensitivity to certain drugs, thus increasing the risk of toxicity. Reduced blood flow, liver functions, and renal function also decrease the metabolism of drugs and further complicate the distribution of drugs during the aging process by causing changes in drug tolerance.

Geriatric patients often have chronic conditions such as heart disease, diabetes, and hypertension, and drugs used for treatment may have untoward effects on these conditions. For example, some medications used to treat glaucoma may not be used by patients with heart arrhythmias, as they will cause a change in the heart rate. Geriatric patients are often prescribed many medications, which increases the risk of undesired drug interactions.

Geriatric patients often have a poor nutritional status owing to lowered food intake or an unbalanced diet. A poor nutritional status often alters the patient's response to a drug. Because of senility or mental confusion, some elderly patients often either forget to take a medication or take a medication incorrectly, resulting in underdosage or overdosage.

Not all the elderly are senile, however. It is important that geriatric patients not be stereotyped as forgetful: forgetfulness happens at any age. Know each patient as an individual. Know how to relate to patients who are fully functional and how to enhance relationships with those who, because of age-related disease, may be forgetful or confused and who may need additional time and explanations.

When a patient cannot be trusted to remember and follow directions, teaching techniques must be altered to maximize compliance. Take into account conditions that include forgetfulness: impaired sight, hearing, and mobility and a decreased ability to understand directions. If necessary, meet with the patient's children or other care providers and share instructions and directions with them. Some information to share includes:

1. Give written teaching instructions and make sure that the patient can physically read the instructions. Side effects, precautions, and other related information should be explained to the patient prior to each initial drug administration.
2. Encourage patients to call the office staff if they no longer feel the medication is working or notice side effects. This will increase the chances that the patient will call the office rather than choose to discontinue treatment.
3. Provide sufficient amounts of fluids to assist in swallowing and help move the medication through the digestive tract.
4. Have the patient sit rather than lie when taking a medication, to prevent aspiration (inhaling the drug into the lungs).
5. For patients who are unable to swallow large tablets (if not contraindicated), crush and mix the tablet with applesauce. Other forms of distasteful medications can also

be mixed with applesauce or other foods. Ask the patient to check with his or her pharmacist before crushing any medication (See also Chapter 3, Drugs That Cannot Be Crushed).

6. During drug therapy, assist the patient to maintain as nutritious a diet as possible.

7. Assess the geriatric patient for signs of fluid buildup such as respiratory changes (difficulty breathing and fluid sounds on breathing) and edema (swelling of the tissues) resulting from impaired cardiac and renal function.

8. Follow-up reports are important. Because of impaired renal function, many elderly patients may require less dosage or less frequent administration. After a patient is stabilized on therapy, often the drug strength and number of doses may be reduced for maintenance. These modifications are decisions the physician will make. However, the health care provider is often the individual relaying information to the physician and the person who educates the patient.

9. Whenever possible, a drug is administered once a day rather than in divided doses to ensure better drug compliance. (It is easier for the patient to remember once-a-day administration.)

10. Drugs that produce a dry mouth as a side effect are best administered at bedtime. Diuretics and laxatives are best taken in the early morning so that increased voiding and bowel evacuation do not disturb the patient's sleep.

11. To avoid confusion, recommend that the patient discard all drugs no longer used or with expired dates. Explain to the patient the purpose of each drug currently being self-administered.

12. Have elderly patients bring in all medications they are taking, especially after release from the hospital. This will ensure that the patient is taking the correct medication(s) and that no medication is being duplicated.

13. Listen carefully to patients' complaints and let them know you care: they may not repeat them, thinking the information must not be important. Let them know that *all* information can be important.

In summary, things to consider when developing patient teaching tools are:

1. Keep it simple.
2. Don't try to teach too much at once (on written materials, white space is important).
3. Use large enough print and easily recognized pictures.
4. Have a logical progression; don't try to be too "arty".
5. Keep the reading level to about 5th to 6th grade.
6. Use color and pictures to make it interesting.

Written Competency 5–1

Performance Competence: Using the simulation, select the one answer or completion that is best in each of the 10 questions, with at least 90 percent accuracy and within 30 minutes. Do not give yourself credit for questions left unanswered. Award 10 points for each correct answer.

Simulation

It is morning office hours. In room No. 1, a 24-year-old woman is experiencing an asthmatic attack. The physician has ordered you to prepare an injectable steroid, epinephrine hydrochloride (Adrenalin) 1:1000, which he will administer.

In room No. 2, a 3-year-old boy with a severe cold and earache is waiting with his mother for you to administer an injection of penicillin, G benzathine (Bicillin L-A).

A third patient, Mr. Allen Jones, has come in for his biweekly allergy shot, his 10th in a long series (for more information, see Figure 9–1).

Ms. Viola Ortez, age 32, also is waiting for her monthly injection of vitamin B_{12} (cyanocobalamin).

---

1. Which of the patients may leave the office after receiving treatment?
   (a) The 3-year-old boy.
   (b) The asthmatic patient.
   (c) Mr. Jones.
   (d) Ms. Ortez.
   (e) None of the above.

2. Gloves should be worn when you:
   (a) Administer the allergy serum.
   (b) Prepare the epinephrine.
   (c) Both a and b.
   (d) Administer the penicillin.
   (e) Both a and d.

3. Which of the drugs can you return to the medication shelf immediately after administration?
   (a) Allergy serum injection.
   (b) Epinephrine injection.
   (c) Penicillin injection.
   (d) Vitamin B_{12} injection.
   (e) None of the above.

4. As you prepare the epinephrine for the asthmatic patient, the medication will be:
   (a) Charted before administration and initialed after.
   (b) Charted and initialed before administration.
   (c) Either a or b.
   (d) Charted and initialed after administration.
   (e) Either a or d.

5. When treating the asthmatic patient, the needle will be in its sheath:
   (a) After administering the medication.
   (b) For disposal into the sharps container in room No. 1.
   (c) Both a and b.
   (d) After withdrawing the epinephrine into the syringe.
   (e) Both a and d.

6. As you prepare the penicillin for the boy, you compare the written order with the medication label for the *third time* as you:
   (a) Read the label before drawing out the medication.
   (b) Withdraw the medication.

(c) Read the label after drawing up the medication.

(d) Take the medication to the room.

(e) Identify the patient.

7. For the boy, special medication considerations include:

(a) Not telling him he is to receive an injection.

(b) Placing a Band-aid at the site as a "badge of courage."

(c) Giving him a lollipop for being brave.

(d) Praising the child for cooperating with you.

(e) Assuming the child will not be cooperative.

8. "Rights" that are checked a second time immediately before administering the allergy serum to Mr. Jones include:

(a) The right drug.

(b) The right dose.

(c) The right time.

(d) The right patient.

(e) All of the above.

9. The epinephrine injection for the asthmatic patient is in which pregnancy risk category?

(a) A

(b) B

(c) C

(d) D

(e) X

10. The vitamin B_{12} for Ms. Ortez is in which pregnancy risk category?

(a) A

(b) B

(c) C

(d) D

(e) X

Score: _____

See Appendix B for answers.

Terminal Performance Objective/Competency

Procedure 5–1: Prepare a Medication

EQUIPMENT Written order:

Smith, Helen	Age: 42
Today's date	No allergies
Rx: Gantrisin 0.5 G; Give: 500 mg	
2 tabs PO (by mouth)	

The ordered medication container (tablets):

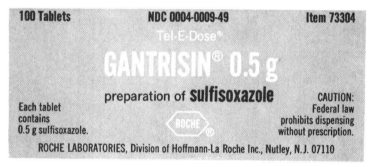

A medication cup
A disposable paper cup with water
Patient chart

Performance Competence: Prepare an ordered quantity of medication for patient administration, by completing every step of the procedure 100 percent accurately, safely, and in the correct order, within 5 minutes.

		V	S	U*
PROCEDURAL STEPS	1. Clear the area of any traffic or activity. Wash hands.	☐	☐	☐
	2. Read the order carefully and understand the order.	☐	☐	☐
	3. Question any unusual orders first. *Rationale:* Questioning first may save the medication from being wasted, if the order needs to be changed.	☐	☐	☐

*V = Value, to be filled in if assigning points or other specific values to each step, or if designating a critical step.
S = Satisfactory completion of the step.
U = Unsatisfactory completion of the step, or step incomplete; needs more practice.

4. Gather the ordered medication and administration materials. ☐ ☐ ☐

5. Check the expiration date and condition of the medication. ☐ ☐ ☐

6. Read the label the *first* of *three* checks and compare with the order: drug name, strength, dosage, and recommended route. ☐ ☐ ☐

7. Remove the cap and empty the correct quantity of medication into the medication cup. ☐ ☐ ☐

8. Read the label the *second* of *three* checks and compare with the order: drug name, strength, dosage, and recommended route. ☐ ☐ ☐

9. Replace the cap. ☐ ☐ ☐

10. Read the label the *third* of *three* checks and compare with the order: drug name, strength, dosage, and recommended route. ☐ ☐ ☐

11. Check the last six of the "seven rights":

    Right patient: Correct name ☐ ☐ ☐

    Right drug and strength: Card matches bottle ☐ ☐ ☐

    Right dose: Chart matches quantity prepared ☐ ☐ ☐

    Right route: Chart matches route on bottle or for this type of drug ☐ ☐ ☐

    Right time/date: Confirm time is now ☐ ☐ ☐

    Right technique: Confirm route procedures correct for this patient ☐ ☐ ☐

12. Return the medication to storage. ☐ ☐ ☐

Date: _____ Competency achieved: Y _____ N _____

Designated reasonable time standard: _____

Actual completion time: _____

Terminal Performance Objective/Competency

Procedure 5–2: Administer a Medication to a Patient

EQUIPMENT	Medicine cup
	2 tablets of Gantrisin, 0.5 G (see Procedure 5–1)
	Disposable cup of water

Audio tape cassette and tape recorder
Patient chart
Medication package insert

REVIEW Procedure 5–1

Performance Competence: Role-play to identify the patient and administer the ordered medication by completing each step of the procedure 100 percent accurately, safely, and in the correct order within 5 minutes. Tape record the role play.

	V	S	U *

PROCEDURAL STEPS

1. If you are not familiar with the drug, take time to read the medication package insert or comparable material in the office medication handbook. ☐ ☐ ☐

2. Identify the patient. Approach the patient and greet by one of the following:

   > "What is your name, please? (pause for response) I'm here to give you your medication. Do you have any drug or food allergies?"

   Rationale: To check the right patient. ☐ ☐ ☐

3. Using the chart (see Procedure 5–1, Written Order), assess the patient's current status and condition.
   Rationale: To check the right drug and strength, dose, and time/date. ☐ ☐ ☐

4. Evaluate the patient's physical and emotional state to determine the ability to take the medication by the prescribed route.
   Rationale: To check the right route. If the patient cannot tolerate the route ordered (e.g., vomiting and nausea), the physician may want to change the route of administration, order another drug, or withdraw the medication order. ☐ ☐ ☐

5. Explain the procedure to the patient.
   Rationale: To check the right technique. ☐ ☐ ☐

6. Explain the name and purpose of the drug.
   Rationale: The patient may have some new assessment information or not understand what to do. ☐ ☐ ☐

7. Administer or hand the medication to the patient to self-administer. ☐ ☐ ☐

8. Remain with the patient until the medication is taken. ☐ ☐ ☐

---

*V = Value, to be filled in if assigning points or other specific values to each step, or if designating a critical step.
S = Satisfactory completion of the step.
U = Unsatisfactory completion of the step, or step incomplete; needs more practice.

9. Collect and dispose of the medication equipment.   ☐ ☐ ☐

10. Observe the patient for any untoward reactions or negative results.   ☐ ☐ ☐

11. Report observations, if any, immediately.   ☐ ☐ ☐

12. Ask the patient to remain in the office for 20 minutes.   ☐ ☐ ☐

13. Record the administration of the medication and the length of time the patient waited in the office.
    Rationale: To check the right documentation.   ☐ ☐ ☐

14. Conduct any education session that should be done.   ☐ ☐ ☐

15. Record the education session on the chart.   ☐ ☐ ☐

Date: _____   Competency achieved: Y _____   N _____

Designated reasonable time standard: _____

Actual completion time: _____

Terminal Performance Objective/Competency

Procedure 5–3: Prepare a Patient Teaching Guide

EQUIPMENT   Reference book or medication
Package insert
Audio tape cassette and tape recorder

Smith, Helen   Age: 42
Today's date, time   No allergies
2nd° burn of R/thumb dressed with Silvadene Cream. Patient instructed to keep the dressing dry and in place for 48 hours. Home care instructions given. Rx: Tylenol with Codeine tabs (No. 1), 1–2 tabs q4h, as needed for pain for 48 hours. Instruction Guide given to pt. Initials.

Performance Competence: Complete a written patient teaching guide, using Fig. 5–3 as a guide, for the medication prescribed with 100 percent completeness and accuracy of information and within reasonable work production time. Tape record the teaching session.

	V	S	U *

PROCEDURAL STEPS

	V	S	U
1. Provided class of drug.	☐	☐	☐
2. Provided understandable description of the way the drug works.	☐	☐	☐
3. Provided name of drug.	☐	☐	☐
4. Provided dose ordered.	☐	☐	☐
5. Povided storage needs.	☐	☐	☐
6. Provided times and how taken.	☐	☐	☐
7. Provided caution about activities.	☐	☐	☐
8. Provided common side effects.	☐	☐	☐
9. Provided information on how long to use and when to stop or not stop the drug.	☐	☐	☐

---

*V = Value, to be filled in if assigning points or other specific values to each step, or if designating a critical step.
S = Satisfactory completion of the step.
U = Unsatisfactory completion of the step, or step incomplete; needs more practice.

Date: _____ Competency achieved: Y _____ N _____

Designated reasonable time standard: _____

Actual completion time: _____

Terminal Performance Objective/Competency

Procedure 5–4: Teach a Patient to Take a Medication

Choose a medication topic and prepare printed patient teaching tool to be used in an office, then teach one of your classmates. You are to explain the information and provide the patient with written material to take with them. The instructor and the student being instructed will evaluate.

Verbal evaluation

1. Introduced self and explained what you were going to do.

2. Presented material in a logical order.

3. Spoke loud enough, clearly and made eye contact.

4. Used understandable vocabulary.

5. Gave specific instructions, and verified understanding of material.

6. Document teaching.

Written material

1. Is pleasing to look at.

2. Print is large enough to read easily.

3. Looks professional.

4. Is simple, and reading level is 5th to 6th grade.

5. Does not have too much information.

6. Has enough white space.

7. Drawings or pictures are easily understood.

8. Has a logical progression.

Date: _____ Competency achieved: Y _____ N _____

Designated reasonable time standard: _____

Actual completion time: _____

Procedure 5–5: Create a Bulletin Board that Instructs Patients About Drug Therapy

Prepare a bulletin board or poster board that will help patients understand anything you think would help them with a pharmacologic issue.

1. Is the topic appropriate and narrow enough?

2. Is the material presented clearly?

3. Are the graphics easily understood?

4. Is the information easy to understand?

Date: _____ Competency achieved: Y _____ N _____

Designated reasonable time standard: _____

Actual completion time: _____

Assignment 5–1: Use Appendix A, the *PDR,* or Other Reference to Create Drug Information Guides

EQUIPMENT

Appendix A; *PDR*; or other drug reference
Lined notepaper or index cards
Drugs: From top 50 most commonly prescribed those ranked 11th–20th.

Performance Competence: Complete a drug guide for each of the drugs listed under Equipment. The ten guides should be completed with 100 percent accuracy and must include the following:

Generic name _____

Brand name (trade name) _____

Classification _____

Controlled substance classification _____

Pregnancy risk category _____

Action _____

Indications/use _____

Contraindications _____

Adverse reactions/side effects _____

Dosage/Route _____

Patient education (in terms the patient will understand)

    Compliance issues _____

    Report to the physician when _____

Special alert _____

Conversion Drill for Skill

Using Table 1–7 and the conversion formula, convert the following within 30 minutes. Do not give yourself credit for partial or incorrect answers. Strive for a score of 100 percent. If you score less than 100 percent, return to Chapter 1 and reread the section on conversions.

1. 2 fl dr   = _____ ml

2. 5 gr   = _____ mg

3. 1 tbs   = _____ ml

4. 140 lb   = _____ kg

5. 2 tsp   = _____ ml

6. 1/60 gr   = _____ mcg

7. 1/200 gr   = _____ mg

8. 34 lb   = _____ kg

9. 128 oz   = _____ gal

10. 24 lb   = _____ kg

11. 220 lbs   = _____ kg

12. 300 cc   = _____ oz

13. 0.5 g   = _____ mg

14. 500 mcg   = _____ mg

15. gr X   = _____ mg

16. 600 cc   = _____ L

17. 45 minims = _____ cc

18. dram V   = _____ cc

19. 0.125 mg   = _____ mcg

20. 750 mg   = _____ g

21. 60 kg   = _____ lbs

22. 15 ml   = _____ oz

23. gr ¾   = _____ mg

24. 450 mg   = _____ g

25. 320 mg   = _____ gr

26. 1.5 L   = _____ cc

27. 3 tsp   = _____ cc

28. gr 1/150   = _____ mg

29. gr 1/300   = _____ mcg

30. 1.5 g   = _____ mg

Score: _____

See Appendix B for answers.

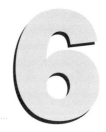

Measuring Medications for Administration

Liquid Medication Equipment
    Droppers
    Teaspoons
    Medicine cups
    Medicine bottles and stock containers
    Rules for stock drugs
    Oral inhalers and nebulizers
Injectable Medication Equipment
    Ampules
    Vials
    Cartridge–needle unit
    Syringes
    Needles
    Syringe measurements

WRITTEN COMPETENCY 6–1: Identify Correct Equipment for Medication Administration

WRITTEN COMPETENCY 6–2: Measure Solutions in a Regular Syringe

WRITTEN COMPETENCY 6–3: Measure Solutions in a Tuberculin Syringe

TERMINAL PERFORMANCE OBJECTIVE/COMPETENCY (PROCEDURE 6–1): Prepare and Administer an Oral Medication Using the EZY-DOSE Oral Syringe

TERMINAL PERFORMANCE OBJECTIVE/COMPETENCY (PROCEDURE 6–2): Prepare and Administer a Liquid Oral Medication

TERMINAL PERFORMANCE OBJECTIVE/COMPETENCY (PROCEDURE 6–3): Open an Ampule Containing a Sterile Medication

CONVERSION DRILL FOR SKILL

ASSIGNMENT 6–1: Use Appendix A, the *PDR,* or Other Reference to Create Drug Information Guides

OBJECTIVES   **WRITTEN COMPETENCY 6–1:** Identify correct equipment for medication administration.

WRITTEN COMPETENCY 6–2: Measure solutions in a regular syringe.

WRITTEN COMPETENCY 6–3: Measure solutions in a tuberculin syringe.

TERMINAL PERFORMANCE OBJECTIVE (PROCEDURE 6–1): Prepare and administer an oral medication using the EZY-DOSE oral syringe.

TERMINAL PERFORMANCE OBJECTIVE (PROCEDURE 6–2): Prepare and administer a liquid oral medication.

TERMINAL PERFORMANCE OBJECTIVE (PROCEDURE 6–3): Open an ampule containing a sterile medication.

CONVERSION DRILL FOR SKILL: Convert grams, milligrams, and micrograms to their metric equivalents.

ASSIGNMENT 6–1: Use drug references to create drug information guides.

A thorough knowledge of the equipment used to measure and administer medications is as important as knowing the routes and techniques of drug administration. It is the equipment that provides for the correct medication measurement, and it is the equipment that, in some instances, keeps a medication sterile and safe for use. In addition to patient care, medication administration involves stocking and replenishing disposable spoons, droppers, and medicine cups for nonparenteral drugs and syringes and needles of various sizes for the administration of parenteral drugs. Correct supplies should be available at all times for proper patient care and in cases of emergency.

Liquid Medication Equipment

Some drugs are available in one strength only and preparation requires only pouring or drawing up a medication to a calibrated mark on a container. Drugs available in one strength do not have a specific weight measure—the physician simply orders the exact amount (volume) to administer to the patient. The calculations of drug weight (strength) to volume, discussed in Chapter 7, are not necessary. Some examples of drugs requiring only measurement include:

Robitussin Syrup 2 tsp q4h
Robitussin Syrup 10 ml q4h
Benadryl Elixir 20 ml stat
Maalox 1 oz

The orders for liquid medications are administered to patients with droppers, spoons, or medicine cups.

DROPPERS

An apothecary or medicine dropper is a pipette or tube with a bulb squeezer used for dispensing liquids in drops (Fig. 6–1). Because 1 drop is considered equivalent to 1 minim in the apothecary measurement system (Chapter 1, Table 1–7), it is commonly assumed that each drop produced by the squeeze of the bulb is the equivalent of 1 minim. Minims may be safely substituted for drops; however, drops should never be substituted for minims, because the size of a drop will vary according to the following:

1. Thickness of the medication
2. Temperature of the solution
3. Angle at which the medication is dropped

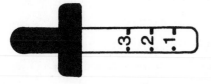

FIGURE 6–1. Calibrated medicine dropper. (From Cornett, EF, and Blume, DM: Dosages and Solutions: A Programmed Approach to Meds and Math, ed 5. F.A. Davis, Philadelphia, 1991, p 69, with permission.)

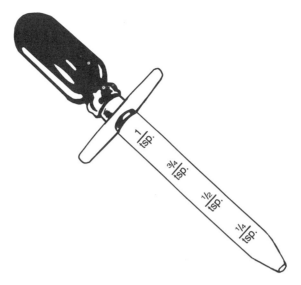

FIGURE 6–2. Spoon dropper.

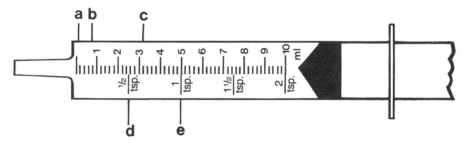

FIGURE 6–3. Oral syringe. (From Cornett, EF, and Blume, DM: Dosages and Solutions: A Programmed Approach to Meds and Math, ed 5. F.A. Davis, Philadelphia, 1991, p 69, with permission.)

4. Force at which the solution is expelled
5. Size of the dropper opening

When measuring minims, use a calibrated container for minims.

A *spoon dropper* (Fig. 6–2) is a plastic tube with a bulb squeezer manufactured in household units and used for measuring liquids by the teaspoonful. Spoon droppers facilitate administering drugs to children and the elderly in the home, and may be useful in the medical facility for the occasional administration of liquid oral medications. They are, however, more expensive to use than the disposable, plastic medicine cup.

The *oral syringe* (Fig. 6–3) works on the same principle as the medicine dropper. It is used for dispensing small amounts of medication, usually up to 10 ml (2 tsp), to infants, small children, and the elderly.

TEASPOONS

At home and in the medical facility, the 4- or 5-ml cooking or household-measure teaspoon (Fig. 6–4) should be used rather than the flatware teaspoon utensil that is used for eating. When using measuring spoons to administer medicine:

1. Choose the deep-bowled type.
2. Do not fill to capacity.
3. Do not dispense the medication until the patient is identified, positioned, and ready to take the medication.

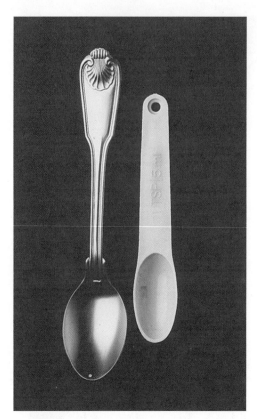

FIGURE 6–4. The cooking teaspoon is consistently more accurate and easier to use than the tableware teaspoon.

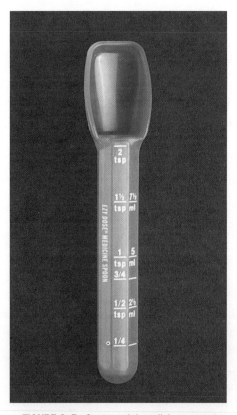

FIGURE 6–5. Commercial medicine spoon.

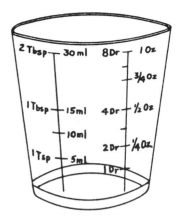

FIGURE 6–6. 1 oz medicine cup. (From Cornett, EF, and Blume, DM: Dosages and Solutions: A Programmed Approach to Meds and Math, ed 5. F.A. Davis, Philadelphia, 1991, p 68, with permission.)

4. Have a paper towel positioned under the spoon to catch any spills.
5. Make available water to the patient in a disposable cup, unless giving water with the medication is contraindicated.

Whenever possible, instruct patients that household measurement spoons are better than commercial oral syringes and medication spoons (see below) for oral suspensions and other thick medications. The larger surface area of all the commercial products becomes coated with medication, sometimes resulting in as much loss as one full dose every 1 1/2 days.

If a patient is using an oral syringe or medication spoon for a thick medication, teach the patient to rinse the utensil thoroughly *before* administration (to wet down the inside surface) and to rinse out all residual medication *after* each administration.

Commercial medicine spoons (Fig. 6–5) are designed to store up to 2 tsp (10 ml) of liquid medication in a cylindric dispenser. This keeps the medication from spilling as the spoon is being moved to the patient's mouth.

MEDICINE CUPS

Medicine cups (Fig. 6–6) are frequently used to administer liquid medications or dispense tablets. Measurement markings on 1-oz medicine cups vary, but most are marked in drams and milliliters (or cubic centimeters) and also include equivalent teaspoon and tablespoon measurements. For quantities less than 5 ml, the oral syringe (shown earlier) is a more accurate measurement.

MEDICINE BOTTLES AND STOCK CONTAINERS

Manufactured medicine bottles come in graduated ounce sizes. The bottles are amber to protect the medication from deterioration by sunlight. Each bottle is embossed with its capacity (Fig. 6–7). On prescriptions, the total amount of the medication is usually ordered in milliliters; for example:

    30 ml = 1-oz bottle
    60 ml = 2-oz bottle
    90 ml = 3-oz bottle
    120 ml = 4-oz bottle

RULES FOR STOCK DRUGS

Drugs commonly stocked for patient use in the outpatient setting usually include syrups and elixirs for immediate patient care and emergencies. These drugs are usually liquid antihistamines, sedatives, antibiotics, antacids, and pediatric preparations. Some drugs in tablet form may also be stocked as starter doses for patients who have not yet had their prescriptions filled. The following rules should be followed for the storage of all drugs:

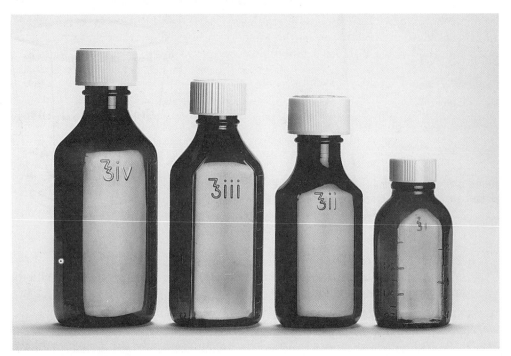

FIGURE 6–7. Medicine bottles of varying capacities: 1 oz approximates 30 ml; 2 oz, 60 ml; 3 oz, 90 ml; and 4 oz, 120 ml.

1. Liquids are stored in cool, dry areas, away from sunlight and safely inaccessible to patients.
2. Each bottle must be labeled with its *original* label.
3. Poison liquids must be marked with skull and crossbones (or otherwise acceptable label, such as Mr. Yuk!) and *stored separately from oral medications.*
4. All liquids should be shaken before dispensing.
5. Caps should be placed inside up on the counter, to prevent contamination of the inner surfaces of the cap. Do not wipe the insides of lids.
6. Liquids are poured away from the label, to prevent label damage from drips down the sides of the bottle. Always wipe bottle after pouring to avoid crusting or sticking.
7. Always pour liquids with containers at eye level, on a flat surface.
8. Measure liquids by placing the medicine cup on a flat surface and read at the bottom of the meniscus at eye level.

ORAL INHALERS AND NEBULIZERS

Other types of nonparenteral equipment include oral inhalers and nebulizers. Bronchodilator aerosols are used by patients with chronic obstructive pulmonary disease (COPD) and in emergencies. The three most common COPD conditions are chronic bronchitis, bronchial asthma, and emphysema. The most common respiratory emergency is the severe asthmatic attack.

Respiratory aerosols may be used for one or more of the following:

1. To widen air passages by relaxing the bronchial smooth muscles that are often in a state of spasm
2. To help clear mucus
3. To reduce swelling of inflamed and congested mucous membranes that line the respiratory tract.

Various devices are available to administer respiratory aerosols (see Fig. 3–2 in Chapter 3). Bulb nebulizers and oral inhalers release measured amounts of liquid spray. Pump-driven nebulizers and intermittent positive pressure breathing (IPPB) machines are available for patients whose respiratory passages are so seriously blocked that they cannot take a deep breath independently. Inhalation solutions do not require a dosage calculation. Administration usually consists of a series of inhalations for the *number of inhalation times ordered* (usually two or three times per administration). For best results, the patient should be instructed to inhale the mist deeply and then to hold his or her breath for several seconds before exhaling slowly through pursed lips, and to take two to three breaths in between inhalations.

> SPECIAL CAUTION: It is often difficult to teach the skill of pursing the lips to the elderly and young children.

Injectable Medication Equipment

Injectable pharmaceutic agents come in sterile, prepackaged plastic or glass containers, in either powdered or liquid form. Powdered injectables must be reconstituted with a specified amount of diluent supplied by the manufacturer or with stock sterile water or sodium chloride (isotonic saline) from another sterile container before injecting. It is important to follow each manufacturer's directions exactly (see also under Chapter 7, Reconstituting Solutions).

Injectables may contain a small amount of antibiotic as a preservative. As all medications have a specific shelf life (expiration date), the expiration date must be checked each time an injectable product is prepared. Once a medication reaches its expiration date, it must no longer be used.

> SPECIAL CAUTION: Antibiotic preservatives and other additives may be a source of patient allergy. It is therefore necessary to know not just the main element of a drug but all other ingredients as well.

AMPULES

An ampule (see Fig. 3–5 in Chapter 3) is a hermetically sealed, single-dose glass flask. It is shaped with a narrow neck that is scored and weakened in the manufacturing process for easy breaking, either with natural hand pressure or by filling the scored line first, to facilitate easier opening. The neck must be cleaned with alcohol before opening and not touched by hands or any other contaminated surface. If the ampule is to be filed, clean with alcohol after filing.

Because of its design, medication will not spill out of an ampule, even when it is turned upside down. Although the glass is designed not to shatter, special filtered syringe needles are available to protect against possible glass contamination of the fluid. An ampule is opened using the following procedure:

1. Wash hands and dry thoroughly to prevent the ampule from slipping in wet hands.
2. Protect hands from cuts, with gauze.
3. Tap the top of the ampule to force all medication to the bottom section of the ampule.
4. File one side of the ampule at the score line, if a file is suggested by the manufacturer or if the ampule is large.
5. Clean the neck area with alcohol and gauze.
6. Sharply tap or bend the top away from the body by snapping both wrists toward the body. The break will make a popping sound.
7. Dispose of the broken ampule in a rigid, puncture-resistant, disposable container (see Chapter 5).

SPECIAL CAUTION: If a clean cut of the glass is in doubt, discard the medication down the sink and dispose of the entire ampule in a rigid, puncture-resistant, disposable container.

VIALS

A vial is a bottle of injectable medication that is vacuum-sealed and sterile. It features a rubber-stopper top through which syringe needles are inserted for withdrawing medication. A sealed plastic or metal cap covering the rubber must be snapped off before use. Each time a vial is used, the rubber stopper must be thoroughly cleaned with alcohol or acetone. This disinfects the rubber stopper so that surface contaminants are not dragged into the vial when the needle is inserted. This is especially important for vials that contain enough medication to be used more than one time.

All vials should be routinely shaken to ensure proper mixing of the contents. The contents of vials should be examined for any precipitate or unusual appearance that might indicate contamination, bacterial growth, or crystallization. Do not use any medication that appears cloudy or contaminated with foreign particles—discard the vial. Check the expiration date of each vial before preparing the injection. Never return unused medication to a vial.

Single-dose vials are becoming more popular than ampules, as they are safer and easier to use. A single-dose vial contains enough injectable material for one patient. Multidose vials contain enough injectable material for use in several patients. With each use, however, the rubber stopper must be carefully disinfected to keep the contents sterile for use with future patients.

Because vials are vacuum-sealed, the internal air–fluid pressure must be maintained. For each amount of fluid withdrawn, an equal amount of air first must be injected into the vial with the syringe. Not replacing fluid with air will result in having to pull hard on the plunger to fill the syringe or, in extreme cases, in the fluid refusing to flow into the syringe (a "tug of war"). Too much air in the vial could result in the fluid surging into the syringe without pulling on the plunger. If the pressure is too great, the plunger may even fly out of the syringe barrel.

CARTRIDGE–NEEDLE UNIT

A cartridge–needle unit resembles a glass syringe and contains a premeasured amount of injectable medication. The cartridge–needle unit fits into a plastic plunger. The cartridges are disposable; the plungers are reused. Figure 6–8 demonstrates how to load a cartridge–needle unit.

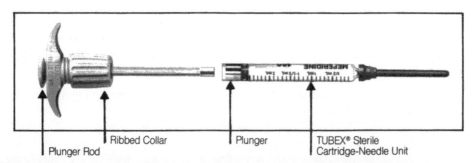

Plunger Rod | Ribbed Collar | Plunger | TUBEX® Sterile Cartridge-Needle Unit

FIGURE 6–8. Loading a cartridge–needle unit syringe. (1) Turn the ribbed collar to the "OPEN" position until it stops, (2) hold injector with the open end up and fully insert the TUBEX sterile cartridge–needle unit. Firmly tighten the ribbed collar in the direction of the "CLOSE" arrow, (3) thread the plunger rod into the plunger of the TUBEX sterile cartridge–needle unit until slight resistance is felt. The injector is now ready for use. To unload and discard, do not recap the needle. Disengage the plunger rod, then hold the injector, needle down over a needle disposal container and loosen the ribbed collar. The TUBEX cartridge–needle unit will drop into the container. The TUBEX injector is reusable: do not discard. (Courtesy of Wyeth-Ayerst Laboratories, Philadelphia, PA.)

SYRINGES

A syringe (Fig. 6–9) is a hollow cylinder that attaches to a needle. The plunger inside the cylinder pushes the medication through the needle and into the patient's tissues. Only the outside of the barrel and the flared end of the plunger may be touched. Touching the end of the syringe or the part of the plunger that is inside the barrel is considered contamination.

Both plastic and glass syringes are manufactured. For patient use, glass syringes are used only in circumstances where medications react with plastic. These circumstances are very rare. Plastic syringes are shipped in boxes of 100, either individually packed in sealed rigid plastic jackets or in sealed paper or plastic envelopes. Syringes may be purchased with needles, or syringes and needles may be purchased separately and assembled when a medication is prepared. Each manufacturer has a color-coding system for easy recognition of syringe and needle size. All syringe units are sterile. Sterility can be guaranteed only if the outer wrappings are intact, free from moisture, and opened properly.

There are three basic types of syringes used for injection: regular syringes, insulin syringes, and the tuberculin syringe. *Regular* syringes for injection come in varying sizes and are calibrated in the metric system (ml) or in the apothecary system (minim), or both. The size of syringe chosen depends on the amount of medication to be injected and the exactness of measurement needed. Figure 6–10 shows the three most commonly used regular syringes, plus the tuberculin syringe.

The *insulin* syringe (Fig. 6–11) is only and always used for administering insulin. Although two other types are available (usually for veterinary medicine), the U-100 syringe is now exclusively used for injecting insulin into humans. The insulin syringe is calibrated in units (see Chapter 9 for insulin preparation and use). The most commonly used U-100 syringe is the low-dose, 1/2-cc, single-use, insulin syringe for 50 U or less. Because the barrel diameter is narrow, calibrations are farther apart, making measurements much more accurate and easier to read because many people with diabetes have impaired vision.

The *tuberculin* syringe (Fig. 6–10D) is designed for administering small amounts of medication. It is measured in both the metric (ml) and apothecary (minim) systems, but the total quantity that can be withdrawn is only 1.0 ml (15 or 16 minims). It is used when the calibration lines of the regular syringe are not exact enough to measure a minute amount of medication.

NEEDLES

Needles for injection are sterile. No part of the needle may be touched or contamination will occur. The needle is constructed with a *hub* that attaches to the tip of the syringe, either as

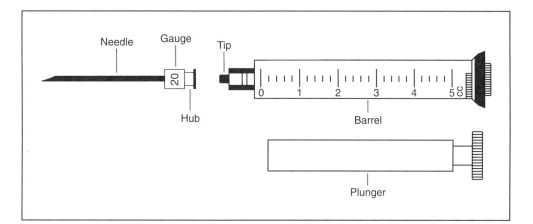

FIGURE 6–9. First count the number of calibrations (lines) in each cc. The first calibration on all syringes is zero. On this 5 cc syringe, there are five calibrations in each cc, which indicates that each calibration is two-tenths (2/10) on this syringe (From Frew, MA, and Frew, DR: Clinical Procedures for Medical Assisting. F.A. Davis, Philadelphia, 1990, p 304, with permission.)

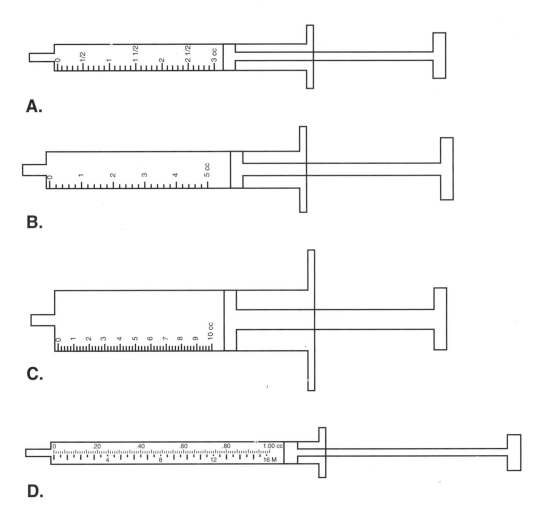

FIGURE 6–10. Syringes. *A,* 3-ml syringe. *B,* 5-ml syringe. *C,* 10-ml syringe. *D,* 1-ml tuberculin syringe. (From Cornett, EF, and Blume, DM: Dosages and Solutions: A Programmed Approach to Meds and Math, ed 5. F.A. Davis, Philadelphia, 1991, p 94, with permission.)

a screw type or slip-on type; a *shaft*; and the *beveled point*, specially sharpened and designed for ease of insertion with minimal pain. The inner opening is called the needle's *lumen*.

The shaft of the needle determines its length. Shaft lengths vary from 3/8 in to 4 in. Needles also vary in diameter, which is measured in *gauge*. The larger the gauge number, the smaller the diameter (lumen or opening). Gauges range from 14, the largest, to 28, the smallest.

The gauge size chosen depends on the thickness of the medication to be injected: thicker medications need a wider opening for pushing through the medication. Although it may appear that a larger needle will cause a patient more pain, this is untrue. Injecting thick medications through a small opening, which means using increased pressure, is what increases the sensation of pain in the tissues.

The length of the needle used depends on the tissue depth desired for depositing the medication, the size of the patient, and the type of medication being administered. Chapter 8 details the different depths (routes) chosen for injections. Table 6–1 summarizes the usual combinations of needles and syringes used for various medications and depths of injection.

Unattached needles are also color-coded by size for easy recognition. As already mentioned, needle and syringe units may be purchased already attached and ready for use, and additional needles may be purchased separately in boxes of 100. If a drug is irritating to the skin, after withdrawing the medication from the vial, a fresh, sterile needle may be exchanged

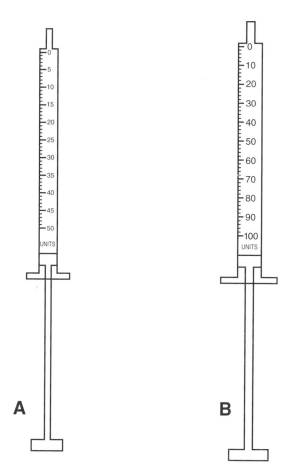

FIGURE 6–11. Insulin syringes. *A,* 0.5 ml syringe. *B,* 1.0 ml syringe. The shading on syringe *A* represents 11 units; the shading on syringe *B* represents 85 units.

TABLE 6–1. **Common Needle–Syringe Combinations**

Gauge	*Length*	*Syringe*	*Use*
18–23	1–3 in	2–5 ml regular	Intramuscular injection of thick fluids
24–25	1/2, 5/8 in	2–3 ml regular, tuberculin, insulin	Subcutaneous injection of aqueous (watery) fluids. Intramuscular aqueous fluids for infants.
26–27	3/8 in	Tuberculin	Intradermal tests for allergies or for
27		Low-dose insulin	administering small amounts of medication

for the needle used to withdraw the medication before injecting the needle into the patient. Sometimes a syringe size and needle size may not be compatible, and a new match must be created; if this occurs choose the syringe size first, then apply a new needle before injecting into the patient.

The procedure for exchanging needles is simple. Needles are exchanged using sterile technique. Remove the original needle from the syringe with the needle *in its original plastic cap.* Never handle an exposed needle. Then open the new needle package by pulling down the paper sides. Tightly affix the new needle to the syringe, and immediately discard the unwanted needle in a rigid, "sharps" container.

SYRINGE MEASUREMENTS

Regular and tuberculin syringes are calibrated in the decimal system, using milliliter as the metric measurement. Larger syringes are not used to measure minute quantities. The 3-ml regular syringe is divided into 30 equal parts, each part indicating *one tenth* of a milliliter (Fig. 6–12). Therefore, drugs are measurable if they can be rounded to an even tenth such as 0.1, 0.2, 0.3, and so on. A medication quantity with two decimal places cannot be measured in this syringe, unless it can be evenly converted to minims.

The smaller-sized regular syringe is also calibrated in minims. One metric milliliter is equal to 15 or 16 minims. The minim calibrations are not frequently used.

Example: The physician orders 0.25 ml (1/4 of a milliliter). There is no 0.25-ml mark on the regular syringe. Convert 0.25 to minims. Figure 6–12 shows a syringe with medication drawn up the 0.25-ml (4-minim) mark.

Known:	1 ml	=	16 minims
	0.25 ml (1/4 of 1 ml)	=	(1/4 of 16 minims)
Therefore:	0.25 ml	=	4.0 minims

The tuberculin syringe (see Fig. 6–10D) also is calibrated in the decimal system, using milliliter as the metric measurement. The tuberculin syringe is divided into 100 equal parts, each part indicating *one hundredth* of a milliliter. Because it is so finely calibrated, the maximum volume of the tuberculin syringe is 1.0 ml. Drugs are measurable to two decimal places—for example, 0.15, 0.25, 0.33, and so on, in the tuberculin syringe, unless the quantity is greater than 1.0 ml.

When the physician orders a parenteral drug by volume (e.g., "Give Tetanus Toxoid 0.5 ml"), the procedure of measuring the drug to the 0.5-ml mark on the regular syringe is a simple and direct one. However, the physician will frequently order a drug by a number of milligrams, grams, or grains rather than by volume. These are weight measures and, before a medication can be drawn into a syringe or other equipment, the weight measures must be converted to milliliters or other units of volume measurement in order to administer the correct dosage. Drug weights (strengths) may be ordered in the following way:

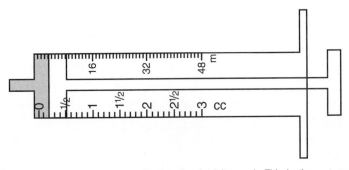

FIGURE 6–12. Medication drawn into a syringe to the 4-minim mark. This is the conversion equivalent to the 0.25 ml ordered in the example.

g/ml	grams per milliliter
mg/ml	milligrams per milliliter
mcg/ml	micrograms per milliliter
gr/ml	grains per milliliter
mEq/ml	milliequivalents per milliliter
U/ml	units per milliliter

Calculating dosage weight by volume before a drug can be measured is a more complicated process. Chapter 7 will discuss this process of calculating dosage by introducing formulas that solve for an unknown volume measurement from values of weight and volume that are known. In preparation for calculating unknown dosages however, it is extremely important that the information in this chapter be first mastered. Before moving on to Chapter 7, practice the written and skill exercises that follow until 100 percent accuracy is accomplished. There can be no room for error when administering medications.

OSHA guidelines now state that gloves and mask must be used when working with certain medications and some medications must be drawn up using a hood to prevent contamination of the person drawing up the medication.

Written Competency 6–1

Performance Competence: Using the simulated equipment below, select the correct materials to use with at least 100 percent accuracy and within 15 minutes. Do not give yourself credit for incorrect, incomplete, or skipped questions.

The following *equipment* is on hand:
- a. Dropper
- b. Spoon dropper
- c. Oral syringe
- d. Measuring teaspoon
- e. Medicine cup

The following *syringes* are on hand:
- a. Regular 2.0 ml
- b. Regular 3.0 ml
- c. Regular 5.0 ml
- d. Tuberculin
- e. Insulin low-dose U-50

The following *needles* are on hand:
- a. 20-gauge 2-in
- b. 21-gauge 1 1/2-in
- c. 25-gauge 5/8-in
- d. 26-gauge 1/2-in
- e. 27-gauge 3/8-in

Conversion Table 1–7, Chapter 1

A *PDR* or other drug reference

---

1. The physician orders 16 minims of Tylenol for an infant. Choose the correct equipment from the box.

2. The physician orders paregoric gtt iii in oz i ss water in a nursing bottle bid × 3d. Choose the correct equipment to teach the mother to make the preparation at home for her infant.

3. The physician orders oral penicillin suspension for a 4-year-old, and asks you to make up a sample first dose with the mother. Which equipment is the best choice?

4. The physician orders allergy testing. Choose the correct needle.

5. The physician orders 0.5 ml of the aqueous solution diphtheria and tetanus toxoids and pertussis vaccine, intramuscularly, for an infant. Choose the correct needle.

6. The physician orders 1.5 ml injectable penicillin, intramuscularly for a 2-year-old. Choose the correct needle.

7. For question 6, choose the correct syringe.

8. The physician orders 0.25 ml of injectable medication subcutaneously. Choose the correct syringe.

9. In question 8, to which line would you draw up the medication in the syringe?

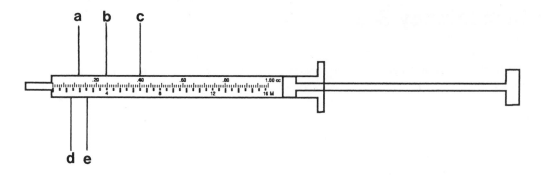

10. Return to question 2. To which line would you draw up the paregoric?

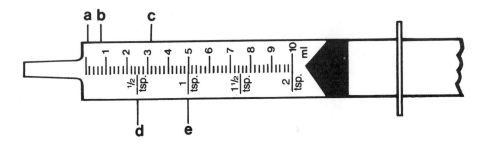

Score: _____

See Appendix B for answers.

Written Competency 6–2

Performance Competence: Using the simulated regular syringes shown here, shade each syringe to the mark to which you would draw up the medication. Mark whether you used the ml scale or the minim scale. If you see the minim scale, also mark whether you used 15 minims or 16 minims to equal 1 ml. Your work must be 100 percent accurate and completed within 15 minutes. Do not give yourself credit for incorrect, incomplete, or skipped questions.

1. 0.1 ml ml _____ minim _____
   15 _____ 16 _____

2. 0.2 ml ml _____ minim _____
   15 _____ 16 _____

3. 0.33 ml ml _____ minim _____
   15 _____ 16 _____

4. 0.50 ml ml _____ minim _____
   15 _____ 16 _____

5. 0.66 ml ml _____ minim _____
   15 _____ 16 _____

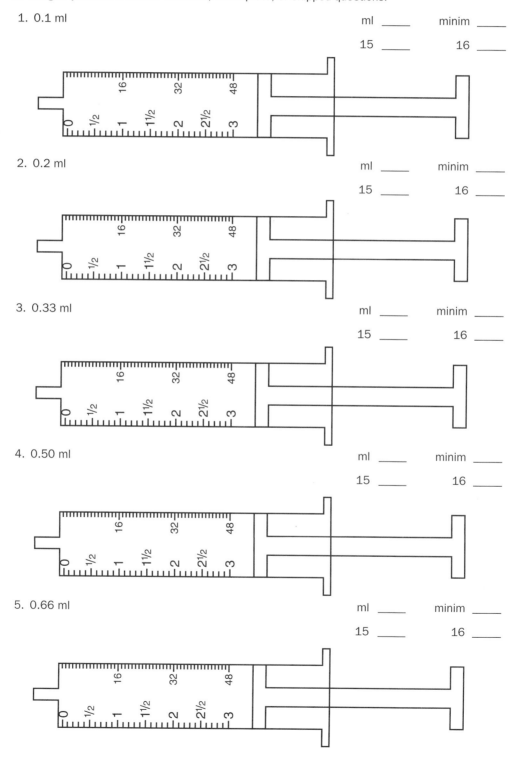

6. 0.75 ml

ml _____   minim _____

15 _____   16 _____

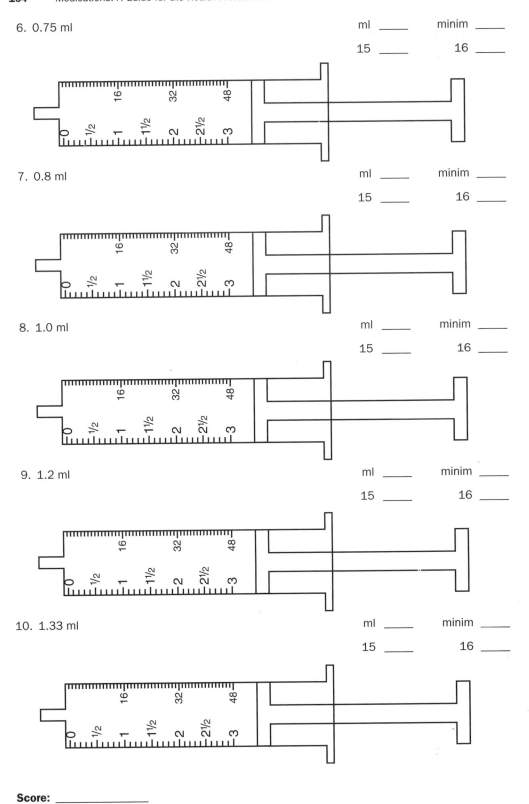

7. 0.8 ml

ml _____   minim _____

15 _____   16 _____

8. 1.0 ml

ml _____   minim _____

15 _____   16 _____

9. 1.2 ml

ml _____   minim _____

15 _____   16 _____

10. 1.33 ml

ml _____   minim _____

15 _____   16 _____

Score: _____

Written Competency 6–3

Performance Competence: Using the simulated tuberculin syringes below, shade in each syringe to the mark you would draw up the medication. Your work must be 100 percent accurate and completed within 15 minutes. Do not give yourself credit for incorrect, incomplete, or skipped questions.

1. 0.1 ml

2. 0.15 ml

3. 0.2 ml

4. 0.25 ml

5. 0.33 ml

6. 0.5 ml

7. 0.66 ml

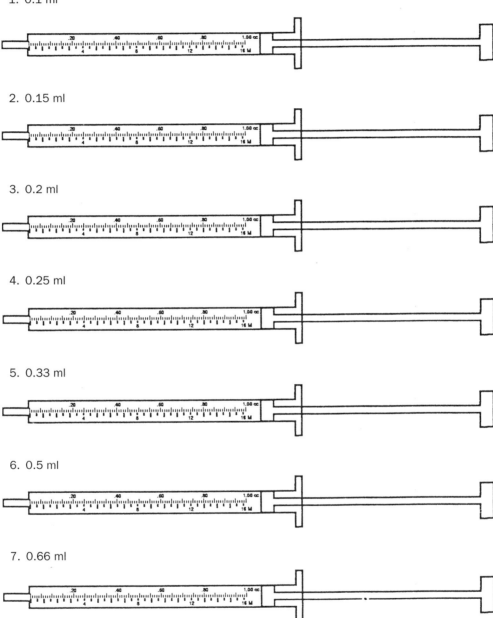

8. 0.75 ml

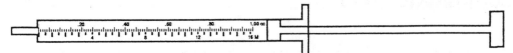

9. 0.8 ml

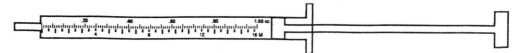

10. 1.0 ml

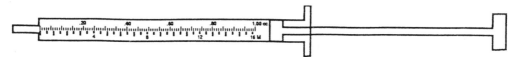

Score: _____

See Appendix B for answers.

Terminal Performance Objective/Competency

Procedure 6–1: Prepare and Administer an Oral Medication Using the EZY-Dose Oral Syringe

EQUIPMENT

EZY-DOSE oral syringe (Apothecary Products, Inc.)
Liquid medication
Rx: Give 1 tsp PO

REVIEW

Procedure 5–1, Chapter 5
Procedure 5–2, Chapter 5

Terminal Performance Objective: Complete each step of this procedure and record your drug administration with exact accuracy, safely, and in the correct order, within reasonable job production time, as stated by your evaluator.

	V	S	U*
PROCEDURAL STEPS (see figure on page 168) 1. Match the written medication order to the medication label (exact name of the drug, available strength, route, ordered amount).	☐	☐	☐
2. Shake the medication.	☐	☐	☐
3. Insert dosage "kork" (cap) into medication bottle with a downward twisting motion until a tight seal is made between the bottle and kork.	☐	☐	☐
4. Remove the cap from the tip of the syringe and draw back the plunger to the last marking on the barrel of the syringe.	☐	☐	☐
5. Open the kork cover and insert the tip of the syringe firmly into the opening in the kork with a twisting motion.	☐	☐	☐
6. Push the plunger down completely, forcing air into the medication bottle.	☐	☐	☐
7. With all pieces attached, turn the entire unit upside down.	☐	☐	☐
8. Withdraw the medication into the syringe by pulling out the plunger.	☐	☐	☐
9. Withdraw slightly more medication into the syringe than ordered. RATIONALE: Excess medication will be forced back into the bottle along with any air bubbles that may cause an inaccurate reading of the medication level.	☐	☐	☐
10. Holding at eye level, return medication to the bottle until the desired level of medication remains in the syringe.	☐	☐	☐
11. Match the medication label against the medication order the second time (exact name of drug, available strength, route, ordered amount).	☐	☐	☐
12. Return the entire unit to the upright position and remove the syringe from the kork with a slow, upward twisting motion.	☐	☐	☐

*V = Value, to be filled in if assigning points or other specific values to each step, or to designate as a critical step.
S = Satisfactory completion of the step.
U = Unsatisfactory completion of the step, or step incorrect; needs more practice.

13. Close the cover on the dosage kork. Advise parents that they may want to replace the kork with a child-proof cap after each use. □ □ □

14. Check the medication for the third time. Return the medication to its storage area.
    RATIONALE: Never leave medications unattended. □ □ □

15. Verbally confirm identification of the patient and match to the name on the written medication order (chart). □ □ □

16. Explain the procedure to the patient. □ □ □

17. Place the tip of the syringe past the patient's lips and teeth. □ □ □

18. Direct the tip of the syringe toward the inner aspect of the cheek.
    RATIONALE: To avoid aspiration and stimulation of the cough reflex. □ □ □

19. Slowly press plunger down to dispense the medication into the patient's mouth. □ □ □

20. Report any reactions or difficulties. □ □ □

21. Offer the patient a cup of water (except after the administration of syrups). □ □ □

22. Record the information on the patient's chart. □ □ □

23. Document any patient education sessions. □ □ □

24. Wash syringe and barrel with warm tap water (if giving the unit to the patient) or dispose of the unit.
    RATIONALE AND PATIENT EDUCATION HINT: Thick medications will leave a residue on the syringe, thereby decreasing the capacity in the barrel on subsequent administrations. □ □ □

Step 1   Step 2   Step 3   Step 4   Step 5

Step 6   Step 7   Step 8   Step 9

Date: _____ Competency achieved: Y _____ N _____

Designated reasonable time standard: _____

Actual completion time: _____

Terminal Performance Objective/Competency

Procedure 6–2: Prepare and Administer a Liquid Oral Medication

EQUIPMENT   Disposable medicine cup   Paper cup filled with water
                 Ordered liquid medication in ounce bottle   Rx: Give 1 tsp PO

REVIEW   Procedure 5–1, Chapter 5
              Procedure 5–2, Chapter 5

Terminal Performance Objective: Complete each step of this procedure and record your drug administration with exact accuracy, safely, and in the correct order, within reasonable job production time, as stated by your evaluator.

		V	S	U *

PROCEDURAL STEPS

1. Check the medication expiration date. If you reconstitute a medication, write the concentration and the date mixed on the label.   ☐ ☐ ☐

2. Match the written medication order to the medication label (exact name of drug, available strength, route, ordered amount).   ☐ ☐ ☐

3. Remove cap from medication and place inside up on the counter.
   RATIONALE: The inside of the cap may not come into contact with any contaminated surfaces.   ☐ ☐ ☐

4. Look at the medicine cup at eye level, with your thumbnail directly on the line of measurement desired.
   RATIONALE: Reading a liquid at eye level on a flat surface allows the correct line of vision for measuring at the bottom of the meniscus.   ☐ ☐ ☐

*V = Value, to be filled in if assigning points or other specific values to each step, or to designate as a critical step.
S = Satisfactory completion of the step.
U = Unsatisfactory completion of the step, or step incorrect; needs more practice.

5. Pour medication to desired measurement with the label up and facing you.
   RATIONALE: Pouring away from the label prevents drips onto the label.   ☐ ☐ ☐

6. Match the medication label against the medication order the second time (exact name of drug, available strength, route, ordered amount).   ☐ ☐ ☐

7. Place the medication bottle on the counter and replace the cap on the medication bottle.   ☐ ☐ ☐

8. Match, for the third time, the medication used against the medication ordered (exact name of drug, available strength, route, ordered amount).   ☐ ☐ ☐

9. Return the medication to its storage area.
   RATIONALE: Never leave medications unattended.   ☐ ☐ ☐

10. Verbally confirm identification of the patient and match to the name on the written medication order (chart). Ask about allergies.
    RATIONALE: The patient could be allergic to any of the component parts of a medication.   ☐ ☐ ☐

11. Explain the procedure to the patient.   ☐ ☐ ☐

12. Stay with the patient while he or she takes the medication. Report any reactions or difficulties.   ☐ ☐ ☐

13. Offer the patient a cup of water (except following the administration of syrups).   ☐ ☐ ☐

14. Dispose of medicine cup.   ☐ ☐ ☐

15. Record the information on the patient's chart.   ☐ ☐ ☐

16. Document any patient education sessions on the chart.   ☐ ☐ ☐

Date: _____ Competency achieved: Y _____ N _____

Designated reasonable time standard: _____

Actual completion time: _____

Terminal Performance Objective/Competency

Procedure 6–3: Open an Ampule Containing a Sterile Medication

EQUIPMENT	Gauze Alcohol Ampule containing sterile water	

REVIEW	Procedure 5–1, Chapter 5 Procedure 5–2, Chapter 5

Terminal Performance Objective: Complete each step of this procedure and record your drug administration with exact accuracy, safely, and in the correct order, within reasonable job production time, as stated by your evaluator.

	V	S	U*

PROCEDURAL STEPS

Step	V	S	U
1. Tap the top of the ampule to force all medication to the bottom section of the ampule.	☐	☐	☐
2. File one side of the ampule at the score line, if a file is suggested by the manufacturer or if the ampule is large.	☐	☐	☐
3. Clean the neck area with alcohol and gauze.	☐	☐	☐
4. Protect your hands with gauze.	☐	☐	☐
5. Sharply tap or bend the top away from your body by snapping your wrists toward your body. You will hear a popping sound.	☐	☐	☐
6. Dispose of broken ampule in a sharps container.	☐	☐	☐

*V = Value, to be filled in if assigning points or other specific values to each step, or to designate as a critical step.

S = Satisfactory completion of the step.

U = Unsatisfactory completion of the step, or step incorrect; needs more practice.

Date: _____ Competency achieved: Y _____ N _____

Designated reasonable time standard: _____

Actual completion time: _____

Conversion Drill for Skill

Using Table 1–7 and the conversion formula, convert the following within 10 minutes. Do not give yourself credit for partial or incorrect answers. Strive for a score of 100 percent. If you score less than 100 percent, return to Chapter 1 and reread the section on conversions.

Convert grams, milligrams, and micrograms to their metric equivalents.

1. 0.25 g   = _____ mg

2. 0.25 mg   = _____ mcg

3. 125 mg   = _____ mcg

4. 125 mg   = _____ g

5. 50 mcg   = _____ g

6. 0.5 g   = _____ mcg

7. 100 mcg   = _____ mg

8. 1000 mcg = _____ mg

9. 1000 mg   = _____ g

10. 1000 g   = _____ kg

Score: _____

See Appendix B for answers.

Assignment 6–1: Use Appendix A, the *PDR,* or Other Reference to Create Drug Information Guides

EQUIPMENT Appendix A; *PDR*; or other drug reference
Lined notepaper or index cards
Drugs: From Top 50 Drugs Most Commonly Prescribed, those ranking 21st–30th

Performance Competence: Complete a drug guide for each of the drugs listed under Equipment. The ten guides should be completed with 100 percent accuracy and must include the following:

Generic name _____

Brand name (Trade name) _____

Classification _____

Controlled substance classification _____

Pregnancy risk category _____

Action _____

Indications/use _____

Contraindications _____

Adverse reactions/side effects _____

Dosage/Route _____

Patient education (in terms the patient will understand) _____

Special alert _____

Calculating Dosages and Solutions

OBJECTIVES **WRITTEN COMPETENCY 7–1:** Translate a medication label

WRITTEN COMPETENCY 7–2: Translate a medication label

WRITTEN COMPETENCY 7–3: Calculate nonparenteral medication orders for liquids and tablets to be administered orally.

WRITTEN COMPETENCY 7–4: Calculate parenteral medication orders for injection.

TERMINAL PERFORMANCE OBJECTIVE (PROCEDURE 7–1): Measure pre-calculated dosages for administration.

ASSIGNMENT 7–1: Use drug reference to create drug information guides.

In Chapter 6, discussion focused on the equipment that makes it possible to determine dosage by measurement. Once the necessary equipment is gathered, the next step is to read the label. Reading the label accurately is absolutely necessary. The label describes how each drug is "packaged," which in turn tells you how it is *available* for usage. If the drug is not available in the same system of measurement as that ordered by the physician, then a *conversion* will be necessary before calculating the exact amount to give to the patient.

Although many pharmaceutical companies are manufacturing drugs in dosages that are immediately measurable, there will be times when the dosage ordered for the patient cannot be directly measured by matching the order to the information on the label. There are two types of calculation problems:

1. Measuring a dose (amount) from an order stated in a *like unit of measurement* as is on the label
2. An order that must be *converted to a new unit of measurement* before the dose (amount) can be calculated

You may want to review pharmacology abbreviations and methods of conversion in Chapter 1 before continuing. The conversion table in Chapter 1 is repeated here (Table 7–1).

TABLE 7–1. **Conversions Between Systems of Measurement**

Metric	*Apothecary*	*Household*
Solids, Mass		
1 g = 1000 mg	15 gr (gr xv)	
60/64/65/66 mg (use what # comes out even)	1 gr (gr i)	
30 mg	1/2 gr (gr iss)	
1 mg = 1000 mcg	1/60 gr (gr 1/60)	
154 g		1.0 lb
1 Kg		2.2 lb
1 g = 1 cc = 1 ml		
Liquids, Volume		
1.0 liter = 1000 ml (or cc)		1 qt (approx)
0.5 liter = 500 ml		1 pt
240 ml	8 fl oz (f℥ viii)	1 c
30–32 ml	1 fl oz (f℥ i)	2 tbs
15–16 ml	4 fl dr (fℨ iv)	1 tbs = 3 tsp
8 ml	2 fl dr (fℨ ii)	2 tsp
4–5 ml	1 fl dr (fℨ i)	1 tsp = 60 gtt
1 ml	15–16 minim (♏ xv–xvi)	15–16 gtt
0.06 ml	1 minim (♏ i)	1 gt

Reading the Label of a Medication

Before you can prepare any medication, you must be able to read and interpret information contained on the medication labels. This skill is necessary to locate drugs and calculate simple dosages.

DRUG NAME

Most labels contain both the trade (brand) name and the generic name. The trade name appears with the first or all letters uppercase and the copyright symbol ®. The generic name usually is printed in lower case letters directly under the trade name. The official name (U.S.P) may also appear (alone or in combination with the trade name) on the label, printed in upper and lower case letters or all uppercase letters.

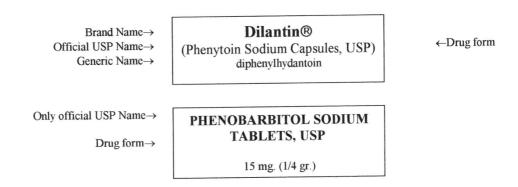

Brand Name→
Official USP Name→
Generic Name→

Dilantin®
(Phenytoin Sodium Capsules, USP)
diphenylhydantoin

←Drug form

Only official USP Name→

Drug form→

PHENOBARBITOL SODIUM TABLETS, USP

15 mg. (1/4 gr.)

THE FORM

The form of the drug is incorporated into the name. Solid drug preparations include tablets, enteric-coated tablets, capsules, and sustained or controlled-release capsules, and suppositories. In the first example above, the drug form is capsules; in the second example, the drug form is tablets. See also Chapter 3, for a review of drug forms.

A medication may contain two or more drug names. Tablets and capsules that contain more than one drug are ordered by trade name rather than by generic names or official names. For example, the drug listed below will be ordered as Dyazide.

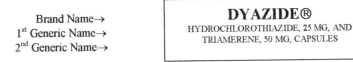

Brand Name→
1ˢᵗ Generic Name→
2ⁿᵈ Generic Name→

DYAZIDE®
HYDROCHLOROTHIAZIDE, 25 MG, AND
TRIAMERENE, 50 MG, CAPSULES

QUANTITY

The quantity refers to the total quantity in a container. *Unit dosage* is common in hospitals and larger care settings. A unit dose is a single-use package in which each tablet or capsule is packaged separately. In this case no quantity is printed on the label; the quantity is understood.

In *multiple-dose* containers, the total number of tablets in a bottle or the total number of ounces in a bottle of oral liquid medication is printed above or below the drug name.

Quantity→

```
        DYAZIDE®
HYDROCHLOROTHIAZIDE, 25 MG, AND
   TRIAMERENE, 50 MG, CAPSULES
─────────────────────────────────
        100 Capsules
```

The labels of solid and parenteral or liquid solutions are similar, but the total volumes used for parenteral medications are much smaller. Parenteral drugs are packaged in a variety of glass ampules, single- and multiple-use, rubber-stoppered vials, and in pre-measured syringes and cartridges. See also Chapter 6.

```
20 mL  multi-dose vial          ←Quantity


        Dilantin®
(Phenytoin Sodium Injection, USP)
       diphenylhydantoin
          50 mg/ml
```

MEDICATION STRENGTH

The medication strength is clearly printed below the drug name. Tablet and capsule strengths are fairly straightforward to understand: the strength printed on the label is the strength in 1 tablet or capsule. The strength may be written in both metric and apothecaries' units of measure or in only one unit of measure.

Both metric and apothecaries' units used→

```
PHENOBARBITOL SODIUM
   TABLETS, USP)
   15 mg. (1/4 gr.)
```

Metric unit only →

```
        Dilantin®
(Phenytoin Sodium Capsules, USP)
      diphenylhydantoin
           30 mg
─────────────────────────────
        100 capsules
```

Metric units used→

```
        DYAZIDE®
HYDROCHLOROTHIAZIDE, 25 MG, AND
   TRIAMERENE, 50 MG, CAPSULES
─────────────────────────────────
        100 Capsules
```

Parental medication strengths, especially those drugs that must be reconstituted, are more confusing. Medications for injection are manufactured so that the average adult dosage will be contained in a volume of between 1 and 3 ml each time it is used. If the total quantity is 1 to 5 ml, the container may be considered a single-dose product. If the quantity is greater, usually 20 to 50 ml, the vial can be assumed to be a multiple-dose product.

5 ml single-dose vial	20 ml multi-dose vial
Dilantin® (Phenytoin Sodium Injection, USP) diphenylhydantoin 50 mg/ml	**Dilantin®** (Phenytoin Sodium Injection, USP) diphenylhydantoin 50 mg/ml

While some drugs are manufactured single strength, other drugs may be prepared in different strengths. The manufacturer will carefully identify strength choices on the label to the right of the trade name.

Dilantin® 30 mg (Phenytoin Sodium Capsules, USP) diphenylhydantoin 100 capsules	**Dilantin®** 100 mg (Phenytoin Sodium Capsules, USP) diphenylhydantoin 100 capsules

LOT NUMBERS AND EXPIRATION DATES

All medications have a shelf life, and it is important to check this each time a medication is prepared. Discard any product that is outdated. Some medications have a long shelf life; others are very short. After the expiration date, the drug's strength and purity are not assured. Medications stocked on shelves as well as in emergency boxes are routinely checked for their expiration dates. It is especially important for emergency drugs, since in an emergency there might not be time to check the expiration date.

Lot numbers are important especially when administering immunization products. On occasion, there have been recalls. Lot numbers are also important to record in the medical record, if a patient has an allergic reaction to an immunization product. Lot numbers and expiration dates usually are printed sideways to the right of the label. Expiration dates begin with "EXP."

Dilantin® (Phenytoin Sodium Capsules, USP) diphenylhydantoin **30 mg** 100 capsules	584 – 399 EXP 6-30-99	Lot Number and Expiration Date

MANUFACTURER NAME

The manufacturer's name will be printed on every label. Each manufacturer uses a style and format that fits the manufacturer's logo.

Dilantin®
(Phenytoin Sodium Capsules, USP)
diphenylhydantoin
30 mg

100 capsules
PARKE-DAVIS

584 – 399   EXP 6-30-99

Manufacturer
Name→

SOLUTIONS MEASURED IN PERCENTAGE

Drugs may be expressed in metric units or apothecary units, as in the examples above, or in percentage and ratio strengths. Drugs labeled as percentage solutions often express the drug strength in metric units as well. The label below states both the percentage and the metric units for the anesthetic lidocaine HCl injection, USP.

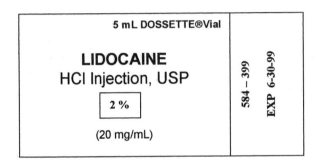

5 mL DOSSETTE®Vial

LIDOCAINE
HCl Injection, USP

2 %

(20 mg/mL)

584 – 399   EXP 6-30-99

If the physician requests 4 ml of 2 percent lidocaine drawn into a syringe, simply choose the vial with the correct percentage and draw up the anesthesia to the 4 ml mark on the syringe. If on the other hand, the physician orders 10 mg of lidocaine, a calculation would be required to determine that 0.5 ml would be drawn into the syringe. This is the type of calculation you will learn to do in the next section of this chapter.

SOLUTIONS MEASURED IN UNITS (U) AND MILLIEQUIVALENTS (mEq)

Some drugs are measured in *International Units* or *milliequivalents*. Insulin, penicillin, and heparin are examples of drugs measured in units; many IV fluids are measured in milliequivalents. The calculations and syringe measurements are the same as for drugs measured in percentages.

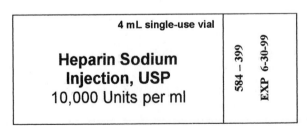

4 mL single-use vial

**Heparin Sodium
Injection, USP**
10,000 Units per ml

584 – 399   EXP 6-30-99

RECONSTITUTED DRUGS

Many drugs are shipped in powdered form. The drug label and package insert will give specific directions for reconstitution of the drug. Reconstitution is difficult and requires careful attention. The label directions appear to the right and left of the label name. Once a drug is reconstituted, the container must be labeled with the date and time of expiration. The person reconstituting the drug should initial or sign the label.

200 mL KEFLEX® CEPHALEXIN FOR ORAL SUSPENSION, USP 125 mg per 5 ml. Oversized bottle provides extra space for shaking. Store in refrigerator. May be kept for 14 days without significant loss of potency. Keep tightly closed. Discard unused portion after 14 days. Shake well before using. Control # 111-11-1111	200 mL (When Mixed) **Keflex®** **Cephalexin for** **Oral Suspension USP** **125 mg per 5 ml** **Dista Products Company** **Division of Lilly** **EXP 12-31-99**	Usual Children's Dose 25 to 50 mg per kg a day in four divided doses. For more severe infections, dose may be doubled. See literature. Contains Cephalexin Monohydrate equivalent to 5 g Cephalexin in a powdered form. Prior to mixing, Store at Controlled Room Temperature 59° to 86° F (15° to 30°C) Directions for Mixing—Add 100 ml of water in two portions to the dry mixture in the bottle. Shake well after each addition. Each 5 ml (approximately one teaspoonful will then contain: Cephalexin Monohydrate equivalent to 125 mg Cephalexin. Date prepared _____ time _____ init.

MULTIPLE STRENGTH RECONSTITUTION

Often drugs may be reconstituted in a variety of strengths. The choice of strength will depend on what is ordered and on patient considerations. The choices are printed on the label and package insert.

Time _____ **Date Prepared** _____ **Strength** _____ **Init.** _____ Shake well before using Control # 111-11-1111	**Geopen®** **Carbenicillin disodium** **Sterile** **equivalent to** **2 g of Carbenicillin** **For IM Use** **Roerig – Pfizer, Inc.** EXP 12-31-99	DIRECTIONS IM Use: Reconstitute with at least 4 ml of Sterile Water for Injection in order to facilitate reconstitution, up to 7.2 ml of Sterile Water for Injection can be used. Amount Of Diluent To Be Added To The 2 G Vial / Volume To Be Withdrawn For A 1 G Dose 4.0 ml — 2.5 ml 5.0 ml — 3.0 ml 7.2 ml — 4.0 ml For dosage information, read accompanying professional information. After reconstitution, discard any unused portion after 24 hours (if stored at room temperature) or after 72 hours (if refrigerated). Store dry powder below 25° C.

PACKAGE INSERTS

Package inserts contain a great deal of additional information about medications. Some manufacturers publish two types of inserts: one for the patient and one for the health professional. Both may be difficult to understand, but it is important for those working in the health care field to be comfortable with the facts on each. It will often be necessary to work with this printed material, since it is the most current, approved information. Some of the most important information includes the administration instructions, patient education needs, and product storage requirements.

RULES OF SAFETY

Reading the label must be mastered before attempting any dosage calculation. Chapter 5 lists the safety precautions for preparing medications. Of the "seven rights" listed there, the "right drug (name and strength)" and the "right dose" require the clear understanding of what is printed on the label. Also, remember that the label is checked three (3) times before giving a medication. Some facilities require as policy that a co-worker verify the calculation and measurement, especially after complex calculations. It may be wise to have a co-worker watch as a drug is reconstituted to verify that it was done correctly. These precautions are most important when giving drugs that can be dangerous.

Terms and Calculation Basics

Before dosage calculations can be solved, there are a few important terms and basic concepts to understand. One of the first tasks to master is reading drug labels. Each label contains all the information needed to (1) choose the correct medication, (2) measure a quantity of medication, and (3) calculate specific quantities for individual patients.

When using liquids, the *solute* is the pure drug that is dissolved in a liquid to form a suspension or solution; the *solvent* is the liquid substance (usually sterile or bacteriostatic water or normal saline) used to dissolve the solute; and the *solution* is the entire mixture. Sometimes, the term *diluent* is also used to mean the solvent.

Strength is the term that describes a drug's potency. Different drug strengths can be stated as follows:

As a percentage (e.g., hydrocortisone 1 percent or 2 percent)
As a solid weight (e.g., grams, milligrams, micrograms, or grains)
As an independent weight measure (e.g., milliequivalent or unit)

Strength is the potency of a drug. It is considered a part of every label. For example, a vial labeled *"Depo-Medrol 20 mg per ml (5 ml)"* is different from another vial labeled *"Depo-Medrol 40 mg/ml (5ml)."* Both vials contain the drug Depo-Medrol; however, the first vial contains 20 mg of the drug in every 1 ml of sterile water and the second, 40 mg of drug in every 1 ml of sterile water. The 40 mg per ml strength (1 ml contains 40 mg) is the stronger solution: it is twice the strength of the 20 mg per ml solution, in which 1 ml contains 20 mg.

Using Figure 7-1, the correct choice to prepare the physician's order "Depo-Medrol 40mg" is Depo-Medrol 40 mg per ml. It would take exactly 1 ml of solution to deliver 40 mg drug strength to the patient. If Depo-Medrol 20 mg were used, it would take 2 ml of solution to equal the same strength—two times the amount. Of course, if the 40 mg per ml strength is not available, the 20 mg per ml would be an acceptable alternative. The amount injected would be two times as much, however.

Dosage is defined as the size (quantity or amount), frequency, and number of doses. *Dose* is the quantity (specified amount) to administer at one time, and it can indicate an amount of solution to inject (milliliters, minims), a number of tablets to give, a number of teaspoons to give, and so on. In the foregoing 40 mg per ml example, the dose is 1 ml.

5 ml single-dose vial	5 ml multi-dose vial
Depo-Medrol® methylprednisolone 20 mg/ml	**Depo-Medrol®** methylprednisolone 40 mg/ml

FIGURE 7–1. The same drug is often manufactured and packaged in different strengths. It is important to read a label's strength as part of the drug's full identification.

Calculating Drugs to Administer to Patients

Not all calculations are obvious. If the physician orders "Depo-Medrol .035 gm," a formula must be used to calculate the dose. When using formulas to calculate dosage, the strength that is on the label is the "*available strength*"; the amount to administer is called the "*ordered strength*," and the amount stated on the label in which a particular strength is contained is the "*available form.*"

We can convert from one system to another in exactly the same way as we converted from one unit of measurement to another in Chapter 1. We multiply what is ordered by a fraction that positions the unit of measurement that is on the label on the top of the fraction and the unit of measurement that is ordered on the bottom of the fraction. This fraction represents equivalent measurements and must always equal 1.

There is a specific formula, with variations, for calculating correct doses to give. This formula is written:

$$\text{ordered strength} \times \underset{\text{(That matches the order)}}{\overset{\text{(To match the label)}}{\frac{\text{New Units}}{\text{Old Units}}}} \times \underset{\text{(On the label)}}{\overset{\text{(On the label)}}{\frac{\text{available form}}{\text{available strength}}}} = \text{Amount to Give}$$

Understanding the elements of the basic formula is half the battle. For example, the first label in Figure 7–1 gives you the available strength (20 mg) and available form (per ml):

$$\text{ordered strength} \times \frac{\text{New Units}}{\text{Old Units}} \times \frac{1 \text{ ml}}{20 \text{ mg}} = x$$

The Conversion Table 7–1 contains the information needed for converting units of measurement, for example, converting grams to milligrams:

$$\text{ordered strength} \times \frac{1000 \text{ milligrams}}{1 \text{ gram}} \times \frac{1 \text{ ml}}{20 \text{ mg}} = x$$

As soon as the physician gives the order, the last piece of the formula can be filled in. In this first example, let's say the physician orders .035 grams:

$$.035 \text{ gram} \times \frac{1000 \text{ mg}}{1 \text{ gm}} \times \frac{1 \text{ ml}}{20 \text{ mg}} = \text{Amt. to give}$$

$$^{*}\frac{.035 \text{ gm}}{1} \times \frac{1000 \text{ mg}}{1 \text{ gm}} \times \frac{1 \text{ ml}}{20 \text{ mg}} = 1.75 \text{ ml}$$

It is important to understand right away how to determine what measurement to use in the answer. Remember that like units of measurement above and below the fraction cancel out. In this case, two sets of measurement cancel out: the gm's and the mg's. This means the answer will be measured in the only remaining measurement: the ml.

---

*A whole number can be written as a fraction with 1 as the denominator.

PRACTICE PROBLEM: *Stop and write the formula at least five times:*

1.

2.

3.

4.

5.

Now, write the formula using Table 7–1, Figure 7–1, and the following orders:

1. Ordered: Depo-Medrol 20 mg.

2. Ordered: Depo-Medrol 50 mg.

3. Ordered: Depo-Medrol 60 mg.

4. Ordered: Depo-Medrol 80 mg.

5. Ordered: Depo-Medrol 15 mg.

CALCULATING LIKE UNITS OF MEASUREMENT

Drug orders are most often calculated using *like* units of measurement (e.g., calculating the number of aspirin tablets to give when the bottle of aspirin is labeled in grains and the physician orders the dose in grains).

Order

The physician orders aspirin 10 gr. The aspirin available is in a bottle labeled, "Aspirin 5 gr/tab" (5 grains per tablet).

Problem Statement

If 5 gr equal 1 tablet (known), then 10 gr will equal how many tablets (unknown)? How many tablets will be administered?

$$\text{(Ordered) Unknown:} \quad 10 \text{ gr} = x$$
$$\text{(Label) Known:} \quad 5 \text{ gr} = 1 \text{ tablet}$$

Formula

$$\text{Ordered Strength} \times \frac{\text{New Units}}{\text{Old Units}} \times \frac{\text{available form}}{\text{available strength}} = \text{Amount to Give}$$

Known/Unknown

Plug the known and unknown factors into the formula:

$$10 \text{ gr} \times \frac{1 \text{ gr}}{1 \text{ gr}} \times \frac{1 \text{ tablet}}{5 \text{ gr}} = x$$

(Note: There is no conversion from Table 7–1 necessary in this problem. Eventually you may feel comfortable omitting the middle step (fraction). For now it is best to leave it in.)

Calculation

Multiply the fractions

$$\frac{{}^*10 \text{ gr}}{1} \times \frac{1 \text{ gr}}{1 \text{ gr}} \times \frac{1 \text{ tab}}{5 \text{ gr}} \times \frac{10}{5} = 2 \text{ tablets}$$

Answer

To administer 10 gr of aspirin from a bottle labeled "Aspirin 5 gr/tablet," *give 2 tablets.*

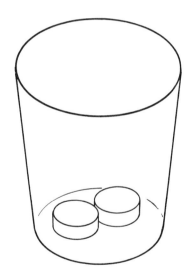

Now, let us return to the Depo-Medrol example from the introduction to this chapter to examine how to calculate a medication *for injection* in *like* units of measurement.

Order

The physician orders Depo-Medrol 56 mg q wk. Depo-Medrol is available in a 5-ml vial labeled "40 mg/ml."

---

*A whole number can be written as a fraction with 1 as the denominator.

Problem Statement

If 1 ml equals 40 mg (known), then 56 mg will equal how many milliliters (unknown)? How many milliliters will be administered?

(Ordered) Unknown: 56 mg = x
(Label) Known: 40 mg = 1 ml

Formula

$$\text{Ordered strength} \times \frac{\text{New Units}}{\text{Old Units}} = \frac{\text{Available Form}}{\text{Available Strength}} = \text{Amount to Give}$$

Known/Unknown

Plug the known and unknown factors into the formula:

$$56 \text{ mg} \times \frac{1 \text{ mg}}{1 \text{ mg}} \times \frac{1 \text{ ml}}{40 \text{ mg}} = x$$

(Note: There is no Table 7–1 conversion necessary for this problem. Eventually you may feel comfortable leaving out the middle step (fraction). For now it is best to leave it in.

Calculation

Multiply

$$^{*}\frac{56 \text{ mg}}{1} \times \frac{1 \text{ mg}}{1 \text{ mg}} \times \frac{1 \text{ ml}}{40 \text{ mg}} = \frac{56}{40} = 1.4 \text{ ml}$$

Answer

To administer 56 mg of Depo-Medrol from a vial labeled "Depo-Medrol 40 mg/ml," *administer (inject) 1.4 ml of medication.*

---

5 ml multi-dose vial

Depo-Medrol®
methylprednisolone
40 mg/ml

CALCULATING DRUGS ORDERED IN BIOASSAY UNITS AND MILLIEQUIVALENTS

There are some drugs whose strengths cannot be weighed in grams, milligrams, grains, and so on. Drugs not measured by weight are measured in *bioassay units* (U), and *milliequivalents* (mEq). A milliequivalent is equal to one thousandth (1/1000 or 0.001) of an equivalent and is based on the number of ionic changes of a compound. Milliequivalents are used mostly with intravenous (IV) fluids and medications.

---

*A whole number may be written as a fraction with 1 as the denominator.

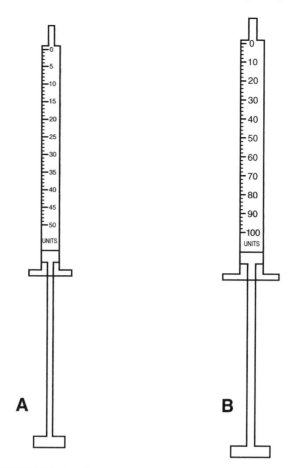

FIGURE 7-2. Insulin syringes. *A*, 0.5 mL (50 U). *B*, 1.0 mL (100 U).

The bioassay unit is based on a standardized amount of drug needed to produce a desired amount. Units standardized by the United States are labeled *USP* (*United States Pharmacopeia*) units; those standardized by international organizations are labeled IU (International Unit). Examples of drug manufactured in units include insulin, certain penicillins, heparin, vitamins, and tetanus toxoid. Units and milliequivalents are calculated with the same formula. Because the unit written as an uppercase "U" or lowercase "u" can be easily mistaken for the symbol μ (micron), it is best to always write out the full word.

Insulin is measured in USP units. The most common strength is 100 units per ml (U-100). Insulin is also manufactured in 40 units per ml (U-40) and 80 units per ml (U-80), but these two strengths are used mostly in veterinarian medicine.

Because insulin is available in 100 units per ml, the amount ordered is the amount to draw up in a 50-unit or 100-unit syringe (Fig. 7-2). To ensure the most accurate dose possible, the U-50 low-dosage syringe should be used for insulin doses to 50 units, and a 1-ml syringe for doses more than 50 units.

Order

The physician orders 70 units of insulin. Insulin is available in a 5-ml vial labeled "100 U/ml."

Problem Statement

If 1 ml equals 100 U of insulin (known), then 70 U will equal how many milliliters (unknown)? How many milliliters will be administered?

$$\text{(Ordered) Unknown:} \qquad 70 \text{ U} = x$$
$$\text{(Label) Known:} \qquad 100 \text{ U} = 1 \text{ ml}$$

Formula

$$\text{Ordered Strength} \times \frac{\text{New Units}}{\text{Old Units}} \times \frac{\text{Available Form}}{\text{Available Strength}} = \text{Amount to Give}$$

Known/Unknown

Plug in the known and unknown factors into the formula:

$$70 \text{ U} \times \frac{1 \text{ U}}{1 \text{ U}} \times \frac{1 \text{ ml}}{100 \text{ U}} = x$$

Calculation

$$^{*}\frac{70 \text{ U}}{1} \times \frac{1 \text{ U}}{1 \text{ U}} \times \frac{1 \text{ ml}}{100 \text{ U}} = \frac{70}{100} = 0.7 \text{ ml}$$

CALCULATING UNLIKE UNITS OF MEASUREMENT

Working with *unlike* units of measurement **requires** the conversion fraction (middle step of the formula).

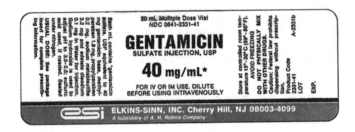

Order

The physician orders Gentamicin 0.04 g. Gentamicin is available in a 20-ml vial labeled "40 mg/ml."

Problem Statement

If 1 ml equals 40 mg (known), then four tenths of a gram (0.04 g) will equal how many milliliters (unknown)? How many milliliters will be administered?

$$\text{(Ordered) Unknown:} \qquad 0.04 \text{ g} = x$$
$$\text{(Conversion Table) Known:} \qquad 1 \text{ g (old)} = 1000 \text{ mg (new)}$$
$$\text{(Label) Known:} \qquad 40 \text{ mg} = 1 \text{ ml}$$

Formula

$$\text{Ordered Strength} \times \frac{\text{New Units}}{\text{Old Units}} \times \frac{\text{Available Form}}{\text{Available Strength}} = \text{Amount to Give}$$

---

*A whole number can be written as a fraction with 1 as the denominator.

Known/Unknown

$$.04 \text{ gm} \times \frac{1000 \text{ mg}}{1 \text{ gm}} \times \frac{1 \text{ ml}}{40 \text{ mg}} = x$$

Calculation

$$^{*}\frac{.04 \text{ gm}}{1} \times \frac{1000 \text{ mg}}{1 \text{ gm}} \times \frac{1 \text{ ml}}{40 \text{ mg}} = \frac{40}{40} = 1 \text{ ml}$$

Answer

To administer 40 mg (originally ordered as 0.04 g) of Gentamycin from a vial labeled "Gentamycin 40 mg/ml," *administer (inject) 1 ml of medication.*

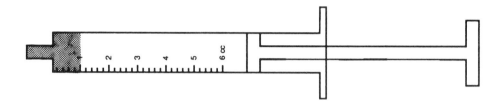

Order

The physician orders ¹⁄₁₅₀ grain of nitroglycerin. The label reads, "0.4 mg/tablet."

Problem Statement

If 1 tablet equals 0.4 mg (known), then ¹⁄₁₅₀ gr will equal how many tablets (unknown)? How many tablets will be administered?

(Ordered) Unknown:	¹⁄₁₅₀ gr $= x$
(Conversion table) Known:	1 gr $=$ 60 mg
(Label) Known:	0.4 mg $=$ 1 tablet

Formula

$$\text{Ordered Strength} \times \frac{\text{New Units}}{\text{Old Units}} \times \frac{\text{Available Form}}{\text{Available Strength}} = \text{Amount to Give}$$

Known/Unknown

Plug in the known and unknown factors into the formula.

$$\frac{1}{150} \text{ gr} \times \frac{60 \text{ mg}}{1 \text{ gr}} \times \frac{1 \text{ tablet}}{0.4 \text{ mg}} = x$$

Calculation

$$^{\dagger}\frac{\frac{1}{150} \text{ gr}}{1} \times \frac{60 \text{ mg}}{1 \text{ gr}} \times \frac{1 \text{ tab}}{0.4 \text{ mg}} = x$$

---

*A whole number may be written as a fraction with 1 as the denominator.
†Note: the 1st numerator contains a fraction (complex fraction). The longer line represents division.

To use this complex fraction in the problem, you first must invert the denominator and multiply.

$$\frac{\frac{1}{150}}{\frac{1}{1}} \quad \text{means} \quad \frac{1}{150} \div \frac{1}{1} \quad \text{or} \quad \frac{1}{150} \div 1 \quad \text{which is} \quad \frac{\frac{1}{150}}{1}$$

The calculation changes to

$$\frac{\frac{1}{150}\,\text{gr}}{1} \times \frac{60\,\text{mg}}{1\,\text{gr}} \times \frac{1\,\text{tab}}{0.4\,\text{mg}} = \frac{\frac{60}{150}}{0.4} = \frac{0.4}{0.4} = 1\,\text{tablet}$$

Answer

To administer 0.4 mg (originally ordered as 1/150 gr of nitroglycerin from a bottle labeled "0.4 mg/tablet,") administer 1 tablet.

PRACTICE PROBLEMS: Work the same three problems just discussed without looking back. Follow each of the seven steps, and take **no** shortcuts. Discipline is required as there can be no margin of error. Write the answer as a full sentence.

1. *Order:* The physician orders aspirin 10 gr. Aspirin is available in a bottle labeled, "Aspirin 5 gr/tab" (5 grains per tablet).

2. *Order:* The physician orders Depo-Medrol 56 mg q wk. Depo-Medrol 40 mg per ml is available in a 5-ml vial.

3. *Order:* The physician orders Gentamicin 0.04 g. Gentamicin is available in a 20-ml vial labeled "40 mg/ml."

MEDICATIONS ORDERED BY BODY WEIGHT

As we discussed in Chapter 5, pediatric dosages are different from those in other age groups. Although factors such as absorption and metabolism are important in determining dosage, the most important factor for children is body size. This method is also used for small adults and to give medications with a narrow margin of safety (e.g., chemotherapy or anesthesia).

Although size is used to determine dosages for children, calculating doses for children by *any* comparison to adult size and dosage is not very accurate. These methods incorrectly assume that all drugs are based exactly on the 150-lb adult.

The most accurate method is to order pediatric doses (as well as any other medication) *per kilogram of body weight* or *per kilogram of body weight per day in divided doses.* The literature that is enclosed with medications contains information on how to administer a drug per kilogram of body weight. It is therefore important to remember the pound per kilogram conversion. The conversion equation for pounds to kilograms is:

$$1 \text{ kg} = 2.2 \text{ lb}$$

For example, a child weighs 33 pounds and the physician orders amoxicillin suspension. The amoxicillin label reads "For adults and children over 20 kg, 250 mg/q8h. For children under 20 kg, 20 mg/kg/day, the total daily dose is divided into 3 doses q8h."

There are three steps to determining the pediatric dose per kilogram of body weight.

Step 1. Determine the child's weight in kilograms.
Step 2. Calculate the number of milligrams per day for the child's weight; then determine the divided doses.
Step 3. Determine the amount to administer.

Step 1—Problem Statement

If 1 kg equals 2.2 lb (known), then 33 lb will equal how many kilograms (unknown)? How many kilograms does the child weigh?

Unknown:	33 lb = x kg
(Conversion Table) Known:	2.2 lb= 1 kg

Formula (see Chapter 1)

$$\frac{\text{New Units}}{\text{Old Units}} \times \text{Available Form}$$

$$\frac{1 \text{ kg}}{2.2 \text{ lb}} \times \frac{33 \text{ lb}}{1} = \frac{33}{2.2} = 15 \text{ kg}$$

Answer

A 33-lb child weighs 15 kg.

Step 2—Order Restated

Determine the number of milligrams of amoxicillin per dose for a child weighing 15 kg.

Problem Statement

If 20 mg is administered for every kilogram per day (known), then 15 kg will equal how many milligrams per day (unknown)? How many milligrams will be administered per day?

$$15 \text{ kg} \times 20 \text{ mg} = 300 \text{ mg}$$

Divided into three equal doses during the day:

$$300 \div 3 = 100 \text{ mg}$$

Answer

For a child weighing 15 kg, *administer 100 mg per dose.*

Step 3—Order Restated

Administer 100 mg to the child. The vial is labeled 250 mg/10 ml.

Problem Statement

If 10 ml equals 250 mg (known), then 100 mg will equal how many milliliters (unknown)? How many milliliters will be administered?

$$\text{(Ordered) Unknown:} \quad 100 \text{ mg} = x$$
$$\text{(Label) Known:} \quad 250 \text{ mg} = 10 \text{ ml}$$

Formula

$$\text{Ordered Strength} \times \frac{\text{New Units}}{\text{Old Units}} \times \frac{\text{Available Form}}{\text{Available Strength}} = \text{Amount to Give}$$

Known/Unknown

Plug the known and unknown factors into the formula:

$$100 \text{ mg} \times \frac{1 \text{ mg}}{1 \text{ mg}} \times \frac{10 \text{ ml}}{250 \text{ mg}} = x$$

Calculation

Multiply

$$\frac{100 \text{ mg}}{1} \times \frac{1 \text{ mg}}{1 \text{ mg}} \times \frac{10 \text{ ml}}{250 \text{ mg}} = \frac{1000}{250} = 4 \text{ ml}$$

Answer

To administer 100 mg amoxicillin from a liquid suspension labeled "Amoxicillin 250 mg/10 ml," *administer 4.0 ml of medication.*

Older, less accurate methods are sometimes used to calculate dosage for children. Each method is based on comparing the child size to adult size and dosage. They are:

1. *Clark's weight rule:* Adjustments based on body weight
2. *West's nomogram:* Adjustments based on body surface area
3. *Fried's law and Young's rule:* Adjustments based on age

Very few physicians calculate dosage based on any of these rules, especially in young children. Weight in children varies too much, no matter what the age. Although growth charts plot average height and weight ranges by age, there is really no such thing as an average dose per child's age.

DOSAGE BASED ON BODY SURFACE AREA

Some physicians believe that the use of body surface area (BSA) is the more accurate method of calculating pediatric dosage, especially in infants weighing less than 10 kg. Although West's nomogram of body surfaces is most often used to determine fluid replacement needs, there is no evidence that the BSA method for calculating dosage is any more effective than the milligram per kilogram of body weight method. In fact, in some cases, the BSA method results in higher, unsafe dosages than those based on the kilograms of body weight method.

The BSA method is based on a nomogram chart (Fig. 7–3), which is first used to calculate the surface area of the body. Using the chart:

1. Plot the height of the far left column.
2. Plot the weight on the far right column.
3. Draw a horizontal line between the two plots.
4. Determine the BSA at the point the line crosses the surface area (square meters [m^2]) column.

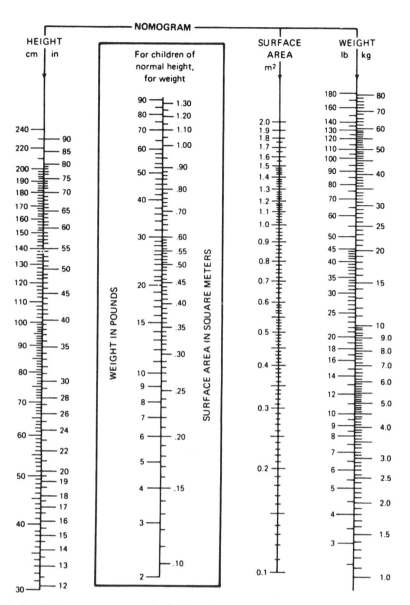

FIGURE 7–3. The West nomogram measuring body surface area (BSA). (From Deglin, JH and Vallerand, AH: Davis's Drug Guide for Nurses. FA Davis, Philadelphia, 1988, p. 707, with permission.)

For children of normal height and weight (determined from growth charts), the boxed area of the chart can be used. It contains preplotted information and is based on weight alone. Using the left side of the boxed-in column, plot the child's weight, then read the BSA (m^2) immediately to the right. The BSA, measured in square meters, is then used with the following formula:

$$\frac{\text{BSA in } m^2 \times \text{Adult dose}}{1.7 \ m^2 \text{ (average adult BSA)}} = \text{Pediatric dose}$$

If drug information specifies the amount of drug to give in square meters of BSA, the formula is not necessary.

CALCULATING FOR A MARGIN OF SAFETY

A few rules and considerations must be taken into account when calculating and measuring medications. You have already learned in a previous chapter that, although conversion tables convert the drop to the minim, you should not, in practice, convert an order in minims to drops. Although they are *mathematically* equivalent, the dropper cannot *physically* dispense an accurate minim. Here are some other important rules for accurate measurement:

> *Rule No. 1.* Do not round off liquid medications for quantities *less than 3 ml*. If a liquid medication cannot be accurately measured in the unit of measurement ordered, the order is converted to a smaller unit and then measured.
>
> *Rule No. 2.* If an order *less than 3 ml* is not measurable in an even 10th of the milliliter, the order is converted to minims.
>
> *Rule No. 3.* For medication quantities *larger than 3 ml*, round off to the nearest 10th of a milliliter.
>
> *Rule No. 4. Do not* increase a medication by more than rounding to 1/10. Only the physician is licensed to increase the dose of a medication more than rounding 1/10 up or down. If a measurement requires a judgment involving more than rounding to the nearest 10th, ask the physician to change the medication order.
>
> *Rule No. 5.* When alternative equivalents are allowed, use the equivalent that works best with the calculation. Certain equivalents are only approximate, and the *United States Pharmacopeia* accepts the use of the following mathematic alternatives for equating adult medications.

$$1 \text{ ml} = 15 \text{ } or \text{ } 16 \text{ minims}$$
$$1 \text{ gr} = 60 \text{ } or \text{ } 64 \text{ } or \text{ } 65 \text{ } or \text{ } 66 \text{ mg}$$
$$1 \text{ oz} = 30 \text{ or } 32 \text{ ml}$$

> *Rule No. 6.* Adult doses may be varied within a *safe range*. The safe range is based on a ± 10 percent (or 0.1) margin of safety. A dose may be multiplied by 0.1, and the answer (1/10 or 10 percent of the amount) may be added to or subtracted from the calculated dose. This gives you a range in which you may safely round off. This rule may not be applied to pediatric dosage calculations.

Example: Administer a calculated dose of 9.12 ml to an *adult* patient.

$$9.12 \times 0.1 = 0.912$$

Added Together	*Subtracted*
9.12	9.12
+0.912	−0.912
10.032	8.208

From 8.208 to 10.032 is considered the safe range. You may round to the nearest 10th or, in this case, to the nearest whole number and stay within a safe range. Because this amount is so large, the range appears wide, but it is only ± 10 percent of the calculated dose.

Answer

For an adult, it is safe to round off this calculated dose to 9 ml. Choose to round to 9 ml, rather than 8.2 ml or 10 ml, because it is closest to the original order and the easiest to measure. When deciding whether to add or subtract the margin of safety range, choose whichever operation leads to the *closest measurable* answer.

RECONSTITUTING POWDERED MEDICATIONS

Some vials contain crystals or powders that must be reconstituted before administration. These medications usually are unstable in liquid form and must be reconstituted before administration. Some medications are packaged with both the liquid diluent and the dry drug premeasured in a single container; other dry forms are reconstituted with stock solutions of sterile isotonic saline or sterile distilled water. If sterile distilled water is used for injection, it must be labeled "for injection."

> SPECIAL CAUTION: Multiple-dose vials of sterile isotonic saline and sterile distilled water contain a bacteriostatic preservative that is now connected to seizures in infants. Single-dose vials do not contain the preservative and should be used with infants less than 3 months of age.

The label instructions give the following information:

1. One or more choices of how much sterile diluent to add. Sterile diluents may include
   a. Sterile water
   b. Bacteriostatic water (has an antibiotic preservative added)
   c. Isotonic (0.9 percent) sodium chloride, also called normal saline or isotonic saline
   d. 1 percent lidocaine
2. How much the total volume will be once you have added the sterile diluent to the powder (Fig. 7–4). It is important to understand that the powdered drug has volume, therefore the total volume will be slightly greater than the amount of the diluent. The volume of the powdered drug is calculated as "displacement."
3. How much medication will be delivered in each milliliter after you have added the exact amount of sterile liquid.

Diluent	Vial	Strength	Calculated Volume	Calculated Displacement
4.2 ml	1 g	200 mg	5 ml	0.8 ml
9.2 ml	1 g	100 mg	10 ml	0.8 ml

Example: The physician orders 250 mg of a drug.

The powdered form of the drug is packaged in a vial labeled "1 g; add 7.5 ml sterile water diluent to make 125 mg/ml"; total volume of available solution will be 8 ml.

Diluent	Vial	Strength	Calculated Volume	Calculated Displacement
7.5 ml	1 g	125 mg	8 ml	0.5 ml

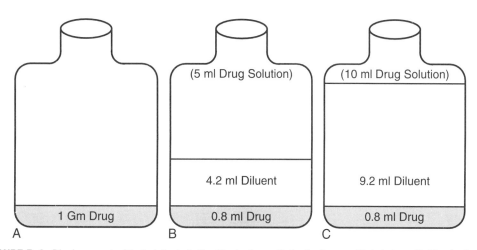

FIGURE 7–4. Displacement of 1 g of drug. *A,* Drug in dry form. *B,* 5 mL of reconstituted drug. *C,* 10 mL of reconstituted drug. (From Cornett, EF, and Blume, DM: Dosages and Solutions: A Programmed Approach to Meds and Math, ed 5. FA Davis, Philadelphia, 1991, p 105, with permission.)

Step 1. Withdraw 7.5 ml of sterile water and inject the sterile water into the vial of medication. The total volume in this vial is now 8 ml, because the powder accounts for a portion of the final volume, in this case, 0.5 ml (7.5 liquid + 0.5 powder = 8 total volume).

Step 2. Shake well. The vial contains 8 ml of medication, and every milliliter contains 125 mg (1/8 of 1 g, or 1000 mg) of medication.

Step 3. Label the vial with the date and time of reconstitution along with the dosage per milliliter. Some facilities require including the initials of the preparer on the label.

Step 4. Calculate the number of milliliters to withdraw to deliver 250 mg (using the formula learned in this chapter). In this case, you would administer 2 ml to deliver 250 mg of medication.

Directions for reconstitution can be found in the product literature and on the vial labels. Directions vary from manufacturer to manufacturer with occasional inconsistencies in the directions. Pharmacists and manufacturers recommend following the directions on the label exactly, even though these inconsistencies exist.

Order

The physician orders 250 mg of a drug.

Available

The powdered form of the drug is packaged in a vial labeled "1 g; add 7.5 ml sterile water diluent to make 125 mg/ml"; total volume of available solution will be 8 ml.

Problem Statement

If, after reconstituting with 7.5 ml of sterile water, 1 ml equals 125 mg (known), then 250 mg will equal how many milliliters (unknown)? How many milliliters will be administered?

(Ordered) Unknown: 250 mg = x
(Label) Known: 125 mg = 1 ml

Formula

$$\text{Ordered Strength} \times \frac{\text{New Units}}{\text{Old Units}} \times \frac{\text{Available Form}}{\text{Available Strength}} = \text{Amount to Give}$$

Known/Unknown

Plug the known and unknown factors into the formula:

$$250 \text{ mg} \times \frac{1 \text{ mg}}{1 \text{ mg}} \times \frac{1 \text{ ml}}{125 \text{ mg}} = x$$

$$\frac{250 \text{ mg}}{1} \times \frac{1 \text{ mg}}{1 \text{ mg}} \times \frac{1 \text{ ml}}{125 \text{ mg}} = \frac{250}{125} = 2 \text{ ml}$$

Answer

To administer 250 mg of a reconstituted drug from a vial labeled "125 mg/ml," *administer (inject) 2 ml of medication.*

DILUTING SOLUTIONS FROM CONCENTRATED LIQUID SOLUTIONS

Solutions are used for irrigations, topical patient treatments, disinfecting surfaces, and sterilizing equipment. Common solutions stocked for medical use include antiseptics such as 70 percent isopropyl alcohol, hydrogen peroxide, and Zephiran Chloride. Disinfectants stocked include 1 : 10 sodium hypochlorite (household bleach) and Cidex. These chemicals are purchased either in concentrated forms or in diluted, ready-to-use, solutions.

If chemicals are ordered in their concentrated form, usually as a very strong (percent) liquid or in the solid form of a powder or tablet (100 percent, pure chemical measured by weight), they must be diluted with water, sterile water, or distilled water before use. Stock solutions are made most easily in 100-ml containers, but pint and gallon containers may also be used.

The strength (concentration) of a solution is stated as a *ratio* or as a *percentage*. Table 7–2 shows the relationships between ratio statements and their percentage equivalents. For instance, a solution stated as either a 1 : 2 or a 50 percent solution contains one part solute (drug) for every two parts of total solution.

The metric system is most often used to express the concentrations of solutions. In the metric system 1 g is considered the weight of 1 ml volume of water. Using the chart, the solute is expressed either as 1 g *dry* drug or 1 ml *liquid* drug dissolved in a volume of solvent (diluent) sufficient to make 100 ml of solution.

The problem to solve, by formula, is how much concentrated liquid will be added to make a certain total quantity of a solution at a needed percentage or ratio. After you solve how much concentrate to add, you then subtract that amount from the total solution. The difference is the amount of solvent to add.

Once again, the same fundamental formula operations are used.

TABLE 7–2. **Solution Concentrations**

Ratio	Percentage Equivalent	Measure of Solvent/Solute	
		Liquid Drug	*Solid Drug*
1 : 1	100	$\dfrac{100 \text{ ml drug}}{100 \text{ ml solution}}$	N/A
1 : 2	50	$\dfrac{50 \text{ ml drug}}{100 \text{ ml solution}}$	$\dfrac{50 \text{ g drug}}{100 \text{ ml solution}}$
1 : 4	25	$\dfrac{25 \text{ ml drug}}{100 \text{ ml solution}}$	$\dfrac{25 \text{ g drug}}{100 \text{ ml solution}}$
1 : 5	20	$\dfrac{20 \text{ ml drug}}{100 \text{ ml solution}}$	$\dfrac{20 \text{ g drug}}{100 \text{ ml solution}}$
1 : 10	10	$\dfrac{10 \text{ ml drug}}{100 \text{ ml solution}}$	$\dfrac{10 \text{ g drug}}{100 \text{ ml solution}}$
1 : 20	5	$\dfrac{5 \text{ ml drug}}{100 \text{ ml solution}}$	$\dfrac{5 \text{ g drug}}{100 \text{ ml solution}}$
1 : 100	1	$\dfrac{1 \text{ ml drug}}{100 \text{ ml solution}}$	$\dfrac{1 \text{ g drug}}{100 \text{ ml solution}}$
1 : 1000	0.1	$\dfrac{0.1 \text{ ml drug}}{100 \text{ ml solution}}$	$\dfrac{0.1 \text{ g drug}}{100 \text{ ml solution}}$
1 : 10,000	0.01	$\dfrac{0.01 \text{ ml drug}}{100 \text{ ml solution}}$	$\dfrac{0.01 \text{ g drug}}{100 \text{ ml solution}}$

N/A = not applicable.

Formula

$$\text{Ordered strength} \times \frac{\text{New Units}}{\text{Old Units}} \times \frac{\text{Available Form}}{\text{Available Strength}} = \text{Amount of chemical to add}$$

Order

Make a 100-ml solution of 1 : 10 chlorine bleach, using household bleach as the solute and water as the solvent.

Problem Statement

If bleach, as purchased, would fill a 100-ml container as a 1 : 1 (100 percent) solution (known), then how much bleach will be required to make a 1 : 10 bleach solution? How many milliliters of bleach and how many milliliters of water (*two* unknowns) are added together?

(Ordered) Unknown:	1 : 10 = x	
(Label) Known:	1 : 1 = 100 ml	
(Table 7–2) Known:	1 : 10 = 10%	

Formula

$$\text{Ordered Strength} \times \frac{\text{New Units}}{\text{Old Units}} \times \frac{\text{Available Form}}{\text{Available Strength}} = \text{Amount of Chemical to add}$$

Known/Unknown

Plug the known and unknown factors into the formula:

$$1 : 10 \times \frac{10\%}{1 : 10} \times \frac{100 \text{ ml}}{100\%} = \text{Amount of bleach to add}$$

Calculation

Multiply:

$$\frac{1 : \cancel{10}}{1} \times \frac{10\%}{1 : \cancel{10}} \times \frac{100 \text{ ml}}{100\%} = \frac{1,000}{100} = 10 \text{ ml bleach}$$

Total solution to make	−	Amount of drug to add	=	Amount of water to add
100 ml	−	10 ml bleach	=	90 ml water

Answer

Measure *10 ml of bleach and 90 ml of water*, and add to an empty 100-ml container.

> *Special Hint: If the container is marked at the 100-ml line, measure and add 10 ml of bleach, then fill with water "quantity sufficient" to reach the 100 ml mark.*

When solving problems of dosage, individuals should work in a quiet area and use a calculator to solve the problem or to double-check a problem worked by hand. For long, difficult calculations, it is safer for two people to solve the same problem independently, and then to check their work with one another.

Patience is important; calculating dosage does not come quickly and shortcuts should never be considered. One last word of advice: Always think about the order and know what problem must be solved. The application of a mathematic solution is only as good as the user's understanding of it.

Written Competency 7–1

Performance Competence: Use the medication labels below to find the following information, with 100 percent accuracy and within ½ hr.

Information to find: A. Generic name

B. Strength

C. Form of the drug

D. Quantity

1. A _____

B _____

C _____

D _____

---

4 mL single-use vial

Heparin Sodium Injection, USP
10,000 Units per ml

584 – 399

EXP 6-30-99

---

2. A _____

B _____

C _____

D _____

---

200 mL (When Mixed)

Keflex®
Cephalexin for Oral Suspension USP
125 mg per 5 ml

**Dista Products Company
Division of Lilly**

EXP 12-31-99

200 mL KEFLEX® CEPHALEXIN FOR ORAL SUSPENSION, USP
125 mg per 5 ml. Oversized bottle provides extra space for shaking. Store in refrigerator. May be kept for 14 days without significant loss of potency. Keep tightly closed. Discard unused portion after 14 days.
Shake well before using.
Control # 111-11-1111

Usual Children's Dose 25 to 50 mg per kg a day in four divided doses. For more severe infections, dose may be doubled. See literature.
Contains Cephalexin Monohydrate equivalent to 5 g Cephalexin in a powdered form.
Prior to mixing, Store at Controlled Room Temperature 59° to 86° F (15° to 30°C)
Directions for Mixing—Add 100 ml of water in two portions to the dry mixture in the bottle. Shake well after each addition.
Each 5 ml (approximately one teaspoonful will then contain: Cephalexin Monohydrate equivalent to 125 mg Cephalexin.
Date prepared _____ time _____ init.

---

3. A _____

B _____

C _____

D _____

```
5 mL DOSSETTE®Vial

LIDOCAINE
HCl Injection, USP

    2 %

(20 mg/mL)
```

584 – 399   EXP 6-30-99

4. A_____

   B_____

   C_____

   D_____

```
Dilantin®
(Phenytoin Sodium Capsules, USP)
diphenylhydantoin
30 mg

100 capsules
PARKE-DAVIS
```

584 – 399   EXP 6-30-99

5. A_____

   B_____

   C_____

   D_____

```
Dilantin®   100 mg
(Phenytoin Sodium Capsules, USP)
diphenylhydantoin


100 capsules
```

6. A_____

   B_____

   C_____

   D_____

```
                5 ml  single-dose vial

Dilantin®
(Phenytoin Sodium Injection, USP)
diphenylhydantoin
50 mg/ml
```

7. A_____

   B_____

   C_____

   D_____

---

20 ml multi-dose vial

Dilantin®
(Phenytoin Sodium Injection, USP)
diphenylhydantoin
50 mg/ml

---

8. A_____

   B_____

   C_____

   D_____

Shake well before using.
Control # 111-11-1111

Strength _____

Date Prepared _____

Time _____   Init. _____

Geopen®
Carbenicillin disodium
Sterile
equivalent to
2 g of Carbenicillin

For IM Use

Roerig – Pfizer, Inc.

EXP 12-31-99

DIRECTIONS
IM Use:
Reconstitute with at least 4 ml of Sterile Water for Injection in order to facilitate reconstitution, up to 7.2 ml of Sterile Water for Injection can be used.

Amount Of Diluent To Be Added To The 2 G Vial	Volume To Be Withdrawn For A 1 G Dose
4.0 ml	2.5 ml
5.0 ml	3.0 ml
7.2 ml	4.0 ml

For dosage information, read accompanying professional information.
After reconstitution, discard any unused portion after 24 hours (if stored at room temperature) or after 72 hours (if refrigerated).
Store dry powder below 25° C.

---

9. Using the labels above, what is the expiration date for
   A. Lidocaine _____
   B. Heparin sodium _____
   C. Keflex _____
   D. Geopen _____

10. Using the labels above, name the manufacturere of
   A. Dilantin _____
   B. Geopen _____
   C. Keflex _____

Score: _____

See Appendix B for answers.

Written Competency 7–2

Performance Competence: Use the medication labels below to answer questions 1–10, with 100 percent accuracy and within 30 minutes.

Time _____ Date Prepared _____ Strength _____ Shake well before using. Control # 111-11-1111 Init. _____	**Geopen®** **Carbenicillin disodium** **Sterile** equivalent to **2 g of Carbenicillin** **For IM Use** **Roerig – Pfizer, Inc.** EXP 12-31-99

DIRECTIONS
IM Use:
Reconstitute with at least 4 ml of Sterile Water for Injection in order to facilitate reconstitution, up to 7.2 ml of Sterile Water for Injection can be used.

Amount Of Diluent To Be Added To The 2 G Vial	Volume To Be Withdrawn For A 1 G Dose
4.0 ml	2.5 ml
5.0 ml	3.0 ml
7.2 ml	4.0 ml

For dosage information, read accompanying professional information.
After reconstitution, discard any unused portion after 24 hours (if stored at room temperature) or after 72 hours (if refrigerated).
Store dry powder below 25° C.

1. If the vial is reconstituted with 4.0-ml sterile water, what amount is used for an IM injection of 1 gram of Geopen? _____

2. How much diluent is added to deliver 1 g of Geopen in 3.0 ml? _____

3. After reconstituting Geopen, what is the refrigeration shelf life? _____

4. Geopen is reconstituted with 7.2-ml diluent. What is the strength of Geopen per ml? _____

200 mL KEFLEX® CEPHALEXIN FOR ORAL SUSPENSION, USP 125 mg per 5 ml. Oversized bottle provides extra space for shaking. Store in refrigerator. May be kept for 14 days without significant loss of potency. Keep tightly closed. Discard unused portion after 14 days. Shake well before using. Control # 111-11-1111	**200 mL (When Mixed)** **Keflex®** **Cephalexin for** **Oral Suspension USP** **125 mg per 5 ml** **Dista Products Company** **Division of Lilly** EXP 12-31-99	Usual Children's Dose 25 to 50 mg per kg a day in four divided doses. For more severe infections, dose may be doubled. See literature. Contains Cephalexin Monohydrate equivalent to 5 g Cephalexin in a powdered form. Prior to mixing, Store at Controlled Room Temperature 59° to 86° F (15° to 30°C) Directions for Mixing—Add 200 ml of water in two 100-ml portions to the dry mixture in the bottle. Shake well after each addition. Each 5 ml (approximately one teaspoonful will then contain: Cephalexin Monohydrate equivalent to 125 mg Cephalexin.

5. How much water is added to Keflex oral suspension to deliver 125 mg/5ml? _____

6. At what times do you mix the Keflex suspension during its reconstitution? _____

7. What is the storage requirement for Keflex in its powdered form? _____

8. After reconstituting Keflex, what is the refrigeration shelf life? _____

9. After reconstituting Keflex, how much Keflex is in each teaspoonful? _____

10. How many times per day is Keflex usually administered to children? _____

Score: _____

See Appendix B for answers.

Written Competency 7–3

Performance Competence: Calculate nonparenteral medication orders for liquids and tablets to be administered orally, with 100 percent accuracy and within 1 hour. The step-by-step process described in this chapter must be used. Show each step of your work on separate sheets of paper. Do not give yourself credit for partial or incorrect answers.

1. Order: Acetaminophen (Cherry) Elixir, *USP*
               120 mg stat
   Label: Acetaminophen (Cherry) Elixir, *USP*
               120 mg per 5 ml in a 120-ml bottle
   Administer: _____

2. Order: Acetaminophen (Cherry) Elixir, *USP*
               180 mg stat
   Label: Acetaminophen (Cherry) Elixir, *USP*
               120 mg per 5 ml in a 120-ml bottle
   Administer: _____

3. Order: Acetaminophen (Cherry) Elixir, *USP*
               60 mg stat
   Label: Acetaminophen (Cherry) Elixir, *USP*
               120 mg per dropperful
   Administer: _____

4. Order: Phenobarbital 15 mg
   Label: Phenobarbital Elixir 20 mg/5 ml
   Administer: _____

5. Order: Pen-Vee K 500,000 units
   Label: Pen-Vee K 250 mg (400,000 U) per 5 ml in a 100-ml bottle
   Give: _____ ml or _____ tsp

6. Order: Paregoric 4 fluid drams stat
   Equipment: 5-ml dropper
   Give: _____ ml or _____ tsp or _____ droppersful

7. Order: Digoxin Elixir Pediatric 0.25 mg
   Label: Digoxin Elixir 50 mcg per ml in a 60-ml bottle
   Give: _____

8. Order: Amoxil Oral Suspension for a 1-year-old child weighing 26 lb, normal height
   Label: Amoxil Oral Suspension 125 mg per 5 ml
               Directions: Adult dose 250 mg q8h; for children under 20 kg, 20 mg/kg/day q8h
   Give: _____

9. Order: Demerol 25 mg
   Label: Demerol 50-mg scored tablets
   Administer: _____

10. Order: Gantrisin 500 mg PO q4h
    Label: Gantrisin 0.5-g tablets
    Administer: _____

11. Order: Erythrocin Stearate 0.75 g
    Label: Erythrocin Stearate 250-mg tablets
    Give: _____

12. Order: Lanoxin 1/250 gr
    Label: Lanoxin 250 mcg (0.25 mg) scored
    Administer: _____

13. Order: Lanoxin 0.75 mg
    Label: Lanoxin 250 mcg (0.25 mg) scored
    Administer: _____

14. Order: Lanoxin 0.125 mg
    Label: Lanoxin 250 mcg (0.25 mg) scored
    Administer: _____

15. Order: Tylenol with Codeine 30 mg
    Label: Tylenol with Codeine tablets: 7.5 mg (No. 1), 15 mg (No. 2), and 60 mg (No. 4)
    Give: _____
    Use tablet strength No. _____

16. Order: Phenobarbital 1/4 gr
    Label: Phenobarbital 15-mg tablets
    Administer: _____

17. Order: Phenobarbital 3/4 gr
    Label: Phenobarbital 30- and 100-mg tablets
    Administer: _____

18. Order: Ferrous Sulfate 15 gr
    Label: Ferrous Sulfate 300-mg tablets
    Administer: _____

19. Order: Aspirin 600 mg
    Label: Aspirin 5 gr per tablet
    Administer: _____

20. Order: Cortone 12.5 mg qid for 9-year-old weighing 65 lb, height 3 ft 10 in
    Label: Cortone 25 mg scored tabs.
                Directions: Adults: Up to 300 mg per day.
    Administer: _____

Score: _____

Incomplete calculations must be corrected using separate worksheets before completing Written Competency 7–4.

See Appendix B for answers.

Written Competency 7–4

Performance Competence: Calculate parenteral medication orders for injection, with 100 percent accuracy within 1 hour. The step-by-step process described in this chapter must be used. Show each step of your work on separate sheets of paper. Do not give yourself credit for partial or incorrect answers.

1. Order: Heparin 800 units subcutaneously (SC)

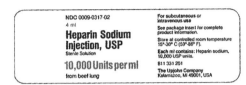

   Give: _____

   Use syringe type: _____

2. Order: Heparin 5000 units SC
   Label: Heparin 10,000 units per ml (4 ml) (see label above)
   Give: _____

3. Order: Tigan 250 mg intramuscularly (IM)

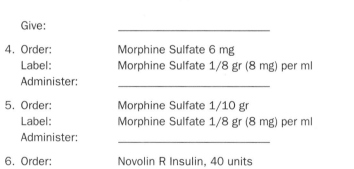

   Give: _____

4. Order: Morphine Sulfate 6 mg
   Label: Morphine Sulfate 1/8 gr (8 mg) per ml
   Administer: _____

5. Order: Morphine Sulfate 1/10 gr
   Label: Morphine Sulfate 1/8 gr (8 mg) per ml
   Administer: _____

6. Order: Novolin R Insulin, 40 units

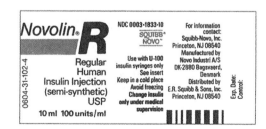

   Using the diagram, choose the correct syringe and shade in the amount of insulin to withdraw for administration:

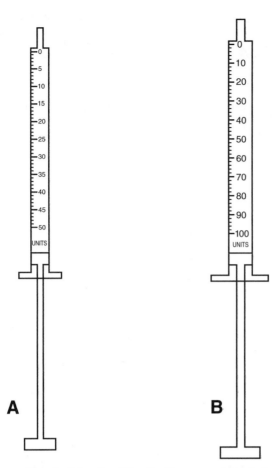

A
B

7. Order: Novolin R Insulin, 60 units (See preceding label)

Using the diagram, choose the correct syringe and shade in the amount of insulin to withdraw for administration:

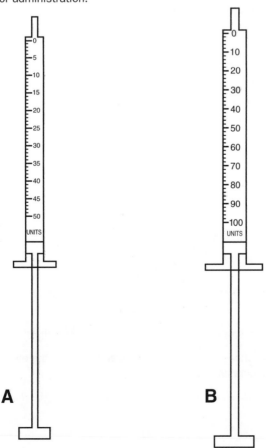

A
B

8. Order: Novolin R Insulin, 80 units (See preceding label)

   Using this diagram, choose the correct syringe and shade in the amount of insulin to withdraw for administration:

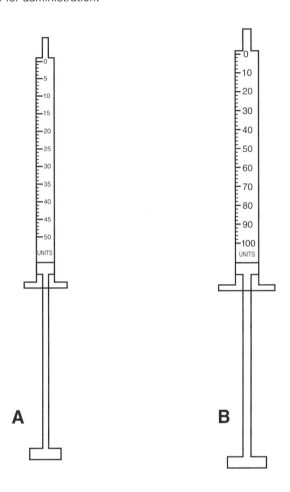

9. Order: Epinephrine 0.2 mg SC stat

   The patient weighs 44 lb and is of normal height.

> 1 mL ampule
>
> **epinephrine HCl**
>
> **1 : 1000**
>
> **contains 1 mg epinephrine as the hydrochloride in each 1 mL**

Administer: _____

   Using the microgram per kilogram method, compare the dosage ordered with the recommended dosage stated on the label directions:

   Label directions: For bronchial asthma give 10 mcg per kg or 300 mcg per m^2 BSA to a maximum of 500 mcg SC.

   Microgram per kilogram recommended dosage: _____

   Using the BSA guideline in the foregoing directions, what is the recommended dosage?

   _____

Make a statement comparing the physician's order with the microgram per kilogram and BSA guidelines:

_____

10. Order: Kefzol 360 mg

    Label: Kefzol 1 gm; reconstitute by adding 2 ml sterile water to make the solution

    Administer: _____

Time   Date Prepared   Strength   Shake well before using. Control # 111-11-1111   Init.

Kefzol®

Cefazolin sodium, USP

Sterile

equivalent to

1 g of Cefazolin sodium

For IM or IV Use

EXP 12-31-99

DIRECTIONS

IM Use:

Reconstitute with at least 2 ml of Sterile Water for Injection in order to facilitate reconstitution, up to 4.0 ml of Sterile Water for Injection can be used.

Amount Of Diluent To Be Added To The 2 G Vial	Volume To Be Withdrawn For A 1 G Dose
2.0 ml	2.0 ml
4.0 ml	4.0 ml

For dosage information, read accompanying professional information.

After reconstitution, discard any unused portion after 24 hours (if stored at room temperature) or after 72 hours (if refrigerated).

Store dry powder below 25°C.

---

11. Order: Penicillin G potassium 50,000 units IM

    Label: Penicillin G potassium 1,000,000 units in dry form

    Label directions: Reconstitute 1,000,000 units as follows:

Diluent	Units per Milliliter
20.0 ml	50,000
10.0 ml	100,000
4.0 ml	250,000
1.8 ml	500,000

Using this syringe, shade in the amount to give:

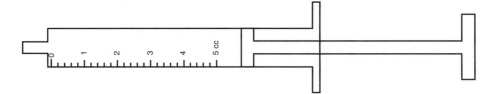

12. Order: Penicillin G 200,000 units, newborn q6h

    Label: Penicillin G 1,000,000 units dry

    Directions: Newborns 500,000 to 1,000,000 per day

    Label directions: Reconstitute 1,000,000 units as follows:

Diluent	Units per Milliliter
20.0 ml	50,000
10.0 ml	100,000
4.0 ml	250,000
1.8 ml	500,000

Using this syringe, shade in the amount to give:

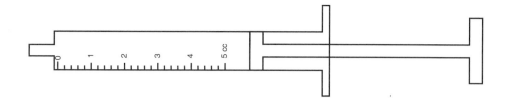

13. Order: Penicillin G potassium 2,400,000 units
    Label: Penicillin G potassium 5,000,000 units dry
    Label directions: Reconstitute 5,000,000 units as follows:

Diluent	Units per Milliliter
18.2 ml	250,000
8.2 ml	500,000
3.2 ml	1,000,000

    Administer: _____

14. Order: Bicillin L-A 2,000,000 units for an adult weighing 186 lb
    Label: Bicillin L-A cartridges labeled: 600,000 units per ml; 1,200,000 units per
                          2.0 ml; 2,400,000 units per 4.0 ml
    Give: _____
    Use cartridge strength: _____
    How would you prepare the cartridge? _____

15. Order: Rocephin reconstituted with 1 percent lidocaine (without epinephrine) IM,
                          first dose for a child weighing 44 lb and of normal height
    Label: Rocephin vials: 0.25 g, 0.5 g, 1 g, 2 g; 50 mg per kg per day, in two di-
                          vided doses q12h.
                          Combine diluent and powder in ratio of 0.9 ml per 0.25 g.
    Use vial strength: _____
    Give: _____

16. Order: M-M-R II Vaccine scheduled for 15 patients
    Label: M-M-R II Vaccine 0.5 ml per dose (5 ml)
    How many vials will you need? _____

17. Order: Heptavax-B 40 mcg and Hepatitis B Immune Globulin for an adult weigh-
                          ing 132 lb
    Labels: Heptavax-B 20 mcg per ml and Hepatitis B Immune Globulin 0.06 ml per kg
    Give: _____ and _____

18. Order: Atropine 1000 mcg
    Give: _____

---

4 mL single-use vial

**Atropine Sulfate
Injection, USP
400 mcg per ml**

584 – 399   EXP 6-30-99

19. Order: Cyanocobalamin 2000 mcg

10 mL single-use vial	
Cyanocobalamin **vitamin b$_{12}$ for injection** **1,000 mcg per ml**	584 – 399 EXP 6-30-99

Give: _____

20. Order: Hydroxyzine HCl 40 mg

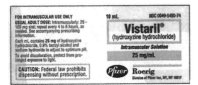 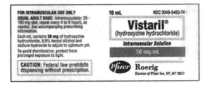

Use vial strength: _____
Give: _____

Score: _____

Incomplete calculations must be corrected using separate worksheets before completing Procedure 7–1.

See Appendix B for answers.

Terminal Performance Objective/Competency

Procedure 7–1: Measure Precalculated Dosages for Administration

EQUIPMENT Answers and work from Written Competencies 7–3 and 7–4
Syringe diagrams provided in this procedure

Performance Competence: Mark each syringe to the correct dosage calculated in Written Competency 7–3 with 100 percent accuracy and within reasonable job production time needed to withdraw medication into a syringe, as stated by your evaluator.

	V	S	U*

1. (See Written Competency 7–4, question 14.)
    Order: Bicillin L-A 2,000,000 units for an adult weighing
                  186 lb
    Performance: Using the following prefilled cartridge, mark to
                  where you will eject the Bicillin before proceeding
                  with the injection.

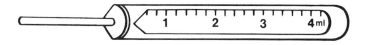

2. (See Written Competency 7–4, question 1.)
    Order: Heparin 800 units
    Performance: Mark the correct amount on the syringe.

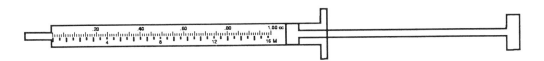

3. (See Written Competency 7–4; question 1.)
    Order: Heparin 5000 units
    Performance: Mark the correct amount on the syringe.

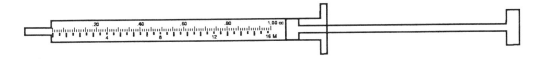

---

*V = Value, to be filled in if assigning points or other specific values to each performance.
 S = Satisfactory completion of the performance.
 U = Unsatisfactory completion of the performance, or performance incomplete; needs more practice.

4.   (See Written Competency 7–4, question 13.)
       Order: Penicillin G potassium 2,400,000 units   □ □ □
       Performance: Mark the correct amount on the syringe.

5.   (See Written Competency 7–4, question 10.)
       Order: Kefzol 360 mg   □ □ □
       Performance: Mark the correct amount on the syringe.

6.   (See Written Competency 7–4, question 16.)
       Order: M-M-R II Vaccine   □ □ □
       Performance: Mark the correct amount on the syringe.

7. and 8. (See Written Competency 7–4, question 17.)
       Order: Heptavax-B 40 mcg   □ □ □
                    Hepatitis B immune globulin   □ □ □
       Performance: Mark the correct amounts on the correct syringes.

9.   (See Written Competency 7–4, question 3.)
        Order: Tigan 250 mg IM
        Performance: Mark the correct amount on the syringe.

10.   (See Written Competency 7–4, question 15.)
        Order: Rocephin reconstituted with 1 percent lidocaine
        Performance: Mark the correct amount on the syringe.

Number Correct: _____

Incorrect Performance No(s).: _____

Incomplete measurements must be corrected before completing this chapter.

See Appendix B for answers.

Date: _____ Competency achieved: Y _____ N _____

Designated reasonable time standard: _____

Actual completion time: _____

Assignment 7–1: Use Appendix A, the *PDR*, or Other Reference to Create Drug Information Guides

EQUIPMENT   Appendix A; *PDR;* or other drug reference
Lined notepaper or index cards
Drugs: From Top 50 Most Commonly Prescribed, those ranked 31st–40th.

Performance Competence: Complete a drug guide for each of the drugs listed under Equipment. The ten guides should be completed with 100 percent accuracy and must include the following:

Generic name _____

Brand name _____

Classification _____

Controlled substance classification _____

Pregnancy risk category _____

Action _____

Indications/use _____

Contraindications _____

Adverse reactions/side effects _____

Dosage/Route _____

Patient education (in terms the patient will understand) _____

Special alert _____

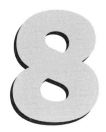

Routes of Administration and Injection Techniques

TERMINAL PERFORMANCE OBJECTIVE/COMPETENCY (PROCEDURE 8–4): Administer a Subcutaneous Injection, Deltoid Region

TERMINAL PERFORMANCE OBJECTIVE/COMPETENCY (PROCEDURE 8–5): Administer an Intramuscular Injection, Vastus Lateralis Region

TERMINAL PERFORMANCE OBJECTIVE/COMPETENCY (PROCEDURE 8–6): Administer a Z-Tract Intramuscular Injection, Ventrogluteal Region

TERMINAL PERFORMANCE OBJECTIVE/COMPETENCY (PROCEDURE 8–7): Administer a Tuberculin Test

ASSIGNMENT 8–1: Use Appendix A, the *PDR,* or Other Reference to Create Drug Information Guides

OBJECTIVES　　**WRITTEN COMPETENCY 8–1:** Select correct routes and techniques for frequently administered medications.

TERMINAL PERFORMANCE OBJECTIVE (PROCEDURE 8–1): Teach a patient to use a nebulizer.

TERMINAL PERFORMANCE OBJECTIVE (PROCEDURE 8–2): Prepare and administer an eye medication.

TERMINAL PERFORMANCE OBJECTIVE (PROCEDURE 8–3): Prepare a medication for injection.

TERMINAL PERFORMANCE OBJECTIVE (PROCEDURE 8–4): Administer a subcutaneous injection, deltoid region.

TERMINAL PERFORMANCE OBJECTIVE (PROCEDURE 8–5): Administer an intramuscular injection, vastus lateralis region.

TERMINAL PERFORMANCE OBJECTIVE (PROCEDURE 8–6): Administer a Z-tract intramuscular injection, ventrogluteal region.

TERMINAL PERFORMANCE OBJECTIVE (PROCEDURE 8–7): Administer a tuberculin test.

As well as being classified according to their effects, drugs are also classified according to their routes of administration. Drug administration routes can be defined as the methods by which drugs are delivered into the body. In this chapter, drug classification focuses on the methods of administration and the patient care and teaching opportunities related to each method.

Chapter 5 pointed out that patient safety starts with the "three checks" and the "seven rights." Before beginning this chapter, it is important to review these two procedures of safe conduct. The "three checks" refers to the practice of checking every medication against the physician's order three times: (1) as you take the medication from the shelf, (2) as you prepare the medication, and (3) as you return the medication to the shelf. The "seven rights" means that each drug administered must be correct in the following: right patient, drug, route of administration, dosage amount, timing, technique, and documentation (recording of the administration).

This chapter will concentrate on the *right routes* and *right techniques* for administering medications. The chapter is divided into discussions on three important concepts for each of the routes and techniques discussed:

- The manner in which a drug is absorbed
- Patient safety during administration
- The opportunities for patient teaching related to administration safety and absorption

Pharmacokinetics

Pharmacokinetics is the study of the movement of drugs in the body, including the processes of absorption, distribution, localization in the tissues, metabolism, and excretion. It is the process by which a drug is handled by the body, from the time it is transported from the site of administration until the body inactivates it and removes all traces of it from the system.

ABSORPTION AND DISTRIBUTION

Absorption is the process of passage of liquids or other chemical substances through a surface of the body into the circulating body fluids and tissues. *Distribution* is the way free drugs are transported by circulating fluids to their tissue sites of action, metabolism, and excretion or to storage sites (e.g., fat tissue or liver). *Localization* occurs when a drug arrives at its intended tissue site and then reaches a critical, or threshold, concentration so that the drug's action can begin producing the desired effects. Drugs are then *metabolized*—that is, they are biotransformed by the liver, kidneys, and blood plasma. Biotransformation is a series of chemical alterations that breaks drugs down into active parts. *Excretion* is the body's process of eliminating drugs from the body. This is accomplished primarily by the kidneys but can also occur through saliva, bile, breast milk, sweat glands, and respiration. Drugs that are not absorbed by the body are eliminated by the bowel.

With few exceptions, drugs are ultimately intended to reach the bloodstream. Drugs then circulate to particular areas of the body where they will be distributed to the tissues and produce their effects. *Bioavailability* is the rate and intent to which an active drug or metabolite enters the general circulation, thereby providing access to the site of action, called the *target organ*. The rate at which a drug is absorbed is determined by two factors:

1. *Where* in the body the drug is deposited (route) for absorption
2. The *time* in which a particular dosage form (see Chapter 3) can break down to be absorbed

The route chosen for administration of a drug plays an important role in pharmacokinetics. The route of administration determines a drug's *onset* (how quickly a drug will take its first effect) and with what *intensity* a drug will begin acting on the body. The route of administration, along with the dosage form being used (e.g., slow-acting, time-release forms), also determines a drug's *duration*—that is, how long a drug will be effective in the tissues before it is metabolized. Finally, the route determines the *excretion rate* (how long a drug takes to be eliminated by the body).

The faster a drug is absorbed into the bloodstream, the more rapid its onset; and the faster the distribution to the body tissues, the more intense its initial effect and usually the shorter its duration. Conversely, the more slowly a drug is absorbed into the bloodstream, the longer its onset, the less intense its effect, and the longer its duration. For example, oral drugs usually reach therapeutic levels within 30 minutes to an hour; injectable drugs, within a few minutes to 20 minutes; and drugs administered via inhalation and intravenously, within seconds. Most drugs reach peak levels in 1–4 hours and last for 4–8 hours.

The presence of a drug in the bloodstream does not necessarily produce a therapeutic effect. For effect, drugs must reach the cellular fluids that bathe the tissues. Drugs must ultimately pass from the site of absorption to the circulating fluids (bloodstream) to the extravascular fluid compartment, and from there into the cells of other body tissues, including the brain tissues. Tissues that naturally receive a large blood supply—such as the heart, brain, liver, and kidneys—are also the first to receive large concentrations of drugs from the bloodstream. Tissues that receive less blood per unit of time—muscle, fat, and bone—accumulate drugs later and in lesser quantities.

Not all drugs can gain access to brain tissues, however. The tissues of the brain have a functional barrier called the *blood–brain barrier*. This barrier blocks out certain compounds that have a high molecular weight or are poorly soluble in fat. Antibiotics are among the drugs that do not effectively penetrate the blood–brain barrier. General anesthesia is able to pass the blood–brain barrier immediately and produces sleep within seconds. Barbiturate sedatives, such as phenobarbital, on the other hand, pass the blood–brain barrier less effectively, and can produce the same amount of sleep only after 30 to 45 minutes.

THERAPEUTIC DRUG LEVEL MONITORING

Bioavailability is determined either by measurement of the concentration of a drug in body fluids or by the magnitude of the patient's response to a drug. Therefore, blood levels of drugs may be used to monitor the achievement or nonachievement of an intended drug therapy (Table 8–1). Determining therapeutic levels of prescribed drugs is especially important for drugs with narrow therapeutic ranges (see Chapter 7) or serious toxic effects. At the time of the initiation of drug administration, serial blood samples may be drawn to determine *peak* (highest) and *trough* (lowest) blood levels of drugs. Peak samples are drawn 30 to 60 minutes after drug administration. Trough levels are drawn immediately before the next dose of the medication is given.

For patients who are taking medications over long periods of time, drug level samples may be required periodically, not only to determine that the dosage prescribed is correct but also to evaluate the patient's degree of compliance with the dosage schedule or accidental overdosing by the patient. Therapeutic drug sampling may be required daily, weekly, or monthly. Blood level screening also may be performed to screen for drug misuse or abuse or to determine levels of toxic substances in the body from environmental exposures or poisoning.

LOCALIZATION

Scientists are still trying to solve the mystery of exactly how drugs produce their effects, as their exact mechanisms are not yet well understood. There are several theories as to how drugs work once localized in the tissues. One is the *receptor theory*. Cells are believed to contain receptive sites on the cell surface or within the cell itself. These receptor sites can be seen as locks that have a specific affinity for specific chemicals shaped to fit into them just as a key would fit into a lock. When a foreign chemical "key" fits into a cellular "lock," the drug is able to set off a chain of effects that leads to increased cellular activity. The cell is the *receptor* and the drug, the *agonist*.

Although current thinking centers on the receptor theory, two other theories exist—the *drug–enzyme interaction theory* and the *physiochemical activity theory*. The drug–enzyme theory suggests that key–lock affinities between drugs and enzymes exist just as they do in receptor-agonist interactions. Enzymes are proteins that bring about all the chemical reactions in the living cell. In drug–enzyme interactions, it is thought that drugs either increase or inhibit enzyme activity rather than receptor activity. The physiochemical activity theory speculates that drugs alter cellular activity by affecting the physical condition of the cell rather than its biochemical processes. Whichever theory predominates, all three are probably correct in certain instances.

METABOLISM AND EXCRETION OF DRUGS

After distribution, use, and some storage by the tissues, drugs are then metabolized for excretion. During metabolism, drugs are converted into harmless substances. This metabolism is known as *biotransformation*. Biotransformation usually results in the formation of new chemicals that are less active than the drug administered and more easily eliminated by the kidneys. It should be noted, however, that drug metabolism sometimes produces new chemicals that are toxic to the patient or cause adverse effects. Occasionally, a drug is administered in an inactive form and then becomes pharmacologically active *after* metabolism. This type of drug is called a *metabolite*.

The liver is largely responsible for the metabolism of drugs. It breaks down active drug molecules into inactive fragments that can be excreted by the kidneys. People differ widely in their ability to metabolize drugs, and effective metabolism depends on the patient's age,

TABLE 8–1. **Blood Levels of Drugs**

Drug	Peak Time	Duration of Action	Therapeutic Level	Toxic Level
Antibiotics				
Amikacin	IM*: 1/2 hr			
	IV†: 15 min	2 days	20–25 μg/ml	35 μg/ml
Gentamicin	IM: 1/2 hr	2 days	4–8 μg/ml	12 μg/ml
	IV: 15 min			
Kanamycin	1/2 hr	2 days	20–25 μg/ml	35 μg/ml
Streptomycin	1/2–1 1/2 hr	5 days	25–30 μg/ml	>30 μg/ml
Tobramycin	IV: 15 min	2 days	2–8 μg/ml	12 μg/ml
Anticonvulsants				
Barbiturates and barbiturate-related				
Amobarbital	IV: 30 sec	10–20 hr	7 μg/ml	30 μg/ml
Pentobarbital	IV: 30 sec	15 hr	4 μg/ml	15 μg/ml
Phenobarbital	15 min	80 hr	10 μg/ml	>55 μg/ml
Primidone	PO‡: 3 hr	7–14 hr	1 μg/ml	>10 μg/ml
Benzodiazepines				
Clonazepam (Clonopin)	1–4 hr	60 hr	5–70 ng/ml	>70 ng/ml
Diazepam (Valium)	1–4 hr	1–2 days	5–70 ng/ml	>70 ng/ml
Hydantoins				
Phenytoin (Dilantin)	3–12 hr	7–42 hr	10–20 μg/ml	>20 μg/ml
Succinimides				
Ethosuximide (Zarontin)	1 hr	8 days	40–80 μg/ml	100 μg/ml
Miscellaneous				
Carbamazepine (Tegretol)	4 hr	2 days	2–10 μg/ml	12 μg/ml
Bronchodilators				
Aminophylline/theophylline	PO: 2 hr	8–9 hr	10–18 μg/ml	>20 μg/ml
	IV: 15 min			
Cardiac drugs				
Disopyramide (Norpace)	PO: 2 hr	25–30 hr	2–4.5 μg/ml	>9 μg/ml
Quinidine	PO: 1 hr	20–30 hr	2.4–5 μg/ml	>6 μg/ml
	IV: immediate			
Procainamide (Pronestyl)	PO: 1 hr	10–20 hr	4–8 μg/ml	>12 μg/ml
	IV: 1/2 hr			
NAPA (*N*-acetyl-procainamide, a procainamide metabolite)	—	—	2–8 μg/ml	>30 μg/ml
Lidocaine	IV: immediate	5–10 hr	2–6 μg/ml	>9 μg/ml
Bretylium	15–30 min	6–8 hr	5–10 mg/kg	30 mg/kg
Verapamil	PO: 5 hrs	8–10 hr	5–10 mg/kg	>15 mg/kg
	IV: 3–5 min	IV: 1/2–1 hr		
Diltiazem	PO: 2–3 hr	3–4 hr	50–200 ng/ml	>200 ng/ml
Nifedipine	1–3 hr	3–4 hr	5–10 mg	90 mg
Digitoxin	4 hr	30 days	5–30 ng/ml	30 ng/ml
Digoxin	2 hr	7 days	0.5–2 ng/ml	>2.5 ng/ml
Phenytoin (Dilantin)	PO: 2 hr	96 hr	10–18 μg/ml	>20 μg/ml
	IV: 1 hr			
Salicylates				
Aspirin	15 min	12–30 hr	20 μg/ml	
			2–30 mg/dl	40 mg/dl
Narcotics				
Codeine	—	—	—	>0.005 mg/dl
Hydromorphone (Dilaudid)	—	—	—	>0.1 mg/dl
Methadone	—	—	—	>0.2 mg/dl
Meperidine (Demerol)	—	—	—	>0.5 mg/dl
Morphine	—	—	—	>0.005 mg/dl

Table continued on following page

TABLE 8–1. **Blood Levels of Drugs** (*Continued*)

Drug	Peak Time	Duration of Action	Therapeutic Level	Toxic Level
Barbiturates				
Phenobarbital	—	—	10 μg/ml	55 μg/ml
Amobarbital	—	—	7 μg/ml	30 μg/ml
Pentobarbital	—	—	4 μg/ml	15 μg/ml
Secobarbital	—	—	3 μg/ml	10 μg/ml
Alcohols				
Ethanol	—	—	—	100 mg/dl
Methanol	—	—	—	20 mg/dl
Miscellaneous				
Acetaminophen	—	—	—	>150 μg/ml 4 hr after ingestion
Phenothiazines	—	—	0.5 μg/ml	1.0 μg/ml

*IM = Intramuscular.
†IV = Intravenous.
‡PO = By mouth.
From Cella, JH, and Watson, J: Nurses Manual of Laboratory Tests. FA Davis, Philadelphia, 1989, pp 283–284.

the presence of liver or kidney disease, the presence of other drugs, and the condition of the patient's cardiovascular functioning and cardiac output.

Among all the routes through which the body excretes drugs, the kidneys play the largest role in drug elimination. The kidneys first filter the broken-down products of drugs. Some drugs are transported directly from the bloodstream into renal tubular fluids where they are excreted, while others undergo tubular reabsorption back into the blood plasma through the membranes of the kidneys. Drugs that are filtered and secreted by the renal tubules without undergoing reabsorption are rapidly eliminated. Most drugs, however, undergo the process of reabsorption and drug excretion is therefore delayed.

The time it takes for a drug to reach and maintain peak levels depends on its rate of elimination. The time it takes for a specific amount of drug in the body to decrease to one-half of the peak previously attained is called a drug's *half-life*. Because penicillin is rapidly excreted by the kidneys, it has a short half-life. Anticoagulants, on the other hand, remain in circulation for a long period of time and have a relatively long half-life. Knowing a drug's half-life makes it possible to calculate dosage schedules not only for patients with normal body functions but also for those with impaired excretory functions.

When it is important to provide peak concentrations of a drug immediately, an initial dose may exceed the body's ability to eliminate it. This is called a *loading dose*. After a peak level is reached, subsequent doses are reduced to the usual daily dose, called the *maintenance dose*. As loading doses are potentially dangerous, patients receiving such a dose must be closely monitored. Occasionally a patient may be given a *megadose*, which is one large loading dose without any further maintenance doses. The biggest danger with "megadosing," of course, is an unsuspected allergic reaction to the medication.

In general, drugs can be said to have either a *systemic effect* or a *local effect*. Systemic drugs may affect the body as a whole, such as muscle relaxant or a general anesthetic, or they may take their action at a specific site (usually other than the site administered), such as a urinary antiseptic or a heart medication. Local drugs, on the other hand, affect the body in one area or part (usually at the site of administration), such as a local anesthetic or an eye medication.

Unfortunately, there are too many exceptions to classifying drugs as either systemic or local. Many systemic drugs are prescribed for one local problem area (e.g., oral medications for athlete's feet), and many local drugs will eventually be absorbed into systemic circulation. It is more specific to classify drugs by their sites of absorption (routes): (1) oral, (2) mucous membrane, (3) topical, and (4) parenteral (literally "beside the digestive tract" and used generally to describe injectable medications).

Oral Administration

Most drugs are manufactured for oral administration, even if they are also manufactured in other dosage forms such as for injection. Drugs that are not available in oral forms must be manufactured for injection because they are inactivated either by gastric secretions or certain food products, or because they are not able to be absorbed adequately through the intestinal mucosa. Oral administration is preferred whenever possible because it is convenient and easy for the patient, as well as being safer, comparatively less expensive, and less painful than by injection.

ABSORPTION

Oral drugs are usually absorbed in the small intestine, although some, such as aspirin and alcohol, begin early absorption in the stomach. Drugs that are absorbed early by the stomach tend to be irritating to the stomach, and for this reason many are specially coated to keep them intact until they pass through the stomach and into the small intestine. During this process, not all of a drug may be absorbed by the small intestine; therefore, oral drugs often must be given in higher doses than drugs administered by injection.

Once absorbed, oral drugs are carried by the bloodstream to the liver, where they are mostly metabolized or broken down and sometimes stored. This is called *first-pass effect*. This is the effect that sometimes makes it necessary to give oral drugs in higher doses than the same drug given by injection. After filtration by the liver, drugs are then carried by the bloodstream for distribution to the intended cells, tissues, or organs.

Most drugs should be taken on an empty stomach; the best times are 1 hour before or 2 hours after meals. An empty stomach allows a drug to be absorbed more rapidly and ensures that food products will not chemically alter the drug and render it less effective. For example, tetracycline chemically binds with calcium and is altered so that it cannot be absorbed in large enough quantities to be effective against infection. For this reason, tetracyclines should not be administered with milk or dairy products or with antacids containing calcium (Table 8–2).

For drugs that are known to be irritating to the stomach, it may be best to take these medications *with food*. Irritating drugs may be administered with crackers, a snack, milk, or meals. The decision to take a medication with food, however, depends on the manufacturer's recommendation, the physician's advice, and whether or not the medication is wrapped in a special coating to protect it from causing stomach discomfort and vomiting.

    PATIENT EDUCATION: **Instruct the patient to observe the following guidelines:**

1. If stomach irritation, nausea, or vomiting occurs, immediately report the condition to the physician *before* taking the next dose. (Dosage levels cannot be calculated without knowing how much of a medication the patient is keeping down. The patient could become overmedicated or undermedicated, or may aspirate the medication when vomiting.)
2. If symptoms such as allergic reactions, swelling of the throat or tongue, headache, or skin rash occur, withhold oral medication and immediately report the signs and symptoms to the physician. (Delay could cause serious complications and, in some instances, death.)
3. Unless otherwise ordered, drink plenty of water after taking an oral medication, to make sure it gets to or through the stomach rapidly and is well diluted for absorption. (Medication is absorbed best when it is "swimming" in water.)
4. If difficulty swallowing tablets is experienced, place the tablet at the back of the tongue, then drink water; place ice on the tongue and lips before taking the medication; or apply ice to the sternal notch or back of the neck before administration. (The physician should be notified, in case there is the possibility of switching to a liquid form of the medication.)
5. Immediately contact the physician if a drug suddenly loses its effectiveness. (The pa-

TABLE 8–2. **Food–Drug Interactions, Key Summary**

Drug	*Food*	*Interaction*
Aspirin Captopril Isoniazid Mercaptopurine Methotrexate Methyldopa Penicillin G and V Phenobarbital Propantheline Rifampin	Any food	Decreased absorption
Carbamazepine Hydralazine Lithium Metoprolol Propanolol	Any food	Increased absorption
Cefuroxime	Any food	Increased absorption
Chlorpropamide Disulfiram Griseofulvin Metronidazole Procarbazine Quinacrine Tolazoline	Alcohol	Antabuse reaction consisting of flushing, headache, nausea, and in some patients, vomiting, and chest and/or abdominal pain
Cyclosporine	Many foods Fatty foods	Decreased absorption Increased absorption
Cyclosporine Felodipine	Grapefruit juice	Increased absorption
Erythromycin stearate	Any food	Increased or decreased absorption
Furosemide	Any food	Decreased rate of absorption, potentially decreasing effect
Levodopa	High-protein diet	Decreased absorption
Lithium	Sodium	Enhanced elimination requiring high doses
MAO inhibitors: Isocarboxazid Phenelzine Procarbazine Tranylcypromine	High-protein foods that have undergone aging, fermentation, pickling, or smoking; aged cheeses, red wines, pods of broad beans and fava beans; bananas, raisins, avocados; caffeine-containing beverages, beer, ale, and chocolate	Elevated blood pressure
Phenobarbital Phenytoin	High doses of vitamin B_6 (pyridoxine) and folic acid	Decreased absorption
Phenobarbital Phenytoin Theophylline Warfarin	Charcoal-broiled foods	Increased metabolism requiring higher doses
Phenytoin	Most foods Pudding	Absorption increased by 25% Absorption decreased by 50%
Quinolones (eg, ciprofloxacin) Tetracycline	Iron, calcium, aluminum, zinc, magnesium (eg, dairy products)	Decreased absorption

Table continued on following page

TABLE 8–2. **Food–Drug Interactions, Key Summary** (*Continued*)

Drug	Food	Interaction
Warfarin	Diets rich in vitamin K such as cauliflower, spinach, broccoli, turnip greens, liver, beans, rice, pork, fish, and some cheeses	Antagonism of effect

Source: Reprinted with permission from Saltiel E, Food-Drug Interactions, *New Developments in Medicine & Drug Therapy*, Physicians & Scientists Publishing Co, Inc, Glenview, IL, 1994, vol 3(4), p 61.

tient could have changed the prescribed way of taking the medication—for example, he or she could have switched to taking a drug with meals when it should be taken on an empty stomach. This type of change in administration would alter absorption and therefore the drug's effectiveness.)

Mucous Membrane Administration

Drugs may be applied to the mucous membranes for systemic or local effects. Common mucous membrane medications are applied in the (1) rectum, (2) vagina, (3) urethra, (4) mouth, (5) nasal passages, and (6) the deeper respiratory passages through inhalation. Systemic application examples include nitroglycerin tablets applied to the mucous membranes under the tongue (sublingual) for rapid absorption into the bloodstream or antinausea suppositories inserted into the rectum for rapid absorption into the bloodstream. Local applications may include rectal and vaginal antibiotics and antifungal agents and throat sprays. Each route will be discussed separately.

ORAL AND NASAL ABSORPTION

Oral and nasal absorption medication forms include rapidly dissolvable tablets placed under the tongue or between the gum and the cheek, soothing liquids that coat the mucous membranes, and liquids that are absorbed by the mucous membranes.

Sublingual and Buccal Tablets

These are placed under the tongue or between the gum and cheek, respectively, where they are rapidly absorbed by the venous capillaries. This route results in very rapid absorption of drugs, usually within 1 minute. Nitroglycerin is the most common medication taken this way. It is used in angina attacks (pain caused by the constricting of vessels leading to the heart).

PATIENT EDUCATION: **Instruct the patient to observe the following guidelines:**

1. Drink water *before* taking the medication to moisten the mucous membranes of the mouth.
2. Place sublingual tablets under the tongue. Do not chew or swallow the tablet. Do not drink water for 20 minutes. (Drinking water or other beverages will interfere with absorption.)
3. Place buccal tablets between the gum and cheek, next to the upper molars. Do not chew or swallow the tablet.

Irrigations and Gargles

These are substances that coat the mucous membranes of the mouth and throat. They may be used to soothe irritated tissues, treat local infection, or cleanse the membranes.

PATIENT EDUCATION: Instruct the patient to observe the following guidelines:

1. Never gargle or rinse with a solution that is warmer than 120°F. Hot solutions can burn and damage the mucous membranes.
2. Gargling with full-strength antiseptics may burn the mucous membranes.
3. Do not use over-the-counter (OTC) irrigations and gargles for oral infections, unless specified by the dentist or physician. (There are no studies to show that OTC preparations are effective and their use would delay the patient's seeking medical advice.)

Sprays, Drops, and Tampons Impregnated with Drugs

These medications are absorbed by the mucous membranes of the nasal cavity and include decongestants to unblock nasal passages or hemostatics to stop nosebleeds.

PATIENT EDUCATION: Instruct the patient to observe the following guidelines:

1. Use paper tissue to clear the nasal passages before instilling nasal medications.
2. Avoid touching the nose with the dropper, as this may cause sneezing.
3. Administer nosedrops directly into the nose with the head tilted back. Wait a few seconds, then lean forward, head down. (This prevents the medication from being swallowed and absorbed systemically.)
4. Administer sprays with head upright. (Tilting the head back will allow the medication to run down into the throat.)
5. Vasoconstrictor drops (including OTC products) should not be used more frequently than ordered or for more than 3 days; otherwise, a rebound effect (nasal membrane swelling) may occur. (It is called rebound effect because the drug causes the exact effect it was intended to relieve.)
6. With physician approval, saline nosedrops may be purchased OTC and used for treating nasal congestion in infants and toddlers.

LOWER RESPIRATORY ABSORPTION (INHALATION)

Patients often administer their own inhalation therapy. The use of this route is increasing and some antibiotics are now being dispensed in inhalant forms. There are many types of inhalers on the market. Each brand works slightly differently, and patients require instruction on the proper use of whichever inhaler is prescribed.

PATIENT EDUCATION: Instruct the patient to observe the following guidelines:

1. Have all the necessary equipment at home to administer the medication accurately. (Teach patients to assemble, disassemble, and clean all equipment.)
2. A seated position permits greater expansion of the diaphragm for optimum inhalation capability.
3. Use nebulizers to administer only one medication at a time, unless otherwise ordered by the physician.
4. Medications that are not premeasured must be measured precisely with a syringe. (The patient must be instructed as to how to obtain accurate measurements.)
5. Medications that must be diluted with saline are diluted *before* placing them in the nebulizer.
6. Do not overuse the medication, and inhale the smallest prescribed amount possible that will provide relief.
7. Limit inhalations to the prescribed times. (Overuse can lead to tolerance or paradoxic rebound bronchospasm and other cardiac and CNS reactions.)

8. Notify the physician immediately if the medication is not working within the prescribed amounts and/or times. Do not increase the dosage or times without the physician's approval.
9. For inhaling "puffs," breathe out and then in with the puff; then hold in the last inspiration for a few seconds. Take a couple of breaths before taking a second puff, if ordered.
10. After each use, rinse mouth with water, especially when using steroid preparations.

RECTAL, VAGINAL, AND URETHRAL ABSORPTION

Drugs are applied to the rectal mucosa in the form of enemas or suppositories. Rectal suppositories are either glycerin- or cocoa butter-based. These substances provide a lubricant and act as a vehicle for transporting the drug. Rectal drugs may be used for local effects (e.g., laxatives) or systemic effects (e.g., antinausea medications). Because time needed for the drug to pass through the upper digestive tract is eliminated, systemic absorption is very rapid by the rectal route. It can therefore be used when medication is needed in cases of emergency. When the patient is unconscious, unable to swallow, or vomiting, or when a drug is destroyed by upper gastrointestinal (GI) secretions, the rectal route is an excellent alternative.

Vaginal and urethral applications are intended for local effects. Vaginal and urethral suppositories are made of either estrogens or anti-infective drugs used to treat vaginitis or local urinary tract infections. Irrigating vaginal douches are used to cleanse or balance the acidity of the vagina. Contraceptive foams and gels, and antibiotic and antifungal creams, usually applied with an applicator, are a few other examples of vaginal drugs used for a local effect.

PATIENT EDUCATION: **Instruct the patient to observe the following guidelines:**

Suppositories

1. Refrigerate suppositories to prevent softening and loss of shape.
2. Use a glove to protect the finger during insertion.
3. For rectal administration, use the index finger for adults; fourth finger for children. Gently and slowly insert the suppository just beyond the internal sphincter. The resistance will cease and the suppository will slip into place. Make sure the suppository is not in fecal material. (A drug deposited into fecal matter cannot be absorbed.)
4. The best time to administer a rectal suppository is just after a bowel movement. The lower bowel may be first evacuated by a Fleet Enema or glycerin suppository. After administration of the suppository, lie down for 20 minutes and refrain from having a bowel movement, even though there is an urge to do so.
5. Insert vaginal suppositories and cream applicators into the vaginal canal with the suppository or applicator directed toward the small of the back.
6. The patient should remain lying down 20 minutes after the administration of vaginal suppositories, creams, and gels. This is why most prescriptions are to be applied at bedtime. During the day, patients should be advised to wear a sanitary pad after vaginal applications.
7. Urethral suppositories must be inserted with sterile technique. The entire urinary tract must be considered a sterile area at all times.

Enemas and Douches

1. Administer enemas slowly and do not exceed 120 ml (4 oz) of solution. The solution temperature should not exceed 100°F or it may burn the tissues.
2. Remain lying down for 30 minutes retaining the fluid, as the fluid must remain in the intestine long enough for the drug to be absorbed through the intestines.
3. Hang enema and douche containers no higher than 12 to 18 in above the patient's hip. This prevents injury to the mucous membranes that may occur from too forceful a flow of the liquid.

Topical Administration

Topical drugs are applied to the skin, the ear canal, and the eyes. Topical drugs are intended for their local effect, but some eventually find their way into systemic circulation. This is the principle for the dermal patch. Drugs such as nitroglycerin, estrogen, and motion sickness products easily reach the bloodstream when applied as slow-release saturated patches to the skin.

Most OTC topical drugs, however, are not absorbed through the skin. Although many OTC drug manufacturers advertise that their topical products can reduce joint and muscle pain, there is little evidence that these drugs affect more than the upper skin layers. Examples of prescription topical drugs include the corticosteroid creams used to relieve skin inflammation, and antibiotic eyedrops and eardrops.

DERMAL (SKIN) MEDICATIONS

The skin is treated with lotions and liniments, or with ointments that are oil- or water-based. Compresses are moist dressings that have been soaked in chemicals and usually have a drying effect on the skin. Compresses are usually applied to sooth oozing lesions or to relieve itching. Moist, warm compresses may also be applied to keep heat on a body part.

> **PATIENT EDUCATION: Instruct the patient to observe the following guidelines:**
>
> 1. Apply dermal medications by patting, not rubbing—unless otherwise instructed by the physician.
> 2. If a medication is to be rubbed in, use a firm stroke rather than dabbing, to minimize itching and pain caused by the application.
> 3. If a preparation will stain clothing, wear old clothes or none at all on the part.
> 4. Remove ointments from jars with a tongue blade; do not use fingers.
> 5. If a drug is easily absorbed through the skin and applied often to another person, or if the area is a wound or rash, wear gloves to prevent personal skin absorption of the drug or contamination.
> 6. Use clean technique if the skin is broken. Always apply topical medications from the center outward, without going back over any skin area.
> 7. Cleanse the skin with an appropriate soap before applying medication (except in burns, of course).
> 8. Unless otherwise directed, apply medications in thin layers.
> 9. Solutions may be painted on with a cotton applicator, using a circular motion, moving from inside to outside.
> 10. Sterile gloves should be worn to apply sterile solutions.
> 11. For dermal patches:
>   - Keep area around patch dry.
>   - Shower with the patch intact.
>   - Apply each new patch at the same time each day.
>   - Rotate sites with each application. Patches can cause contact dermatitis.
>   - Apply to the upper parts of the arms and legs or to the torso. Estrogen patches are applied to the gluteus muscle.
>   - If the patch is worn 24 hours per day, apply a new patch approximately 30 minutes before removing the old patch.
>   - Keep out of the reach of children. Discarded patches resemble Band-aids and can be toxic to children. After use, patches continue to have some available medication.

OPHTHALMIC (EYE) MEDICATIONS

The eyes are treated with sterile solutions or sterile ointments. Solutions are instilled for diagnostic testing (e.g., dilating the pupils for examination), treatment of infections and inflammation, flushing out foreign particles, and for the treatment of eye diseases, such as glaucoma. Because the eye is so susceptible to infection, all ophthalmic medications must be kept sterile.

PATIENT EDUCATION: Observe the following guidelines. Instruct the patient to adapt these same guidelines for administering medications at home.

1. Wash hands before administering eye medications. Never share eye administration equipment.
2. Keep eyedrop medication containers stored inside a protective container.
3. Do not touch the dropper or place the dropper on nonsterile surfaces.
4. When treating both eyes, be careful not to touch the dropper to either eye or either eyelid. This would cause cross contamination from one eye to the other.
5. Administer eyedrops so that the flow is *away* from the nose.
6. Place the dropper close to the eye, to reduce the shock or pain of the medication hitting the eye.
7. Administer drops onto the lower conjunctiva (area between the eyeball and the lower lid) (Fig. 8–1). Drops should *not* hit the cornea, as this could tear the cornea.
8. Apply slight pressure for a few seconds to the inner canthus of the eye to prevent absorption of the medication into the bloodstream.
9. Administer ointment as a fine line onto the lower conjunctiva (area between the eyeball and the lower lid), then gently massage the eye with a cottonball to distribute the ointment.
10. The patient's vision may be temporarily blurred. Make sure the patient is able to see before he or she leaves the facility. Safeguard against patient falls.

OTIC (EAR) MEDICATIONS

Eardrops may be antibiotic, antifungal, anti-inflammatory, or locally anesthetic in their effect. Eardrops should be warmed to body temperature before installation to prevent any "shocks" to the auditory nerve, which could cause vertigo (dizziness).

PATIENT EDUCATION: Observe the following guidelines. Instruct the patient to adapt these same guidelines for administering medication at home.

1. Warm the medication to body temperature by holding the bottle in your hand for a few minutes.

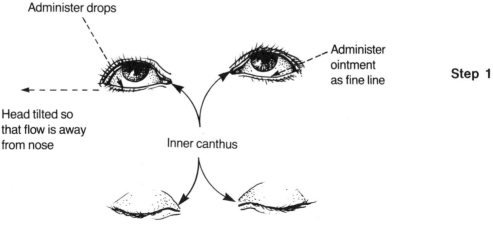

FIGURE 8–1. Administering ophthalmic medications.

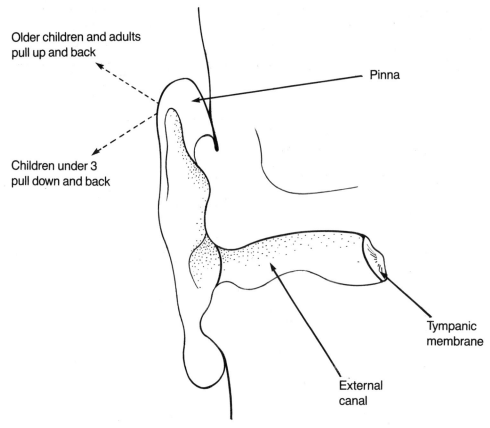

FIGURE 8–2. Straightening the external ear canal for the administration of otic medications.

2. Have the patient lie down with the ear to be treated facing upward.
3. Pull the external part of the ear:
   • Up and back for adults (Fig. 8–2).
   • Up and back for children over 3 years of age.
   • Down and back for children under 3 years of age. (In children under 3 years of age the ear canal is underdeveloped and shaped differently.)
4. Have the patient remain lying down for a few minutes to facilitate absorption around the area of the eardrum.
5. Never tightly pack a wick (earplug of cotton or gauze) of medication in the ear. A wick should be loose and removed as soon as it is dried out or soiled.

Parenteral (Injectable) Administration

Injections are ordered for the following reasons:

• Medications given by injection are rapidly absorbed by the body, and are often used when a rapid onset is desired. (Of course, a rapid onset often means a short duration, and the effects of drugs administered by the rapid-acting routes are often very short in duration.)
• Some medications are destroyed or inactivated by gastric secretions, or cannot be absorbed through the lining of the digestive tract.
• Injectable medications are very useful for patients who are unconscious, unable to swallow, or nauseated or vomiting.

The disadvantages of injections are that they are expensive, they are only available when there is a person skilled enough to administer them, and they are more hazardous and less likely reversible if the patient is overdosed or given the wrong medication. In addition, injections are painful and intimidating, and they may even cause local tissue damage or permit the entrance of micro-organisms into the sterile tissues of the body.

The injectable routes include the following:

1. Intradermal (ID): Into the upper skin layers—namely, the dermis and epidermis
2. Subcutaneous (SC): Within the subcutaneous layers of the skin
3. Intramuscular (IM): Within a muscle

Drug administration by the following routes is limited to specially trained and licensed personnel. These routes bypass all absorption barriers and produce an instantaneous drug onset. These are the most dangerous routes of administration, and are usually reserved for emergency medications or surgery.

1. Intravenous (IV) or intra-arterial: Within a vein or artery
2. Intrathecal: Into the subarachnoid spaces of the spine
3. Intraspinal: Into the spinal fluid
4. Intra-articular: Into a joint
5. Intralesional: Into a lesion

INTRADERMAL ROUTE

Intradermal medications are deposited directly into the skin layer (Fig. 8–3). The ID site is used for sensitivity testing such as allergy testing and testing for tuberculosis, histoplasmosis, and mumps. Allergy is the specialty in which the ID route is used most routinely. The other frequent use of the ID site is in tuberculin testing. Mantoux serum or purified protein derivative, "PPD," is used for tuberculin testing, and is available in multidose vials (Fig. 8–4). The Mantoux test is the standard method by which tuberculin skin sensitivity is defined. The standard dose is 0.1 ml.

Any doubtful reaction to the Mantoux test should be rechecked before a follow-up chest x-ray is ordered. When administering the Mantoux test, a solution of 0.1 ml of PPD-

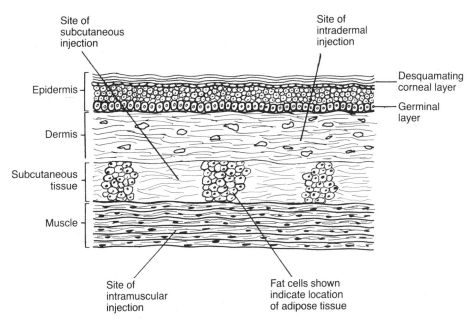

FIGURE 8–3. Cross section of skin showing subcutaneous, intradermal, and intramuscular injection sites. (From Saperstein, AB, and Frazier, MA: Introduction to Nursing Practice. FA Davis, Philadelphia, 1980, p 612, with permission.)

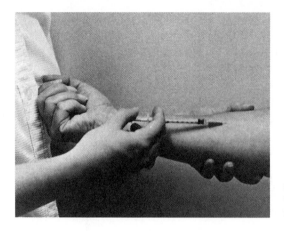

FIGURE 8–4. Injection technique for Mantoux test. (Courtesy of Lederle Laboratories, Wayne, N.J.)

tuberculin containing 5 tuberculin units is injected ID into either the anterior or the posterior surface of the forearm. The test is read in 48 to 72 hours. The result is considered positive if the induration (raised area) at the test site is more than 10 mm in diameter (Fig. 8–5).

INTRADERMAL ADMINISTRATION PRECAUTIONS

The sites chosen for ID administration are the forearm or the hairless areas of the upper back. Acetone is preferred over alcohol for cleansing the skin, because acetone immediately dries and will not chemically interfere with the testing material.

Intradermal sensitivity tests are administered with a 3/8-in, 26- to 27-gauge needle attached to a tuberculin syringe. The ID needle is inserted almost parallel to the skin surface. ID injections will form a wheal or bleb (fluid-filled bump) and may sting. For skin testing, each ID site (Fig. 8–6) should be carefully marked as to which allergen is injected. Multiple injections should be exactly mapped for reference on the patient's chart. Skin reactions to the test materials should be read 24 to 72 hours later by an experienced person at the medical facility.

SUBCUTANEOUS ROUTE

Subcutaneous injections (Fig. 8–7) are also called hypodermic injections; both terms mean literally "under the skin." The SC route is commonly chosen for soluble drugs less than 2 ml. Therefore, the drugs that are administered this way must be highly soluble (absorbable) and potent enough in small quantities to be effective. SC injections commonly administered include insulin, local anesthesia, and epinephrine.

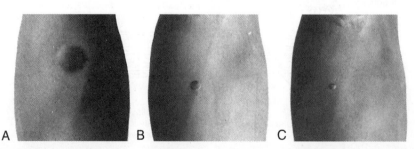

FIGURE 8–5. (*A*) Unequivocally positive Mantoux test reaction; diameter of induration is 30 mm. (*B*) Minimum positive Mantoux test reaction; diameter of induration is 10 mm. (*C*) Negative Mantoux test reaction; diameter of induration is less than 5 mm.

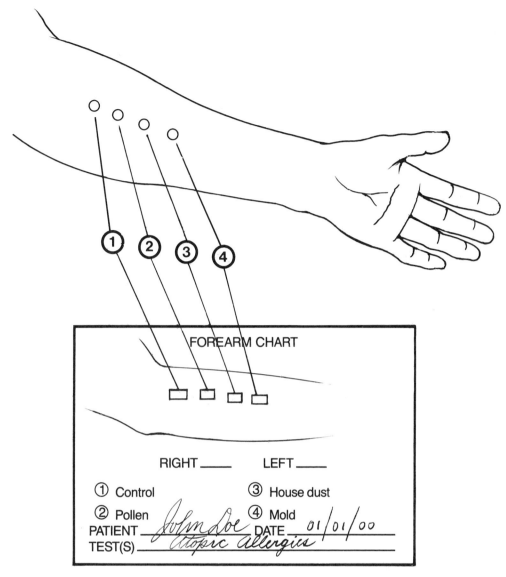

FIGURE 8–6. Intradermal skin tests are used for the diagnosis of infectious diseases (e.g., tuberculosis, diphtheria, and fungal and parasitic infections) or to determine sensitivity to a specific allergen or group of allergens.

SUBCUTANEOUS ADMINISTRATION PRECAUTIONS

SC drugs are administered with a 1/2- or 5/8-in, 24- to 28-gauge needle (Table 8–3) attached to a regular (2- to 3-ml), insulin, or tuberculin syringe. Amounts of medication range from 0.1 to 2 ml for adults. For children, amounts should be limited to no more than 0.5 ml.

For older children and adults, the sites chosen are the upper arm, upper thigh, or abdomen; for infants, sites should be limited to the thigh and abdomen. The SC needle is inserted at a 45-degree angle. The angle will have to be increased (60 to 90 degrees) for patients with large amounts of fatty tissue. Insulin syringes with the 28-gauge 1/2-in needle are usually administered at a 90-degree angle.

SC drugs are often painful because most medications are irritating to the never endings in the area. SC drugs may be irritating to the soft tissues and may even cause an abscess or scar formation. Repeated injections must be rotated to prevent tissue damage (see Chapter 9, Fig. 9–4, for a chart of rotating insulin injections).

Before injecting, aspirate the fluid in the syringe by pulling the plunger back, to ensure that the needle is in SC tissue and not in a blood vessel. Do not aspirate when giving insulin or heparin, however.

TABLE 8–3. **Choosing the Correct Needle Length**

Patient Body Size	Subcutaneous	IM Deltoid	IM Vastus Lateralis	IM Ventrogluteal	IM Dorsogluteal
Under age 7	24–28g 1/2 in		5/8–1 in		
Children	24–28g 1/2 in		5/8–1 in		
Frail or underweight adults, 70–90 lb	24–28g 1/2 in		1 in	1 in	1 in
Adults with small muscles, 91–115 lb	24–28g 1/2 in	1 in	1 1/4 in	1 1/4 in	1 1/4 in
Average adult, 116–174 lb	24–28g 5/8 in	1 in–1 1/2 in	1 1/2 in	1 1/2 in	1 1/2 in
Adults with well-developed muscles, 175–200 lb	24–28g 5/8 in	1 1/2 in	1 1/2 in	2–3 in	2–3 in
Obese, >200 lb	24–28g 1/2 in	1 1/2 in	1 1/2 in	3 in (sometimes 4 in)	3 in (sometimes 4 in)
Elderly, <140 lb or ↓ muscle mass	24–28g 1/2 in	1 in	1 1/4 in	1 1/4 in	1 1/2 in

Choosing the proper length hypodermic needle will depend on the size of the muscle mass, the tissue depth desired for depositing the medication, and the volume of fluid injected.

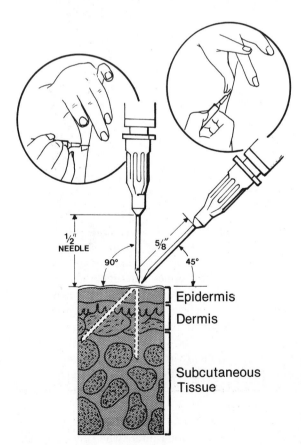

FIGURE 8–7. Subcutaneous and deep subcutaneous injections. The 5/8-in needle is injected at a 45° angle to the skin. The 1/2-in needle is inserted at a 90° angle to the skin. Because of the shortness of the needle, it remains within the subcutaneous tissue rather than the muscle. (Note the inserts depicting angles of needle to subcutaneous tissue of upper arm and proper grasping techniques.) (From Saperstein, AB, and Frazier, MA: Introduction to Nursing Practice. FA Davis, Philadelphia, 1980, p 637, with permission.)

INTRAMUSCULAR ROUTE

IM injections penetrate past the SC tissues and are used to deposit drugs into the deep muscular layers of the body. The IM route is desired if larger amounts of medication or an absorption rate more rapid than that of the SC route are necessary. The muscles also provide a repository for the long-acting insoluble substances that are slowly absorbed over 24 to 48 hours, or even for weeks.

The IM route is commonly chosen for drug amounts from 1 to 5 ml. If more than 5 ml is to be administered, the dose should be divided into two injections. IM drugs commonly administered include tetanus toxoid, the long-acting corticosteroid drugs, and long-acting penicillin G procaine.

INTRAMUSCULAR ADMINISTRATION PRECAUTIONS

IM drugs are administered with a 1- to 3-in, (Table 8–3) 20- to 23-gauge needle attached to a regular syringe (2- to 5-ml). The sites chosen are the mid-deltoid area of the upper arm, the vastus lateralis muscle of the upper thigh, or the ventrogluteal area of the buttocks (Figs. 8–8, 8–9, and 8–10).

The vastus lateralis, the safest route for infants and children, is becoming a popular site for adults as well. Use of the buttocks as a site for IM injections in children can result in sciatic nerve damage and possible leg muscle paralysis. For adults, the ventrogluteal and the

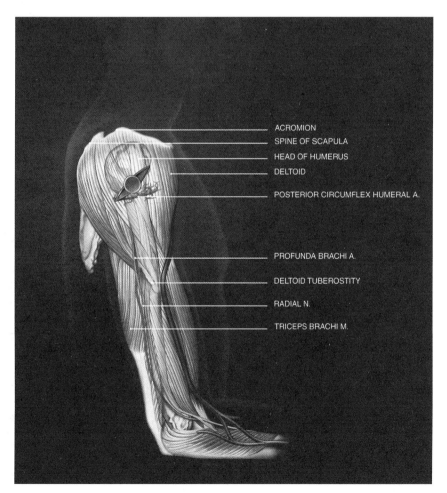

ACROMION
SPINE OF SCAPULA
HEAD OF HUMERUS
DELTOID
POSTERIOR CIRCUMFLEX HUMERAL A.

PROFUNDA BRACHI A.

DELTOID TUBEROSTITY

RADIAL N.

TRICEPS BRACHI M.

FIGURE 8–8. Mid-deltoid area intramuscular injection site. The mid-deltoid area boundaries are located by forming a rectangle bounded by the lower edge of the acromion on the top to a point on the lateral side of the arm opposite the axilla or armpit on the bottom. The two side boundaries are parallel lines one-third and two-thirds of the way around the outer lateral aspect of the arm. The deltoid area is considered small and cannot tolerate repeated or large quantities of medication. (Courtesy of Wyeth-Ayerst Laboratories, Philadelphia, PA.)

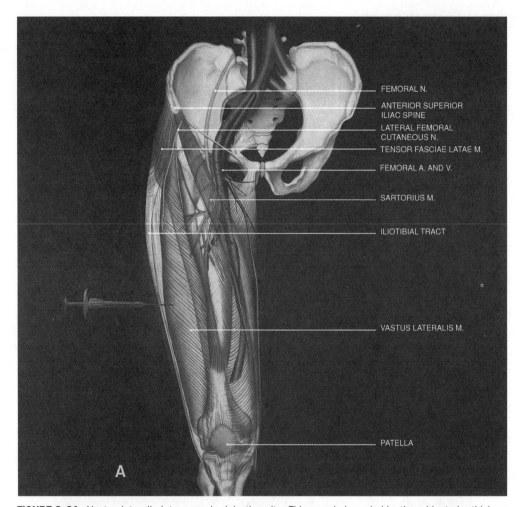

FIGURE 8–9A. Vastus lateralis intramuscular injection site. This area is bounded by the midanterior thigh on the front of the leg, the midlateral thigh on the side, and is one hand's breadth below the greater trochanter at the proximal end and another hand's breadth above the knee at the distal end. (Courtesy of Wyeth-Ayerst Laboratories, Philadelphia, PA.)

dorsogluteal sites are considered safe for use, but the gluteus maximus site is no longer considered safe. Long considered the classic site for the majority of deep IM injections, the dorsogluteal injection has recently aroused controversy, primarily because of an increase in injury to the sciatic nerve (Fig. 8–11). The ventrogluteal and vastus lateralis sites offer comparable muscle mass with relatively greater margins of safety. Despite the reservations expressed, many drug manufacturers continue to specify on package inserts "deep IM injection into the upper outer quadrant of the buttocks." Although the site is acceptable for most adults, it should never be considered for children.

In adults, amounts of medication range from 1 to 2 ml in the deltoid region to 1 to 5 ml in the vastus lateralis and gluteal regions. For infants and children, amounts should be limited to 2 ml in either the vastus lateralis or the ventrogluteal region. The IM needle is inserted at a 90-degree angle (see Figs. 8–8 and 8–9A, for example); longer shafts are necessary for patients with large amounts of fatty tissue.

IM drugs are usually not painful or irritating to muscle tissues. If a drug is known to be irritating or the amount is unusually large, the medication may be manufactured in combination with an anesthetic to help reduce pain. At the muscle level, nerve damage is always a risk, unless utmost care is taken in marking off landmarks for proper positioning of the needle.

The danger of blood vessel penetration is greater in the muscle tissue, and blood vessel penetration is especially risky with oily suspensions of insoluble materials. Before injecting,

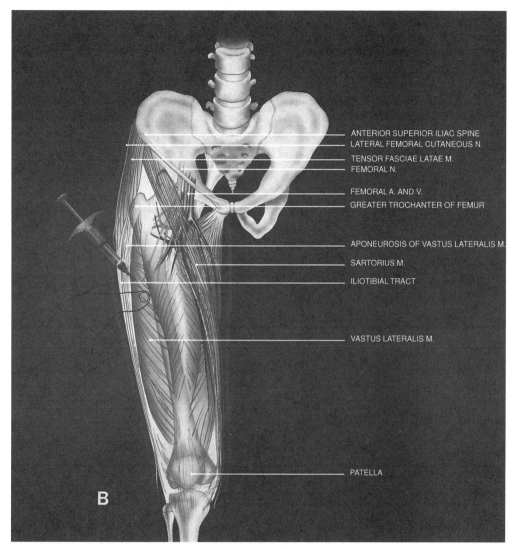

ANTERIOR SUPERIOR ILIAC SPINE
LATERAL FEMORAL CUTANEOUS N.

TENSOR FASCIAE LATAE M.
FEMORAL N.

FEMORAL A. AND V.
GREATER TROCHANTER OF FEMUR

APONEUROSIS OF VASTUS LATERALIS M.
SARTORIUS M.
ILIOTIBIAL TRACT

VASTUS LATERALIS M.

PATELLA

B

FIGURE 8–9B. Vastus lateralis intramuscular injection site for infants and children. Direct the needle at a 45° angle (toward the knee) to reduce the possibility of the needle traversing the muscle and endangering major blood vessels. (Courtesy of Wyeth-Ayerst Laboratories, Philadelphia, PA.)

aspirate by pulling the plunger back, to ensure that the needle is in the muscle and not in a blood vessel. If blood appears in the syringe, immediately remove the entire unit and prepare a new medication with new equipment. Blood in the needle or syringe represents a foreign material that would contaminate the medication.

Z-TRACT INTRAMUSCULAR ROUTE

The Z-tract IM route is actually not a distinctly different route but rather an alternative technique for administering an IM injection. Certain medications such as iron preparations are extremely irritating to the skin and SC tissues, and using the Z-tract technique prevents the deposited medication from seeping back to the skin layers.

Before the medication is drawn up, the plunger is pulled back to the 0.1 ml mark. This provides an "air bubble" that will additionally seal the drug in the muscle after injection. After the medication is drawn up, the needle used to withdraw the medication is replaced with a new one. During injection, the skin is pulled to one side, the needle is inserted at a 90-degree angle and the drug deposited. After a wait of 10 seconds, the skin is released *as the needle is withdrawn*. This way, the drug is sealed in the muscle tissues.

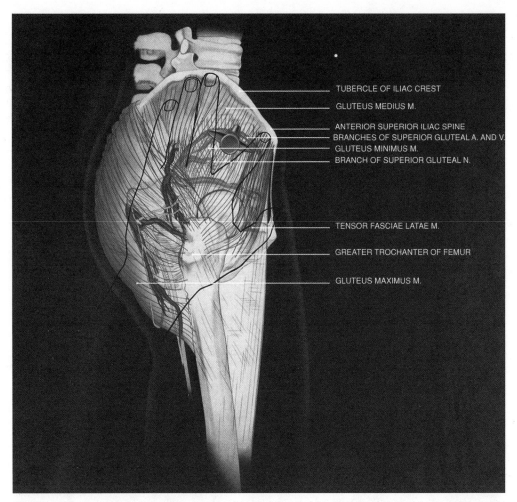

TUBERCLE OF ILIAC CREST
GLUTEUS MEDIUS M.
ANTERIOR SUPERIOR ILIAC SPINE
BRANCHES OF SUPERIOR GLUTEAL A. AND V.
GLUTEUS MINIMUS M.
BRANCH OF SUPERIOR GLUTEAL N.
TENSOR FASCIAE LATAE M.
GREATER TROCHANTER OF FEMUR
GLUTEUS MAXIMUS M.

FIGURE 8–10. Ventrogluteal area intramuscular injection site. To identify the anatomical landmarks, palpate to find the greater trochanter, the anterior superior iliac spine, and the iliac crest. When injecting into the left side of the patient, place the palm of the right hand on the greater trochanter and the index finger on the anterior superior iliac spine. (Use the left hand to delineate the site when injecting into the patient's right side.) Spread the middle finger posteriorly away from the index finger as far as possible along the iliac crest, as shown in the inset. A "V" space or triangle between the index and middle finger is formed. The injection is made in the center of the triangle with the needle directed slightly upward toward the crest of the ilium. (Courtesy of Wyeth-Ayerst Laboratories, Philadelphia, PA.)

INTRAVENOUS ROUTE

Intravenous (IV) means "directly into a vein." The effects of drugs given directly into the circulatory system are immediate. Drugs or sterile solutions may be injected directly into a vein to secure an immediate result as in cases of hemorrhage, shock, or collapse. Many liquid preparations, such as isotonic saline and potassium chloride, are used (see Chapter 9). The quantity depends on the needs of the patient. Intravenous fluids or drugs are usually administered in the arm, but veins at other site may be used.

The injection of a single drug dose is called a *bolus*. It is delivered in a syringe through an IV *port* (a rubber stopper attached to an IV *line*). This is also called an *IV push* because it is injected manually using the syringe plunger. A drug may be mixed with another solution in a bag and administered continuously over several hours. This is called an *IV drip*. A drug in a small bag or bottle may also be attached to an existing IV line. This is referred to as an IV *piggy-back* line. An *IV infusion pump* is a special pump designed to provide a constant and adjustable rate of flow of IV solutions.

Other vascular routes include intra-arterial, sometimes referred to as *A-lines*, and umbilical artery or vein catheter techniques for administering fluids to newborn infants. These methods are usually reserved for critical care use or the administration of anticancer drugs.

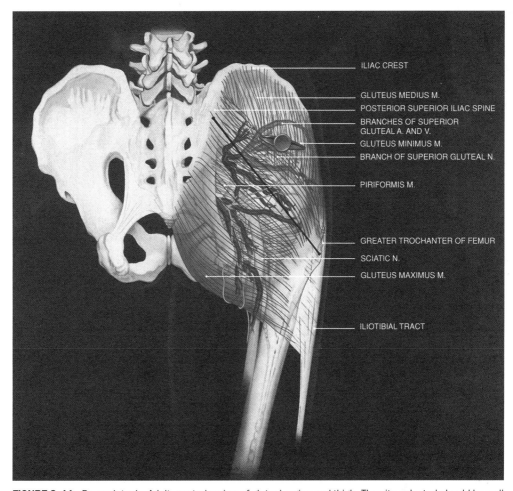

ILIAC CREST

GLUTEUS MEDIUS M.

POSTERIOR SUPERIOR ILIAC SPINE

BRANCHES OF SUPERIOR
GLUTEAL A. AND V.

GLUTEUS MINIMUS M.

BRANCH OF SUPERIOR GLUTEAL N.

PIRIFORMIS M.

GREATER TROCHANTER OF FEMUR

SCIATIC N.

GLUTEUS MAXIMUS M.

ILIOTIBIAL TRACT

FIGURE 8–11. Dorsogluteal—Adult, posterior view of gluteal region and thigh. The site selected should be well into the upper outer mass of the gluteus maximus and away from the central region of the buttocks. To avoid the central region of the buttocks or slanting the needle downward and inward toward the sciatic nerve, angle the needle 90° to the flat surface upon which the prone patient is lying. (Courtesy of Wyeth-Ayerst Laboratories, Philadelphia, PA.)

INTRA-ARTICULAR ROUTE

In the outpatient setting, patients may be treated with intra-articular medications (usually adrenocorticosteroids) injected directly into an inflamed joint. Adrenocorticosteroids are natural or synthesized hormones of the adrenal gland. They are extremely useful as anti-inflammatory agents but can produce serious side effects, no matter which route is used.

The physician is responsible for administering these drugs. Intra-articular injections may also be called intrasynovial injections. The same techniques may be used for injecting medications into the bursa (intrabursal route), into the tendon sheaths, or into lesions (intralesional route).

INTRA-ARTICULAR ADMINISTRATION PRECAUTIONS

Skin areas to be used for intra-articular injections should be carefully prepared, using the same techniques as for minor surgery. The site may be first anesthetized. The patient will experience local discomfort for a few hours until the medication takes effect and relieves the pain and inflammation of the joint. The patient should remain in the office for 30 minutes following injection, as the adrenocorticosteroid drugs used in this treatment are reported to cause fainting (syncope) and anaphylactic reactions.

The patient should limit the use of the joint and be careful not to overuse it, once pain has subsided. The patient may experience transient flushing and dizziness following injection. Discoloration at the site of injection is common a few days after treatment. This usually diffuses. Any increase in swelling and pain may indicate a septic joint. Sepsis is severe infection due to contamination of tissue by blood or pathogenic microorganisms. The patient should report this immediately. If the patient is receiving long-term therapy, the patient should be instructed to increase protein intake, as the adrenocorticosteroids may cause gradual weight loss owing to loss of appetite and muscle wasting. Since there are many side effects from long-term adrenocorticosteroid therapy, the patient should be told to report any changes in health status, such as increased bleeding, slow healing, and fatigue.

Preparing and Administering Drugs for Injection

When preparing a medication for injection, you must carefully put together all the rules of safety you have learned so far: safety in the medication room; safe sterile technique; the three medication checks; the "seven rights"; and continuous patient assessment. If you need a review of any of these safety factors, please review Chapter 5.

Preparing and giving injections is a multifold task that requires logical coordination and attention to detail. Much of the process is "standard procedure," and each person responsible for administering injections must develop a controlled pattern of preparation and safety checks.

Skill and practice are required to become proficient at giving injections. Certain attitudes are also required. First, come to terms with the fact that patients fear injections and may sometimes exaggerate their discomfort and blame the health care provider for it. Injections may be somewhat uncomfortable, but if quality equipment is used and the task is performed expertly, then injections need not be painful. Take time and care with each patient and learn the time-proved techniques. Patients will compliment good technique and may even show surprise at the "tender touch."

Skill includes an aseptic conscious—that is, attention to sterile technique and recognition when contamination has occurred. Although injections are extremely useful in patient

---

TABLE 8–4. **Techniques to Be Followed with Every Injectable Medication You Prepare**

1. Use sterile technique.
2. Select each needle gauge and length according to the route desired, the patient's weight (amount of fatty tissue), and the thickness of the medication.
3. Select each syringe size according to the amount of medication to be prepared.
4. Gather all equipment, including alcohol or other antiseptic, cottonballs or wipes, and the written order for the medication beforehand.
5. Compare the patient name and the medication name, strength (dose), route, and time with those on the order *three times.*
6. Inspect each medication for expiration date and quality. Make sure all medications are well mixed.
7. Clean all ampules and vial stoppers with antiseptic, using a firm circular motion before exposing the medication container to the needle.
8. Always replace an amount of air in the vial equal to the amount of medication to be withdrawn into the syringe. Withdraw air into the syringe before you remove the needle cap. This minimizes movement when the needle is exposed to air.
9. Never place the needle cap on a surface, or in any other way contaminate the cap.
10. Withdraw medications with the vial upside down and the needle tip submerged. Slowly withdraw the medication into the syringe. These techniques will reduce the amount of air drawn into a syringe. Withdrawing the medication too quickly causes a "fizzing" effect, which results in air bubbles being dispersed throughout the syringe.

    Special Hint: Tiny air bubbles are not a danger to the patient; however, every air bubble displaces medication that the patient should be given. Accurately measured medications depend on your keeping air bubbles to a minimum.

11. To further keep air bubbles to a minimum, withdraw more medication than the amount ordered. Tapping the syringe will dislodge any air bubbles formed. The bubbles should float and form a single air space at the top (hub) where it can be eliminated before removing the syringe from the vial or ampule.
12. Measure all medications exactly, at eye level.
13. When replacing the needle cap, never touch the needle to the lip or sides of the cap.

TABLE 8–5. **Techniques to Be Followed with Every Injectable Medication You Administer**

1. Review the "seven rights" each time you confirm you have the right patient.
2. Keep all equipment visible and above your waist height, to ensure sterility is maintained.
3. Select each site according to the amount of medication to be injected and the size of the patient. Inspect each body site to be injected. Palpate each area to ensure that a site is not tender or becomes firm when grasped. Drugs should never be injected into an inflamed area, scar tissue, or an area with reduced circulation.
4. For long-term injection therapy, rotate sites and keep a record of the rotation by marking the exact sites used on the patient's chart; for example, left deltoid (LD) or right ventrogluteal (RVG), right arm (R/A), left arm (L/A), right abdomen (R/ABD), left abdomen (L/ABD).
5. Assist patient to relax the area being used for the injection. Position patient to reduce strain on the part to be used:
   • Never give an injection with the patient standing.
   • Rest patient's arm on a flat and comfortable surface.
   • Have the patient lie down.
   • Have the patient point toes inward to relax the buttocks.
6. Cleanse injection sites thoroughly using 70 percent alcohol or acetone, always using a circular motion from the point site outward.
7. Use diversion tactics with the patients:
   • Ask patient to take a deep breath just as you inject.
   • Have patient count to three or count backwards from 10.
   • If you cannot get a patient to relax, gently touch your little fingernail to the skin outside but near the cleansed area. The patient usually thinks that the touch of your nail is the injection and immediately relaxes the muscle.
8. Inject SC medications by picking up and holding the skin tissue between your fingers until the needle has passed into the SC space at a 45-degree angle or, depending on the order, at a 90-degree angle.
9. Inject IM medications into patients of normal weight and structure by stretching the tissue until the needle has passed into the muscle at a 90-degree angle. For thin patients and small children, firmly grasp a muscle bundle and squeeze while the needle is inserted at a 90-degree angle.
10. Insert needles swiftly, with the beveled tip of the needle pointing upward. The best technique is to use a motion much like that of throwing a dart.
11. Aspirate before injections (except for SC heparin and insulin injections), to ensure that the needle is not in a blood vessel. Pull back enough with the plunger to see if blood can be drawn into the syringe. If blood appears in the syringe, the needle is in a vessel and the entire unit must be withdrawn and discarded. Start again with uncontaminated materials (blood is a contaminant to sterile tissues).
12. After aspirating, keep needles motionless while medications are injected. Movement may cause the needle to enter a blood vessel. The proper depth and position should be determined by the appropriate needle length.
13. Deposit medications slowly to allow tissues to adjust to the volume of drug being deposited. Too forceful a flow will cause tissue tearing and pain.
14. Withdraw needles quickly and dispose of them immediately into a rigid, sharps container (right there, at the site).
15. Briskly massage injection sites to help increase circulation and decrease pain. For certain repository drugs and Z-tract drugs massage is contraindicated, however. Always check massage orders when using long-acting IM medications or the Z-tract technique.

treatment, they may cause tissue damage or allow the invasion of bacteria. The patient is kept safe only when the medication is sterile, the equipment is sterile, and the site for the injection has been properly cleansed. Tables 8–4 and 8–5 list the techniques that must be followed when preparing and administering drugs by injection.

Skill includes being familiar with the absorption and effects of drugs and in calculating correct dosage for administration. Injection of a miscalculated dose can be disastrous: there is no way to retrieve the medication and it is very difficult to prevent an injected medication from being absorbed.

> SPECIAL ALERT: If an incorrect medication has been injected or too much of a medication has been injected, the physician may order emergency first-aid measures or an antidote. The physician must directly manage this type of emergency procedure. For this reason, *no* medication should be injected without a physician on site. In some states, this is regulated by law.

What Can Go Wrong?

Any injection can cause two types of injury: injury or infection to the skin penetrated by the hypodermic needle; and local or systemic injury or allergic reaction caused by the medication deposited in the tissues. The size of the patient, the angle and depth of the injection, and the characteristics of the injected material all greatly determine the type of complication that can occur. Practically speaking, there are three techniques that can minimize most site injuries. These three techniques are (1) pulling back slightly on the plunger for 2 to 3 seconds while observing for any discoloration, (2) leaving at least a small portion ($\cong$ 1/8 in) of the needle shaft above the skin, and (3) keeping the needle steady while depositing the medication. Aspiration helps to determine whether the needle is in a blood vessel; leaving a portion of the shaft visible allows the needle to be retrieved, should a needle ever break off at the hub; and a steady hand avoids traumatizing the tissue.

The importance of knowing the anatomical landmarks for every type of injection cannot be stressed enough. Severe injury or allergic reaction, or even death, can be caused by inadvertently injecting a medication intended for subcutaneous tissue or muscle into or too near a blood vessel. For example, accidentally injecting certain antibiotics into an artery has resulted in severe neurovascular injuries, such as spinal cord lesions, paralysis, and gangrene. These types of side effects have occurred most often in children.

In addition to accidental injection in or too near an artery, repeated injections of penicillin or large amounts of medication at a single site may cause nerve damage resulting in permanent neurological deficit. Multiple injections have also caused the formation of scar tissue in the muscle, permanent muscle contractions, intramuscular hemorrhage, and muscle atrophy.

Injuries can happen even with the most superficial injections. Possible complications common to subcutaneous injections include skin pigmentation changes, sterile abscesses forming below the skin, cellulitis, tissue necrosis, gangrene, and cyst or scar formation. Accidental injection into a joint space or bone has resulted in joint injury or infection and periostitis.

There is potential danger in every injection given. Discontinue any type of injection if the patient complains of severe, immediate pain at the injection site or if infants or young children show immediate signs suggesting severe pain.

Written Competency 8–1

Performance Objective: Using the information in this chapter and the PDR, answer the following 10 questions with 100 percent accuracy and within 30 minutes. Do not give yourself credit for incorrect or omitted answers.

Choose the correct route and site to administer the orders in questions 1 through 3.

1. DTP (diphtheria, tetanus, and pertussis) No. 1, 3-month-old infant
   a. ID, forearm
   b. SC, deltoid
   c. SC, vastus lateralis
   d. IM, deltoid
   e. IM, vastus lateralis

2. Tuberculin tine test, 18-year-old
   a. ID, forearm
   b. SC, deltoid
   c. SC, vastus lateralis
   d. IM, deltoid
   e. IM, vastus lateralis

3. Bicillin L-A, 600,000 units, 24-month-old
   a. ID, forearm
   b. SC, deltoid
   c. SC, vastus lateralis
   d. IM, deltoid
   e. IM, vastus lateralis

Choose the correct syringe and needle size to administer the orders in questions 4 through 6.

4. DTP No. 1, 3-month-old infant
   a. 26-gauge, 3/8-in
   b. 24-gauge, 5/8-in
   c. 25-gauge, 5/8-in
   d. 22-gauge, 1-in
   e. 22-gauge, 1-1/2-in

5. Bicillin L-A, 600,000 units, 24-month-old
   a. 26-gauge, 3/8-in
   b. 24-gauge, 5/8-in
   c. 25-gauge, 5/8-in
   d. 22-gauge, 1-in
   e. 22-gauge, 1-1/2-in

6. Bicillin L-A, 1,200,000 units, 28-year-old
   a. 26-gauge, 3/8-in
   b. 24-gauge, 5/8-in
   c. 25-gauge, 5/8-in
   d. 22-gauge, 1-in
   e. 22-gauge, 1-1/2-in

7. The patient in question 6 should be instructed to notify the physician *immediately* if which of the following should occur?
   (1) Swelling of the throat or tongue
   (2) Fever
   (3) Skin rash
   (4) Vomiting
       a. 1,2,3
       b. 1,3
       c. 2,4
       d. 4 only
       e. all of the above

8. Products that must be considered sterile include:
   (1) Eyedrops.
   (2) Nebulizer solutions.
   (3) Urethral suppositories.
   (4) Ear wicks.
       a. 1,2,3
       b. 1,3
       c. 2,4
       d. 4 only
       e. all of the above

9. Standing-order medications may be administered if:
   a. The physician is available by telephone.
   b. The physician is present.
   c. Either a or b.
   d. The medical personnel are trained in cardiopulmonary resuscitation (CPR).
   e. Either a or d.

10. When treating the patient's right eye with drops, the patient should be:
   a. Seated, looking up.
   b. Lying, with the head turned right.
   c. Either a or b.
   d. Lying with the head turned left.
   e. Either a or d.

Score: _____

See Appendix B for answers.

Terminal Performance Objective/Competency

Procedure 8–1: Teach a Patient to Use a Nebulizer

EQUIPMENT

Audio cassette and tape recorder
Nebulizer
Tissues
Patient record
Procedure handout

Rx: Metaprel Inhalant Solution 5 percent (10 ml)
Sig: two to three inhalations of undiluted solution every 3 or 4 hours, up to 5 to 15 inhalations (usually 10) per day.

Performance Competence: Complete each step of this patient teaching sequence by completing each step of the procedure in correct order and within reasonable job production time, as stated by your evaluator, and record the session on the patient's medical record. Tape record the teaching session.

	V	S	U*

PROCEDURAL STEPS

Wash hands and check medication expiration date.

1. Explain that you will allow the patient to prepare the first dose with guidance. ☐ ☐ ☐

2. "Place your medication in your nebulizer." ☐ ☐ ☐

3. "Exhale slowly through pursed lips." ☐ ☐ ☐

4. "Place the nebulizer in your mouth, without sealing your lips around it." ☐ ☐ ☐

5. "Take a deep breath through your mouth as you squeeze the bulb of the nebulizer." ☐ ☐ ☐

6. "Hold your breath for 3 to 4 seconds, as soon as you've taken as full a breath as possible." ☐ ☐ ☐

7. "Exhale slowly through pursed lips."
   RATIONALE: This will increase pressure in the air passages, which in turn will better circulate medication through the bronchial tree. ☐ ☐ ☐

8. "Repeat the inhalation/squeeze/exhalation cycle for the number of times ordered at each administration." ☐ ☐ ☐

9. Have the patient clean the equipment, using the manufacturer's directions. ☐ ☐ ☐

10. Record the session in the patient's record on the following page. ☐ ☐ ☐

---

*V = Value, to fill in if assigning points or other specific values to each step, or if designating a critical step.
S = Satisfactory completion of the step.
U = Unsatisfactory completion of the step, or step incomplete; needs more practice.

DATE			SUBSEQUENT VISITS AND FINDINGS	B.P.	WGT.
MO.	DAY	YR.			

Date: _____ Competency achieved: Y _____ N _____

Designated reasonable time standard: _____

Actual completion time: _____

Terminal Performance Objective/Competency

Procedure 8–2: Prepare and Administer an Eye Medication

EQUIPMENT	Two sterile droppers Two tissues, two cottonballs Gloves	Sterile medication Cleansing solution Patient record with order: Rx: gt i both eyes.

REVIEW   Procedure 5–1, Chapter 5
Procedure 5–2, Chapter 5

Terminal Performance Objective: Instill an ordered amount of drops into a patient's eyes by completing each step accurately, safely, and in the correct order, within reasonable job production time.

	V	S	U*
PROCEDURAL STEPS Wash hands and check medication expiration date.			
1. Position the patient lying down or sitting with head tilted backward.	☐	☐	☐
2. Hand the patient a separate tissue for each eye.	☐	☐	☐
3. Wipe each eyelid and eyelashes clean with a single, gentle downward and outward motion, using the solution and a separate cottonball for each eye.	☐	☐	☐
4. Draw the exact amount of medication needed for one eye into the eyedropper.	☐	☐	☐
5. Hold the dropper close to but not touching the eye.	☐	☐	☐
6. Expose the lower conjunctival sac.	☐	☐	☐
7. Instill the drops into the center of the conjunctival sac. RATIONALE: To avoid having the drops fall on cornea, which is an unpleasant feeling and could damage the cornea.	☐	☐	☐
8. Ask the patient to close the eyes gently and not to squeeze the lids shut. Let the patient blink a few times before instilling more drops in the same eye.	☐	☐	☐
9. If the drug has possible toxic systemic effects, gently press on the inner canthus for 10 to 15 seconds. RATIONALE: Pressure here will prevent the drug from entering the lacrimal duct and being absorbed systemically.	☐	☐	☐
10. For the second eye, repeat steps 4 through 9.	☐	☐	☐
11. Observe the patient and assist the patient out of position.	☐	☐	☐
12. Document the administration on the record shown here.	☐	☐	☐

*V = Value, to fill in if assigning points or other specific values to each step, or if designating a critical step.
S = Satisfactory completion of the step.
U = Unsatisfactory completion of the step, or step incomplete; needs more practice.

13. Verify that the patient can see clearly before letting him or her leave the office. ☐ ☐ ☐

DATE			SUBSEQUENT VISITS AND FINDINGS	B.P.	WGT.
MO.	DAY	YR.			

Date: _____ Competency achieved: Y _____ N _____

Designated reasonable time standard: _____

Actual completion time: _____

Terminal Performance Objective/Competency

Procedure 8–3: Prepare a Medication for Injection

EQUIPMENT	Stock of sterile syringe-needle units Two cottonballs Alcohol 70 percent	Vial sodium chloride (isotonic) Medical record with order: Rx: Sodium chloride 0.5 ml SC for a 24-yr-old, 125-lb patient.

REVIEW   Techniques to be followed (with rationales) for every injectable medication you prepare, this chapter and Table 8–2.

Terminal Performance Objective: Prepare an ordered amount of sterile injectable solution by completing each step accurately and in the correct order without a break in sterile technique and within reasonable job production time.

V   S   U*

PROCEDURAL STEPS   Wash hands and check medication expiration date.

1. Use sterile technique: Touch only the barrel, the flared portion of the plunger, and the outside of the needle cap. Do not touch the vial's rubber stopper.   ☐ ☐ ☐

2. Select the needle gauge and length according to the route desired, the patient's weight (amount of fatty tissue), and the thickness of the medication.   ☐ ☐ ☐

3. Select the syringe size according to the amount of medication to be prepared.   ☐ ☐ ☐

4. Gather the alcohol (as antiseptic), two cottonballs, and written order for the medication.   ☐ ☐ ☐

5. Take the medication from the shelf and compare the medication name and strength (dose) with that on the order.   ☐ ☐ ☐

6. Inspect the medication for quality; then mix the medication by rotating the vial.   ☐ ☐ ☐

7. Clean the rubber-stoppered vial with alcohol and the first cottonball, using a firm circular motion.   ☐ ☐ ☐

8. Pull back the plunger to the milliliter or minim line that marks the amount of medication to be withdrawn into the syringe, without removing the needle cap.   ☐ ☐ ☐

9. Remove the needle cap and, without putting it down or in any other way contaminating cap or needle, insert the needle through the rubber stopper.   ☐ ☐ ☐

10. Inject the air into the vial.   ☐ ☐ ☐

---

*V = Value, to fill in if assigning points or other specific values to each step, or if designating a critical step.
S = Satisfactory completion of the step.
U = Unsatisfactory completion of the step, or step incomplete; needs more practice.

11. Turn the vial upside down and slowly withdraw the medication into the syringe.

     RATIONALE: Withdrawing the medication too quickly causes a "fizzing" effect, which results in air bubbles forming in the syringe.   ☐ ☐ ☐

12. Draw up a little more of the medication than the amount ordered.   ☐ ☐ ☐

13. Tap the syringe to dislodge any air bubbles formed. They should all float to the top (the hub area).   ☐ ☐ ☐

14. Eject the medication back into the vial until you have the exact amount of milliliters or minims ordered.   ☐ ☐ ☐

15. If you ejected too far and must again withdraw more medication into the syringe, repeat steps 11 through 13.   ☐ ☐ ☐

16. Read the medication label, compare it with the order, and confirm that you are using the correct medication.   ☐ ☐ ☐

17. Remove the syringe from the vial and immediately replace the cap on the needle, without touching the sides of the cap or in any other way contaminating the needle.   ☐ ☐ ☐

18. Read the medication label and order a third time, then replace the medication back on the shelf.   ☐ ☐ ☐

19. Saturate the second cottonball with alcohol in readiness for administration.   ☐ ☐ ☐

Date: _____ Competency achieved: Y _____ N _____

Designated reasonable time standard: _____

Actual completion time: _____

Terminal Performance Objective/Competency

Procedure 8–4: Administer a Subcutaneous Injection, Deltoid Region

EQUIPMENT	Stock of sterile syringe–needle units Two cottonballs Gloves Alcohol 70 percent Vial sodium chloride (isotonic)

Rigid sharps container
Medical record with order: Rx: Sodium chloride
   0.5 ml SC, deltoid region for a 30-yr-old,
   210-lb patient.

REVIEW   Techniques to be followed (with rationales) for every injectable medication you administer, this chapter and Table 8–3.

Terminal Performance Objective: Administer an ordered amount of a sterile injectable solution by completing each step accurately and in the correct order, without a break in sterile technique and within reasonable job production time.

	V	S	U*

PROCEDURAL STEPS   Wash hands and check medication expiration date.

	V	S	U
1. Visually reinspect your equipment.	☐	☐	☐
2. Greet the patient and verify the patient's name. Ask the patient, "Do you have any allergies to food or drugs?"	☐	☐	☐
3. Explain the procedure to the patient.	☐	☐	☐
4. Position the patient to reduce strain on the part to be used.	☐	☐	☐
5. Identify and palpate the body site to be used. RATIONALE: To be sure that the site is not tender or becomes firm when grasped.	☐	☐	☐
6. Cleanse the site thoroughly using 70 percent alcohol, in a circular motion from the site point outward.	☐	☐	☐
7. Talk to the patient or otherwise divert the patient's attention.	☐	☐	☐
8. Grasp the tissues of the deltoid region and hold between your fingers (see Fig. 8–7 inset).	☐	☐	☐
9. Insert the needle at a 45- to 90-degree angle, with the beveled tip upward, leaving 1/8″ of the needle shaft above the skin. RATIONALE: Should a needle break off at the hub, it can be retrieved by the shaft exposed above the skin.	☐	☐	☐
10. Insert needle swiftly. Use a motion much like that of throwing a dart. Keep your hand close to the site to steady the needle.	☐	☐	☐
11. Release the tissues and pull back enough with the plunger to see if blood can be drawn into the syringe (except for heparin and insulin).	☐	☐	☐

*V = Value, to fill in if assigning points or other specific values to each step, or if designating a critical step.
  S = Satisfactory completion of the step.
  U = Unsatisfactory completion of the step, or step incomplete; needs more practice.

12. If blood appears in the syringe, withdraw and discard the entire unit. Start again with uncontaminated materials.
    or
    If no blood appears in the syringe, deposit the medication slowly to allow the tissue to adjust to the volume of drug being deposited.   ☐ ☐ ☐

13. Keep the needle motionless in the tissues while you inject the medication.
    RATIONALE: If moved, the needle may enter a blood vessel after aspiration.   ☐ ☐ ☐

14. Withdraw the syringe quickly and dispose of it immediately into a rigid sharps container. Do not recap the needle.   ☐ ☐ ☐

15. Briskly rub the area, unless contraindicated.   ☐ ☐ ☐

16. Observe the patient for adverse reactions and assist the patient out of position.   ☐ ☐ ☐

17. Record the administration and the site used on the patient's chart shown below.   ☐ ☐ ☐

18. Document patient teaching on the chart.   ☐ ☐ ☐

DATE			SUBSEQUENT VISITS AND FINDINGS	B.P.	WGT.
MO.	DAY	YR.			

Date: _____   Competency achieved: Y _____   N _____

Designated reasonable time standard: _____

Actual completion time: _____

Terminal Performance Objective/Competency

Procedure 8–5: Administer an Intramuscular Injection, Vastus Lateralis Region

EQUIPMENT

Stock of sterile syringe–needle units
Two cottonballs
Alcohol 70 percent
Gloves
Vial sodium chloride (isotonic)

Rigid sharps container
Medical record with order: Rx: Sodium chloride 0.5 ml IM, vastus lateralis region for an 18-yr-old, 120-lb patient.

REVIEW

Techniques to be followed (with rationales) for every injectable medication you administer, this chapter and Table 8–3.

Terminal Performance Objective: Administer an ordered amount of a sterile injectable solution by completing each step accurately, safely, and in the correct order, without a break in sterile technique and within reasonable job production time.

	V	S	U*

PROCEDURAL STEPS

Wash hands and check medication expiration date.

	V	S	U
1. Visually reinspect your equipment.	☐	☐	☐
2. Greet the patient and verify the patient's name. Ask the patient, "Do you have any allergies to food or drugs?"	☐	☐	☐
3. Explain the procedure.	☐	☐	☐
4. Position the patient to reduce strain on the part to be used.	☐	☐	☐
5. Identify and palpate the body site to be used. RATIONALE: To be sure that the site is not tender or becomes firm when grasped.	☐	☐	☐
6. Cleanse the site thoroughly using 70 percent alcohol, in a circular motion from the site point outward.	☐	☐	☐
7. Talk to the patient or otherwise divert the patient's attention.	☐	☐	☐
8. Mentally map out the vastus lateralis landmarks (see Fig. 8–9).	☐	☐	☐
9. Stretch the tissues at the site. RATIONALE: Stretching the skin will make the skin taut, facilitating needle insertion. For thin adults and children, when there is not sufficient muscle to spread, the muscle must be grasped to increase the amount of penetrable muscle mass. For obese patients, a combination of stretching *and* grasping may be required.	☐	☐	☐

*V = Value, to fill in if assigning points or other specific values to each step, or if designating a critical step.
S = Satisfactory completion of the step.
U = Unsatisfactory completion of the step, or step incomplete; needs more practice.

10. Insert the needle at a 90-degree angle just to the hilt, with the beveled tip upward, leaving 1/8″ of the needle shaft above the skin.
    RATIONALE: Should the needle break off at the hub, it can be retrieved by the shaft exposed above the skin. ☐ ☐ ☐

11. Insert needle swiftly. Use a motion much like that of throwing a dart. Keep your hand close to the site to steady the needle. ☐ ☐ ☐

12. Release the tissues and pull back enough with the plunger to see if blood can be drawn into the syringe. ☐ ☐ ☐

13. If blood appears in the syringe, withdraw and discard the entire unit. Start again with uncontaminated materials.
    or
    If no blood appears in the syringe, deposit the medication slowly to allow the tissue to adjust to the volume of drug being deposited. ☐ ☐ ☐

14. Keep the needle motionless in the tissues while you inject the medication.
    RATIONALE: If moved, the needle may enter a blood vessel after aspiration. ☐ ☐ ☐

15. Withdraw the syringe quickly and dispose of it immediately into a rigid sharps container. Do not recap the needle. ☐ ☐ ☐

16. Briskly rub the area, unless contraindicated. ☐ ☐ ☐

17. Observe the patient and assist the patient out of position. ☐ ☐ ☐

18. Record the administration and the site used on the patient's chart shown below. ☐ ☐ ☐

19. Document any patient teaching on the chart. ☐ ☐ ☐

DATE			SUBSEQUENT VISITS AND FINDINGS	B.P.	WGT.
MO.	DAY	YR.			

Date: _____ Competency achieved: Y _____ N _____

Designated reasonable time standard: _____

Actual completion time: _____

Terminal Performance Objective/Competency

Procedure 8–6: Administer Z-Tract Intramuscular Injection, Ventrogluteal Region

EQUIPMENT

Stock of sterile syringe–needle units
Two cottonballs
Alcohol 70 percent
Vial sodium chloride (isotonic)
Gloves

Rigid sharps container
Medical record with order: Rx: Sodium chloride 0.5 ml IM, Z-tract, ventrogluteal region for a 20-yr-old, 130-lb patient.

REVIEW

Techniques to be followed (with rationales) for every injectable medication you administer, this chapter and Table 8–3.

Terminal Performance Objective: Administer an ordered amount of a sterile injectable solution by completing each step accurately, safely, and in the correct order, without a break in sterile technique and within reasonable job production time.

	V	S	U*

PROCEDURAL STEPS

Wash hands and check medication expiration date.

	V	S	U
1. Visually reinspect your equipment.	☐	☐	☐
2. Greet the patient and verify the patient's name. Ask the patient, "Do you have any allergies to food or drugs?"	☐	☐	☐
3. Explain the procedure.	☐	☐	☐
4. Position the patient to reduce strain on the part to be used.	☐	☐	☐
5. Identify and palpate the body site to be used. RATIONALE: To be sure that the site is not tender or becomes firm when grasped.	☐	☐	☐
6. Cleanse the site thoroughly using 70 percent alcohol, in a circular motion from the site point outward.	☐	☐	☐
7. Talk to the patient or otherwise divert the patient's attention.	☐	☐	☐
8. Mentally map out the ventrogluteal landmarks (see Fig. 8–10).	☐	☐	☐
9. Stretch the tissues at the site. RATIONALE: The gluteal muscles are more difficult to grasp and there is a thinner layer of subcutaneous tissue than at other sites. The muscle mass is usually sufficient for stretching.	☐	☐	☐
10. Insert the needle at a 90-degree angle just to the hilt, with the beveled tip upward and angled slightly toward the iliac crest. Leave 1/8″ of the needle shaft above the skin. RATIONALE: Should the needle break off at the hub, it can be retrieved by the shaft exposed above the skin.	☐	☐	☐

*V = Value, to fill in if assigning points or other specific values to each step, or if designating a critical step.
S = Satisfactory completion of the step.
U = Unsatisfactory completion of the step, or step incomplete; needs more practice.

11. Insert needle swiftly. Use a motion much like that of throwing a dart. Keep your hand close to the site to steady the needle. □ □ □

12. Release the tissues and pull back enough with the plunger to see if blood can be drawn into the syringe. □ □ □

13. If blood appears in the syringe, withdraw and discard the entire unit. Start again with uncontaminated materials.
    or
    If no blood appears in the syringe, deposit the medication slowly to allow the tissue to adjust to the volume of drug being deposited. □ □ □

14. Keep the needle motionless in the tissues while you inject the medication.
    RATIONALE: If moved, the needle may enter a blood vessel after aspiration. □ □ □

15. Withdraw the syringe quickly and dispose of it immediately into a rigid sharps container. □ □ □

16. Observe the patient and assist the patient out of position. □ □ □

17. Record the administration and the site used on the patient's chart shown below. □ □ □

18. Document any patient teaching on the chart. □ □ □

DATE			SUBSEQUENT VISITS AND FINDINGS	B.P.	WGT.
MO.	DAY	YR.			

Date: _____ Competency achieved: Y _____ N _____

Designated reasonable time standard: _____

Actual completion time: _____

Terminal Performance Objective/Competency

Procedure 8–7: Administer a Tuberculin Test

EQUIPMENT	Tuberculin test vial, 0.1 ml of PPD (5TU)
	Tuberculin syringe with 26-gauge or 27-gauge
	  needle
	Cottonball
	Acetone or alcohol
		Gloves
		Rigid sharps container
		Medical record with order: Rx: Tuberculin
		  Mantoux test

REVIEW   Techniques to be followed (with rationales) for ID testing, this chapter.

Terminal Performance Objective: Administer a tuberculin skin test to form a wheal by completing each step accurately, safely, and in the correct order, without a break in sterile technique and within reasonable job production time.

	V	S	U*
PROCEDURAL STEPS Wash hands and check for expiration dates.			
1. Visually reinspect your equipment.	☐	☐	☐
2. Greet the patient and verify the patient's name. Ask the patient, "Do you have any allergies to food or drugs?"	☐	☐	☐
3. Explain the procedure.	☐	☐	☐
4. Position the patient to expose the volar surface of the forearm, about 4″ below the bend of the elbow.	☐	☐	☐
5. Identify and palpate the body site to be used. RATIONALE: To be sure that the site is not tender or becomes firm when grasped.	☐	☐	☐
6. Cleanse the site thoroughly using acetone, in a circular motion from the site point outward. Allow the surface to dry.	☐	☐	☐
7. Talk to the patient or otherwise divert the patient's attention.	☐	☐	☐
8. Mentally map out the hairless anterior surface of the forearm, 4 in below the elbow.	☐	☐	☐
9. Stretch the tissues at the site.	☐	☐	☐
10. Insert the needle, bevel upward, just beneath the surface of the skin and inject the 0.1 ml of Tuberculin, PPD.	☐	☐	☐
11. A wheal 6 mm to 10 mm in diameter should appear if the injection has been performed properly.	☐	☐	☐
12. Dispose of the needle and syringe unit immediately into a rigid sharps container.	☐	☐	☐
13. Do not rub the area. The wheal will usually disappear within minutes. No dressing is required.	☐	☐	☐

*V = Value, to fill in if assigning points or other specific values to each step, or if designating a critical step.
 S = Satisfactory completion of the step.
 U = Unsatisfactory completion of the step, or step incomplete; needs more practice.

14. Observe the patient and assist the patient out of position. □ □ □

15. Instruct the patient to return to the office for a reading in 48 to 72 hours, or teach the patient how to read the test at home and call in the results. □ □ □

16. Record the administration and the site used on the patient's chart shown here. □ □ □

| DATE | | | SUBSEQUENT VISITS AND FINDINGS | B.P. | WGT. |
MO.	DAY	YR.			

Date: _____ Competency achieved: Y _____ N _____

Designated reasonable time standard: _____

Actual completion time: _____

Assignment 8–1: Use Appendix A, the *PDR*, or Other Reference to Create Drug Information Guides

EQUIPMENT Appendix A; *PDR;* or other drug reference
Lined notepaper or index cards
Drugs: From Top 50 Most Commonly Prescribed, those ranked 41st–50th.

Performance Competence: Complete a drug guide for each of the drugs listed under Equipment. The ten guides should be completed with 100 percent accuracy and must include the following:

Generic name _____

Brand name_____

Classification _____

Controlled substance classification _____

Pregnancy risk category _____

Action _____

Indications/use_____

Contraindications _____

Adverse reactions/side effects _____

Dosage/Route _____

Patient education (in terms the patient will understand) _____

Special alert _____

Drugs Commonly Administered or Prescribed in the Medical Office

Pulmonary and Upper Respiratory Preparations
  Antihistamines
  Antitussives and Expectorants
  Bronchodilators
  Decongestants
Gastrointestinal Drugs
  Antacids
  Antidiarrheal drugs
  Antiemetric drugs
  Antiulcer beta-histamine (H_2) blockers
  Helicobacter pylori treatments
  Laxatives
Neurologic Drugs
  Alzheimer's agents
  Anticonvulsants
  Antimigraine drugs
  Antipsychotic drugs
  Antidepressants
  Parkinsonian Agents

WRITTEN COMPETENCY 9–1: Apply Drug Information to the Assessment of the Patient in the Clinical Setting

TERMINAL PERFORMANCE OBJECTIVE/COMPETENCY (PROCEDURE 9–1): Teach a Patient to Administer Insulin

OBJECTIVES   **WRITTEN COMPETENCY 9–1:** Apply drug information to the assessment of the patient in the clinical setting.

TERMINAL PERFORMANCE OBJECTIVE (PROCEDURE 9–1): Teach a patient to administer insulin.

Each medical facility stocks drugs and other pharmaceutic agents that are administered on a regular basis. Drug company representatives visit medical practices periodically to supply updated information on drugs being used, to inform the physician about new drugs, and to offer sample medications for physicians to use in patient care, either for administration in the office or as starter doses for the patients to use at home. It is common for a particular practice to stock 20 to 30 drugs that may be used in the day-to-day treatment of patients. Some emergency care centers may stock even more. This chapter discusses a *sampling* of drugs that may be encountered in a general or family practice. The sampling includes basic emergency drugs, products for immunization, pain medications, antibiotics, and local anesthetics.

Drug Samples

Pharmaceutical companies provide physicians with product samples. Samples should be stored in a secure area not accessible to patients and the general public. The area should be locked when not in use. Because regulations for over-the-counter (OTC) samples are minimal, the physician may determine the method of dispensing OCT drugs. The physician should not charge the patient for them, however. With regard to product samples available only by prescription, there are a number of rules to follow.

1. The physician must sign for the receipt of product samples. The office staff may not sign for samples.
2. The drug company representative may not remove samples from the office once the physician signs for them.

3. It is the responsibility of the office staff to ensure that samples are not outdated.
4. Prescription samples must be considered the same as a purchased prescription. A note is placed in the patient's chart each time a sample medication is given.
5. The office staff may not use prescription samples without the authorization of the physician.
6. Sample drugs may not be repackaged.
7. The patient may not be charged for sample drugs.
8. Drug company representatives do not handle narcotic samples. Narcotic samples are shipped directly to and signed for by the physician.

Office Dispensing Systems

Many medical facilities are including pharmacy services. Some large practices hire pharmacists to operate limited pharmacies on site. Other practices that are satellites of corporately owned medical centers often repackage and stock frequently prescribed medications. A licensed pharmacist employed by the corporation does this.

Each stock prescription is labeled with the center's name and the necessary directions for patient usage. A patient may choose to have a prescription filled at an independent pharmacy or at the time of the office visit. This service can be very convenient for patients.

Drugs stocked for on-site dispensing may be generic or brand name drugs. Arrangements are made with insurance companies to reimburse patients in the same way as the insurance plan would reimburse the independent pharmacy. The medical assistant may be responsible for completing the patient's information on the label, ordering and inventorying stock, processing payments, and submitting claims for insurance reimbursement.

Emergency Drugs

Emergency drugs are needed to treat mild to moderate allergic reactions or shock. There are five classifications of circulatory shock: low-volume (hypovolemic) shock; cardiogenic shock; septic shock; allergic shock (anaphylaxis); and neurogenic shock. Every drug inventory will include emergency drugs. An emergency kit or cart must be stocked with fresh supplies and must be quickly accessible. Emergency supplies include tourniquets and ice packs for delaying further absorption of drugs or allergens from injection sites; endotracheal tubes and a tracheotomy set for maintaining an open airway; oxygen; needles and syringes; and emergency drugs, such as antihistamines, epinephrine, ephedrine, aminophylline, and corticosteroids. Table 9–1 summarizes general treatments used in emergencies.

TREATMENT FOR MILD TO MODERATE ALLERGIC REACTIONS

Mild to moderate allergic reactions may result from patient exposure to certain drugs, to household chemicals, or to toxins such as poison ivy or jellyfish stings. Atopic (inherited) allergies such as hay fever and bee stings affect approximately 10 percent of the population and are also often treated in the medical office.

℞ Common Corticosteroids (generic name: Tradename)

cortisone acetone: Cortone	prednisone: Deltasone, Orasone
dexamethasone: Decadron	prednisolone: Delta Cortef
fludrocortisone acetate: Florinef	methylprednisolone: Medrol, Solu-Medrol, Depo-Medrol
hydrocortisone: Cortef, Hydrocortone, Solu-Cortef	triamcinolone: Aristocort, Kenacort, Kenalog

---

℞ **Common Antihistamines (generic name: Tradename, *Over-the-Counter*)**

brompheniramine: *Dimetane*	dimenhydrinate: *Dramamine*
chlorpheniramine: Chlor-Trimeton	ephenhydramine: Benadryl
clemastine: *Tavist*	hydroxyzine: Atarax, Vistaril
cyproheptadine: *Periactin*	promethazine: *Phenergan*

Long-term treatment of allergic reactions begins with a thorough patient history and documentation in the patient record of known or suspected allergies; but when a patient presents with these conditions in the medical office, certain emergency drugs such as antihistamines, epinephrine, and corticosteroids first may be necessary for immediate treatment.

Mild to moderate allergic reactions include acute and *chronic urticarias* (hives, nettle rash), *contact dermatitis, atopic (chronic) dermatitis*, and *angioneurotic edema*. Most often, oral antihistamines are used to control these symptoms, along with local applications of cold and topical medications to relieve itching and soothe the skin. Among the oral antihistamines that are most effective are those that also have a strong sedative effect, such as diphenhydramine (Benadryl). Other drugs used to treat acute skin reactions include hydroxyzine (Atarax, Vistaril), which combines an antihistamine with a mild tranquilizer.

Chronic dermatitis may sometimes be treated with antihistamines, but topically applied corticosteroid drugs are usually the treatment of choice. Here, the relief of itching is controlled by antipruritic action rather than by antihistaminic action. Anesthetics may be used to treat acute urticarias and dermatitis may be treated with anesthetics. Anesthetics are not recommended for long-term use in cases of chronic dermatitis because allergy-prone patients may become sensitized to the anesthetic. Thus, drugs that contain both an antihistamine and an antipruritic, such as cyprotheptadine (Periactin), are most effective when given orally.

Angioneurotic edema affects the subcutaneous (SC) tissues rather than the skin and is marked by fluid accumulation and sometimes giant hives. Typical sites of eruption include the eyelids, lips, hands, feet, and, less often, genitalia. Because giant hives erupt quickly and can involve the tissues of larynx and cause asphyxia, angioedema should be quickly prevented or treated with SC injections of epinephrine, as is described under anaphylactic shock.

> **PATIENT EDUCATION: •** Every patient with known allergies should be thoroughly instructed about the nature of the allergy and taught what actions to take in the case of an allergic reaction. **•** Patients with atopic allergies should be instructed to wear medical alert jewelry at all times. **•** Any patient with a history of severe systemic reaction to an allergen should be prescribed an emergency kit containing diphenhydramine (Benadryl), a syringe and needle, and a vial of epinephrine. **•** Patients who have received injections of penicillin, other drugs known to cause hypersensitivity, or allergenic extracts must be kept under observation for 20 to 30 minutes before being allowed to leave the office or clinic.

TREATMENT FOR CIRCULATORY SHOCK CONDITIONS

As stated earlier, there are five types of circulatory shock. Shock is the sudden disturbance of circulation, characterized by hypotension, coldness of the skin, tachycardia, and anxiety. Untreated, shock can be fatal. Certain drugs may be useful (or contraindicated) in each case.

Hypovolemic shock results from blood loss due to internal or external injury. The treatment for hypovolemic shock is emergency first aid and the replacement of lost blood, when applicable. The use of drugs in the early stages of treatment is usually *contraindicated*.

Allergic (anaphylactic) shock, although rare, may occur in the medical office after the injection of certain medications. In this type of allergic reaction, the blood vessels and respiratory tissues are directly affected by the allergic reactions. Within minutes, the patient's blood pressure falls and severe difficulty in breathing develops. Left unattended, sudden death will result.

TABLE 9–1. **General Treatments for Emergencies**

	Mild to Moderate Allergy	Angioedema	Hypovolemic Shock	Anaphylactic Shock	Septic Shock	Cardiogenic Shock	Neurogenic Shock
Condition	Hives, rash	Temporary edema, giant hives	Hemorrhage	Life-threatening allergic reactions	Severe bacterial infections	Myocardial infarction, heart failure, arrhythmia	Fainting
Drugs	Oral antihistamines, topical soothing creams	Vasoconstrictors	Contraindicated	Bronchodilators, sometimes vasoconstrictors	Antibiotics, steroids, vasoconstrictors	Adrenergic vasopressors, antianxiety agents, analgesics, anticoagulants	Contraindicated
Physical treatment	Cold application	Cold application	First-aid, volume expanders	Maintain airway, oxygen, volume expanders	Maintain airway, oxygen, volume expanders	Immediate hospitalization, oxygen, volume expanders	Keep safe, head lower than body
Rx	Benadryl, Atarax, Vistaril, cortisone creams	Epinephrine 1 : 1000	Contraindicated	Epinephrine 1 : 1000	Carbenicillin, hydrocortisone	Varies	None

---

℞ Common Volume Expanders (generic name: Tradename, *Over-the-Counter*)

albumin: Albuminar

cryoprecipitate

dextran: D5W, D5

packed red blood cells: PRBC

plasma protein fraction: Plasmanate

hetastarch: Hespan

hypertonic saline: 2% saline, 3% saline

lactate Ringer's: LR

normal saline 0.9%: NS (contains sodium/chlorine), NS w/Potassium

parenteral nutrition: TPN (total parenteral nutrition)

pediatric rehydration: *Lytren, Pedialyte, Rehydrate, Resol*

Localized, mild anaphylaxis involving the skin can be treated with antihistamines, local cold to minimize swelling, and topical medications to soothe the skin. These reactions should be watched closely for at least 30 minutes, as they may escalate into a systemic response.

Systemic anaphylaxis involves generalized itching, swelling, and urticaria of the skin or mucous membranes, or both, and progresses to impair respiration owing to bronchospasm and laryngeal edema. In these cases, the airway must be maintained and supplemental oxygen provided.

In severe anaphylaxis, the drug of choice is epinephrine, administered subcutaneously, sublingually, or intravenously. Epinephrine acts as a bronchodilator, relieves laryngeal spasm, and elevates blood pressure. Epinephrine 1 : 1000 solution is usually administered in a dose of 0.3 ml, and the injection site is massaged to increase absorption. Injections may be repeated every 15 to 30 minutes during the first hour of treatment and less frequently during subsequent hours. Patients who have suffered *vascular collapse*, however, may not respond to epinephrine. Vasoconstrictors must be used only briefly and in as small a dose as possible, however, because they increase the blood flow to the brain and heart only at the expense of the other organs, especially the kidneys.

Steroid therapy may be started to counteract further the affects of histamine. Steroids act as anti-inflammatory agents that prevent further release of histamine chemicals. Further supportive measures include giving intravenous fluids, plasma, and drugs to increase or maintain blood pressure.

Septic shock results from a severe bacterial infection that spreads systemically and releases bacterial toxins that impair the muscular functioning of the blood vessels. Septic shock resulting from gram-negative bacteria is being recognized with increasing frequency. The treatment for septic shock is the same as for anaphylactic shock, but includes massive doses of antimicrobials (antibiotics) in addition to the first measures of shock treatment. Patients seriously ill with life-threatening infections may be treated with steroids to suppress possible hypersensitivity to the antimicrobials being administered.

Cardiogenic shock results from a failure of the heart to function properly as a pump, possibly resulting from myocardial infarction (heart attack), severe heart failure, and severe arrhythmias. Cardiogenic shock is treated with adrenergic vasopressor drugs and life support measures. Because no single drug is ideal in all types of shock syndromes, each specific case must be individually assessed before the correct emergency measure is ordered. Adrenergic drugs used in cardiogenic shock are administered intravenously; in general, patients in cardiogenic shock should not receive drugs by intramuscular (IM) or SC routes.

Because time is a critical factor in cardiogenic shock, patients should be transported to

---

℞ Common Vasopressors (generic name: Tradename)

dobutamine HCl: Dobutrex

dopamine HCl: Dopastat, Intropin

ephedrine

epinephrine: Adrenaline chloride

isoproterenol HCl: Isuprel

norepinephrine: Levophed, Levarterenol barbiturate

phenylephrine HCl: Neo Synephrine (IV)

---

the emergency room of a hospital as soon as possible. Drugs used on admission will include drugs for anxiety and pain (such as morphine), anticoagulants, and oxygen.

Neurogenic shock, the sudden disturbance of mental equilibrium, may be caused by severe pain, trauma, anxiety, sudden frights, or various other strong stimuli that overtax the nervous system. The most usual manifestation of this type of shock is fainting. Emergency measures include placing the patient's head lower than the body and keeping the patient comfortable. *Spirits of ammonia (or ammonium capsules) are no longer recommended* as an inhalant to revive a patient who has fainted. Spirits of ammonia provides only a noxious odor and has no medical value. In mild cases, drug therapy is usually contraindicated; the patient is kept safe and allowed to recover naturally. Pain medications may be used to treat the symptoms causing the neurogenic shock, and if the anxiety or fear is suspected to continue for a long time, antianxiety, sedative, or hypnotic drugs may be administered.

Fluid Replacement Therapy

The regulation of the amount of water in the body is necessary to sustain life. This balance is upset when fluids are lost or not enough fluids are taken in. Fluid deficits may occur due to physiological reasons, such as dehydration following heat exposure, exercise, or failing to drink enough fluids. Serious body fluid loss can occur in disease states (e.g., diabetic ketosis, acute respiratory distress syndrome, or chronic renal failure). More often, body fluids are lost due to severe vomiting and diarrhea, bleeding, or septic shock.

ELECTROLYTES

Electrolytes are ionized salts in the blood, tissue fluids, and cells. The major electrolytes include sodium (Na), potassium (K), chloride (Cl), and bicarbonate (HCO_3). These four major electrolytes are usually tested together, since changes in the concentration of one of them are almost always accompanied by changes in the concentration of one or more of the others. The other electrolytes include calcium (Ca), magnesium (Mg), sulfate (SO_4), and phosphate (PO_4). The kidneys and lungs are the organs that furnish most control over the body's electrolyte concentration. When body fluids are lost, it naturally follows that the electrolyte balance in the plasma, interstitial fluids, and intercellular fluids also will be disrupted.

FLUID AND ELECTROLYTE BALANCE

Fluid balance is determined by measuring the amount of intake and output, abbreviated *I/O*, of fluids. The total fluids taken in by mouth or given by intravenous solutions are measured against the amount of urine voided in the same period:

Intake	1500 cc
Output	1200 cc
I/O Balance	300 cc

A fluid balance is desirable. If the balance is a positive number, the fluid balance is said to be "positive." If the output subtracted from the input is a negative number, the balance is said to be "negative." A large positive balance is an indication that fluids are being retained, due to excess salt in the body or disease; during intravenous fluid therapy, it could be an indication of fluid "overload." Electrolyte balance is determined by a group of laboratory tests called an *electrolyte panel*, consisting of measurement of levels of sodium, potassium, chloride, and bicarbonate. These tests are usually performed using plasma or serum.

The goal of fluid therapy is therefore twofold: (1) to correct fluid depletion in the body, and (2) to correct the electrolyte imbalance. The oral route is the preferred replacement route. Examples include forcing fluids, or having patients drink Gatorade or Pedialyte. Flu-

TABLE 9–2. **Intravenous Fluid Replacement Composition**

Type	*Use*	*Examples*
Isotonic	Isotonic to body fluids, used to replenish body water in dehydration, restoring blood volume during shock or hemorrhage; irrigating mucous membranes and wounds	Normal saline (NS), consisting of 0.9% sodium chloride in distilled water: 1 tsp. table salt in 1 pint water
Hypotonic		Less than 0.9% saline
Hypertonic		NaCl 2%, NaCl 3%
Crystalloid additives	Electrolyte replacement	Sodium, potassium, chloride, calcium, KCl
Colloid (osmolar) additives	Plasma volume expander	Glucose, protein, starch, D5W, Ringer's lactated
Synthetic plasma volume expanders	Plasma volume expander	Dextran, hetastarch
Blood products	Restoring blood components of blood volume during shock or hemorrhage, anemia	Packed red blood cells (PRBCs), fresh frozen plasma (FFP), whole blood

ids may be replaced using the intravenous, subcutaneous, or intraperitoneal routes as well. Of these three, the intravenous route is used most often (Table 9–2).

Immunizations

One aspect of general, family, and pediatric practices is the primary immunization of children and administration of immunologic products to adolescents and adults at risk of serious infections. Although some people are born with the innate ability to resist infections, most people are not immune to common infectious diseases. People therefore *acquire* the ability to resist infectious diseases.

Immunity is classified as either *active* or *passive*. Active immunity is produced by the body's ability to produce immune antibodies in response to viruses and bacteria. Immune antibodies remain and circulate in the gamma globulin fraction of blood serum, ready to fight off infection at any time. This response is usually produced in a person by actually having had a clinical or subclinical case of the infection or by artificially being exposed to the same infectious organisms through immunization—that is, being inoculated with a vaccine or toxoid.

Immunity introduced through inoculation may last a lifetime, especially if the immunization is produced by a primary series of injections, and then reinforced through booster inoculations to restimulate effective levels of antibody response. The routine use of immunizations has reduced the mortality rates of diphtheria, tetanus, measles, mumps, rubella (German measles), whooping cough (pertussis), influenza, and poliomyelitis almost to the vanishing point in this country, and some infections (such as smallpox) have virtually been eliminated worldwide. Other immune products such as those for rabies, typhoid, paratyphoid, influenza, hepatitis B, pneumonia, yellow fever, and plague are now widely used for high-risk populations, and new vaccines continue to be produced each year.

Oral or injected antigenic products for producing active immunity are either of the vaccine type or of the toxoid type. *Vaccines* are made from the organisms that cause the disease, usually viruses and bacteria. They may be either "killed" (chemically inactivated) or "live, attenuated" (alive but reduced in their potency). Vaccines are relatively safe because they are strong enough to stimulate antibody production but too weak to cause the actual disease. Live, attenuated vaccines are no more dangerous than killed vaccines, the former can pro-

> ## ℞ Immunizations (generic name: Tradename)
>
> | | |
> |---|---|
> | diphtheria–tetanus toxoid (DT) (children <7 yrs) | measles, mumps, and rubella vaccine: M-M-R II |
> | diphtheria–tetanus toxoid (Td) (children >7 yrs) | measles and rubella vaccine (MR) |
> | diphtheria–tetanus–pertussis (DTP) | mumps vaccine |
> | diphtheria, tetanus, and acellular pertussis vaccine (DTaP): Acel-Imune | pneumococcal vaccine: Pneumovax |
> | | poliovirus trivalent vaccine (OPV) (Sabin): Orimune |
> | diphtheria, tetanus, and whole cell pertussis vaccine (DTwP): | rabies vaccine: Imovax |
> | haemophilus B conjugate vaccine: ProHIBiT, HibTITER, PedvaxHIB | tetanus toxoid (adsorbed) |
> | | tetanus toxoid (fluid) |
> | hepatitis A vaccine: Havrix | tuberculin PPD: Tubersol |
> | hepatitis B vaccine: Engerix-B, Recombivax HB | varicella vaccine: Varivax |
> | influenza vaccine: Fluogen, Fluzone, Fluvirin | yellow fever vaccine: YF-Vax |

duce immunity after a single dose, whereas the latter usually have to be administered in a series of doses at appropriately spaced intervals. Both types may require periodic booster doses to keep antibodies at protective levels.

Vaccines may be grown in artificial media or in animal media such as chick or duck embryos or horse serum. Those grown in artificial media are safer because they are free of secondary foreign animal proteins that might cause allergic reactions. In addition, some vaccines are packaged with a small amount of antimicrobial as a preservative. It is important to know the components of every vaccine administered and to question each patient about a history of immediate-type (anaphylactoid) reactions to any of the components of vaccines.

Toxins are the gaseous substances secreted by micro-organisms. In organisms of this type it is the toxin that causes disease. Toxins are attenuated and manufactured as *toxoids*. The length of toxoid effectiveness (immunity) may be enhanced by adsorbing a toxoid with chemicals such as aluminum hydroxide or aluminum phosphate. Adsorbed toxoids remain in human tissues longer, providing long-term immunity. Because of this partial insolubility, however, toxoids tend to cause local reactions, such as redness (erythema), hardness (induration), swelling, and pain. Toxoid reactions may be more pronounced in adolescents and adults; therefore, older patients are often started on smaller amounts of toxoids than are infants and young children. Table 9–3 is the schedule for initial immunization. Table 9–4 is a sample immunization checklist.

Products for Passive Immunity

Passive immunity is immunity that is "borrowed" for a short amount of time; it is not permanent. Passive immunity includes the natural immunity that is passed from mother to neonate. Because it is borrowed, however, the immunity will lose its effectiveness by the end of the first year. Because of this natural immunity, the live, viral vaccines are not started until the infant is at least 12 months old. Viral vaccines are not effective as active immunization until the child's natural immunity has worn off.

Passive immunity can also be accomplished by the transfer of gamma globulin from the immune serum of an animal or human who has been actively immunized against a disease. In essence, these products are borrowed from the animal or other human. The borrowed antibodies begin to work immediately: that is why we use immune serum when we need antibodies in an emergency. The drawback, however, is that these borrowed antibodies are very short-lived. Immune sera should be used only *after* a patient has been exposed to an infection that is considered serious or life threatening. Immune serum will not provide long-term immunity and may not even prevent the clinical infection at all, even if given in time.

Immune sera derived from animals, like vaccines grown in animal media, can cause severe complications. Animal immune sera may cause *hypersensitization*, often called *serum sick-*

TABLE 9–3. **Recommended Schedule for Immunization of Healthy Infants and Children***

Recommended Age[†]	Immunizations[‡]	Comments
2 mo	DTP, HbCV,[§] OPV	DTP and OPV can be initiated as early as 4 wk after birth in areas of high endemicity or during epidemics
4 mo	DTP, HbCV,[§] OPV	2-mo interval (minimum of 6 wk) desired for OPV to avoid interference from previous dose
6 mo	DTP, HbCV[§]	Third dose of OPV is not indicated in the U.S. but is desirable in other geographic areas where polio is endemic
15 mo	MMR,[‖] HbCV[¶]	Tuberculin testing may be done at the same visit
15–18 mo	DTP,[**]/[††] OPV[#]	(See footnotes)
4–6 y	DTP,[§§] OPV	At or before school entry
11–12 y	MMR	At entry to middle school or junior high school unless second dose previously given
14–16 y	Td	Repeat every 10 y throughout life

*For all products used, consult manufacturer's package insert for instructions for storage, handling, dosage, and administration. Biologics prepared by different manufacturers may vary, and package inserts of the same manufacturer may change from time to time. Therefore, the physician should be aware of the contents of the current package insert.

[†]These recommended ages should not be construed as absolute. For example, 2 mo can be 6 to 10 wk. However, MMR usually should not be given to children younger than 12 mo. (If measles vaccination is indicated, monovalent measles vaccine is recommended, and MMR should be given subsequently, at 15 mo.)

[‡]DTP = diphtheria and tetanus toxoids with pertussis vaccine; HbCV = *Haemophilus* b conjugate vaccine; OPV = oral poliovirus vaccine containing attenuated poliovirus types 1, 2, and 3; MMR = live measles, mumps, and rubella viruses in a combined vaccine; Td = adult tetanus toxoid (full dose) and diphtheria toxoid (reduced dose) for adult use.

[§]As of October 1990, only one HbCV (HbOC) is approved for use in children younger than 15 mo.

[‖]May be given at 12 mo of age in areas with recurrent measles transmission.

[¶]Any licensed *Haemophilus* b conjugate vaccine may be given.

[**]Should be given 6 to 12 mo after the third dose.

[††]May be given simultaneously with MMR at 15 mo.

[#]May be given simultaneously with MMR and HbCV at 15 mo or at any time between 12 and 24 mo; priority should be given to administering MMR at the recommended age.

[§§]Can be given up to the seventh birthday.

Source: Reprinted with permission, from the *Report of the Commission on Infectious Diseases*, ed 22, p 17. Copyright © 1991.

ness, a phenomenon in which a patient may be made prone to allergic reactions. Eight to 12 days following the administration of immune serum, the patient may develop a rash, edema, adenitis, joint pain, high fever, and prostration. Reactions to immune globulin derived from horse serum are the most common. Once a person has had a serum reaction, the serum type responsible must not be used again. A second reaction will be more severe, possibly leading to anaphylaxis.

Before administering a passive immunization, carefully question the patient about any previous exposure to animal sera and past allergic reactions. Patients who have other allergy susceptibilities are at higher risk for serum sickness. It is customary to test a patient's sensitivity with a small amount of serum applied to the skin before injecting the full dose. If the seriousness of the infection warrants the risk of treatment, emergency equipment such as oxygen, epinephrine 1 : 1000, corticosteroids, and antihistamines must be available.

Human immune serum globulin is a newer product that is obtained from the pooled plasma of human donors and contains antibodies against a variety of diseases including measles, rubella, poliomyelitis, and infectious hepatitis. Human sera are free of the foreign animal proteins causing serum sickness and are much safer to use. This product is often administered to women of childbearing age who have been exposed to rubella and may be both pregnant and susceptible to the disease.

Other human immune globulin products are specific to one disease (e.g., measles, pertussis, polio, hepatitis, Rh, and tetanus-specific sera).

TABLE 9–4. Sample Immunization Checklist

Age	DPT	OPV*	MMR	Hib	Td	Hep B	Hep A	Varicella	Influenza	Pneumonia
0–2 mos						X				
1–4 mos						X				
2 mos	X	X		X						
4 mos	X	X		X						
6 mos	X			X						
6–18 mos						X				
12–15 mos			X	X						
12–18 mos		X								
15–18 mos	X		X							
4–6 yrs										
11–16 yrs					X (& Q10 yr)					
Adults if not previously			1 dose		2 doses 1 mo apart; 3rd dose 6 mos later	2 doses 1 mo apart; 3rd dose 5 mos later	2 doses 6–12 mos apart	2 doses 1 mo apart		
At risk patients									Every fall	1 dose anytime

This checklist is only a guide and is subject to change.
See Table 9–3 for explanation of abbreviations.
*Special alert: Before administration, determine the immune status of the patient and close household members. The vaccine virus is excreted in stool as a live virus. Warn that the vaccine can cause vaccine-related paralysis in recipients and close contacts, especially in immunosuppressed household members.

℞ **Immunoglobulins (generic name: Tradename)**

hepatitis B immune globulin: H-BIG

immune globulin: Gamastan, Gammar (for hepatitis A, hepatitis non-A-non-B, rubeola)

rabies immune globulin (human): Imogam, Hyperab

RHO immune globulin: RhoGAM

tetanus immune globulin: Hyper-tet

varicella zoster immune globulin

Immunotherapy

An alternative to allergy reaction drug treatment is immunotherapy, which is desensitization of the patient to the allergen. This is done through a series of injections that expose the patient to the allergen so that he or she develops an immune-response resistance to it. This process usually requires weekly injections over a period of years (Fig. 9–1). Some patients are cured; others experience only a reduction in the severity of symptoms.

Immunotherapy is most widely used in the management of respiratory allergies such as allergic rhinitis and bronchial asthma and has been proved effective for respiratory reactions to pollen allergies. However, the effectiveness of immunotherapy is still questioned by some who suggest that there is little evidence that patients actually improve from prolonged treatment. Immunotherapy for other allergies such as food and animal allergies has not been proved.

Immunotherapy is an expensive method of treatment and is inconvenient and often painful for patients. Moreover, immunotherapy itself can cause dangerous reactions such as anaphylactic shock. It is therefore reserved for use in cases when patient symptoms are both severe and poorly controlled with antiallergy drugs alone.

Pain Medications

NARCOTIC ANALGESICS (CONTROLLED SUBSTANCE PRESCRIPTIONS)

Narcotic analgesics depress the central nervous system (CNS) and are used to relieve pain, depress the cough reflex, and decrease the peristaltic movement of the gastrointestinal (GI) tract. The narcotic analgesics include opium and its derivatives, morphine, codeine, propoxyphene (Darvon), and various synthetic substances, the most common of which is meperidine (Demerol).

Narcotic analgesics are usually prescribed for severe pain, including that of acute coronary attacks, bone fractures, extensive burns, cancer, and following surgery. As GI antispasmodics, narcotics are useful in treating severe diarrhea, dysentery, and peritonitis. As cough suppressants, narcotics are useful for treating coughs accompanied by pain, as occurs with rib fractures.

It is most important to remember that all narcotic analgesics are addictive. Dependence can be psychologic and physical, and tolerance can develop quite quickly. *Tolerance* is characterized by the need for larger doses in shorter periods of time for pain relief. Other effects of narcotics include euphoria, drowsiness, mood changes, diminished mental capacity, and deep sleep.

Narcotics depress the vital signs, may have a nauseant and emetic effect, constrict the pupils, and are constipating. Toxicity is usually manifested by respiratory depression, stupor or coma, and pinpoint pupils. Chronic narcotic use also results in skin infections, allergies, and itching. These drugs pass the placental barrier and depress the respiration of the neonate if taken by the mother just before the neonate's birth.

Narcotics are contraindicated in asthmatic and other pulmonary conditions, convulsive states, hepatic disease, endocrine disease, pulmonary heart disease, urinary tract disease, and children under 6 months of age. Narcotics are used with caution in patients with head injury

MICHAEL R. MARDINEY, JR., M.D., P.A.
9380 BALTIMORE NATIONAL PIKE
ELLICOTT CITY, MARYLAND 21043
—
DIPLOMATE AMERICAN BOARD OF ALLERGY AND IMMUNOLOGY
—
TELEPHONE 301 - 461-7660

PLEASE REFRIGERATE ALLERGY SOLUTION
READ INSTRUCTIONS CAREFULLY!!
PAGE 1 OF 2

PATIENT: _____   DATE: _____

DATE OF BIRTH: _____   HOME TELEPHONE NUMBER: _____

Will you please have your physician carry out as closely as possible the treatment of your **ALLERGY** as outlined below. You should receive your treatment **TWO TIMES A WEEK.** After **Dose 38** please continue to take **0.9 cc** of the 1:10 solution **ONE TIME A WEEK.** It is **ESTIMATED** that this **CURRENT SERIES OF INJECTIONS** should be **COMPLETED BY**

THE PATIENT SHOULD REMAIN IN AREA OF IMMUNOTHERAPIST FOR 15 MINUTES AFTER INJECTION SO THAT PATIENT CAN BE EVALUATED FOR REACTION!! IMMUNOTHERAPIST SHOULD REVIEW PATIENT AND INJECTION SITE AT THAT TIME!! ENTER DOSAGE ADMINISTERED ON SEPARATE IMMUNOTHERAPY RECORD SHEET. FOR SAFETY REASONS, DOSAGE IS REDUCED WITH EACH RENEWED SOLUTION.

ALLERGY SOLUTION FORMULATION - SERIES # 1

____	RAGWEED	____	DUST
____	PLANTAIN	____	TOBACCO
____	TIMOTHY	____	CAT
____	ORCHARD	____	DOG
____	TREES	____	MOLD SPORES (1-4)
____	_____	____	MOLD SPORES (5-8)
____	_____	____	_____
____	_____	____	_____
____	_____	____	SALINE

GREEN LABEL VIAL
SOLUTION 1:10,000   FOR SAFETY, DO NOT
START HERE > Dose 1 - 0.1 cc   REMOVE LABEL FROM
            Dose 2 - 0.2 cc   TOP OF VIAL UNTIL
ADMINISTER   Dose 3 - 0.3 cc   READY TO USE!
EACH DOSE BY Dose 4 - 0.4 cc
SUBCUTANEOUS Dose 5 - 0.5 cc
INJECTION.   Dose 6 - 0.6 cc   CHECK VIAL TO
             Dose 7 - 0.7 cc   BE USED CAREFULLY!
ACTIVE   Dose 8 - 0.8 cc
ADRENALIN   Dose 9 - 0.9 cc
MUST BE
AVAILABLE!!

YELLOW LABEL VIAL
SOLUTION 1:1000
Dose 10 - 0.1 cc
Dose 11 - 0.2 cc
Dose 12 - 0.3 cc
Dose 13 - 0.4 cc
Dose 14 - 0.5 cc
Dose 15 - 0.6 cc
Dose 16 - 0.7 cc
Dose 17 - 0.8 cc
Dose 18 - 0.9 cc

RED LABEL VIAL
SOLUTION 1:100
Dose 19 - 0.1 cc
Dose 20 - 0.2 cc
Dose 21 - 0.3 cc
Dose 22 - 0.4 cc
Dose 23 - 0.5 cc
Dose 24 - 0.6 cc
Dose 25 - 0.7 cc
Dose 26 - 0.8 cc
Dose 27 - 0.9 cc

WHITE LABEL VIAL
SOLUTION 1:10
Dose 28 - 0.05 cc
Dose 29 - 0.1 cc
Dose 30 - 0.15 cc
Dose 31 - 0.2 cc
Dose 32 - 0.3 cc
Dose 33 - 0.4 cc
Dose 34 - 0.5 cc
Dose 35 - 0.6 cc
Dose 36 - 0.7 cc
Dose 37 - 0.8 cc

ONCE DOSE 38 IS REACHED, MAINTAIN
0.9 cc FOR REMAINDER OF VIAL 1:10. > Dose 38 - 0.9 cc

Should any constitutional reaction (characterized by sneezing, asthma or hives) occur after an injection, you should be given at once an injection of Adrenalin Chloride solution 1:1000 subcutaneously (0.3 to 0.5 cc). Your physician should **NEVER** treat you unless an active solution of Adrenalin Chloride 1:1000 is available immediately. **IF A CONSTITUTIONAL REACTION OCCURS, FURTHER INJECTIONS OF ALLERGY SERUM SHOULD NOT BE RECEIVED AND DOCTOR MARDINEY SHOULD BE CONSULTED.**

61 E. PADONIA ROAD TIMONIUM, MD 21093 561-4488   9650 SANTIAGO ROAD COLUMBIA, MD 21045 964-0066
7010 GOVERNOR RITCHIE HIGHWAY GLEN BURNIE, MARYLAND 21061 789-9282

FIGURE 9-1. Schedule and patient instructions for allergy desensitization. (Courtesy of Michael R. Mardiney, Jr., M.D., Baltimore, MD.)

MICHAEL R. MARDINEY, JR., M.D., P.A.
9380 BALTIMORE NATIONAL PIKE
ELLICOTT CITY, MARYLAND 21043

—

DIPLOMATE AMERICAN BOARD OF ALLERGY AND IMMUNOLOGY

—

TELEPHONE 301 - 461-7660

PLEASE REFRIGERATE ALLERGY SOLUTION
READ INSTRUCTIONS CAREFULLY!!
PAGE 2 OF 2

If a large local reaction occurs, marked by redness and swelling at the site of injection, your physician should go back to a previous dose which failed to give a reaction: for instance, if 0.7 cc of a solution 1:10 causes large local swelling shortly after injection, the next dose should be 0.6 cc of 1:10; the subsequent dose should then be 0.7 cc. Should this last dose again cause marked swelling, it would then be necessary to return to 0.6 cc and then gradually continue the treatment according to schedule.

GENERAL RULES CONCERNING THE SCHEDULE OF
IMMUNOTHERAPY AS RELATES TO UNAVOIDABLE MISSES,
ILLNESS, LOCAL AND GENERALIZED REACTIONS

If one week of Immunotherapy is missed, proceed to the next dose. If two weeks are missed, repeat the last dose. If three weeks are missed , go back to one dose below the last dose. If four or more weeks are missed, call this office for specific instructions.

If you are ill, Immunotherapy should not be given. In case a large local reaction occurs, i.e., 3 inches of swelling, go back to the dose which elicited no reaction (SEE ABOVE!).

If a systemic or generalized reaction occurs Immunotherapy should not be continued under any circumstance until review of the patient and circumstances of reaction are evaluated by Doctor Mardiney (SEE ABOVE!).

Finally, in case of continued doubt concerning the dose of Immunotherapeutic that should be given, do not receive Immunotherapy and call Doctor Mardiney for specific instructions.

Keep an accurate record of any **ALLERGY SYMPTOMS** which you might have on the enclosed **SYMPTOM SHEET.** Please bring the **SYMPTOM SHEET** into this office, when being reviewed by Doctor Mardiney. **CALL DR. MARDINEY, IF YOU ARE HAVING PROBLEMS.**

PLEASE CALL THIS OFFICE TO ORDER ADDITIONAL ALLERGY SERUM. THIS SHOULD BE DONE, WHEN YOU HAVE APPROXIMATELY THREE WEEKS OF THE CURRENT SERUM LEFT. TREATMENT SHOULD NOT BE DISCONTINUED WITHOUT PROFESSIONAL RECOMMENDATION. HMO AND IPA OFFICES SHOULD CONSULT SPECIAL INSTRUCTION SHEET BEFORE ORDERING ALLERGY SERUM.

SERUM .1
07-15-90

_____
Michael R. Mardiney, Jr., M.D.

61 E. PADONIA ROAD TIMONIUM, MD 21093 561-4488   9650 SANTIAGO ROAD COLUMBIA, MD 21045 964-0066
7010 GOVERNOR RITCHIE HIGHWAY GLEN BURNIE, MARYLAND 21061 789-9282

FIGURE 9–1. *Continued.*

or hemorrhage, or both; in urinary tract complications; during labor and delivery; in alcoholic patients; and in the elderly.

> **PATIENT EDUCATION:** • Patients should not hesitate to use a prescribed medication if they feel uncomfortable; it is important to use the medication before the pain becomes severe. • Patients should be instructed not to take more than the dosage prescribed without checking with the physician first, as narcotics can cause respiratory depression. • If GI upset occurs, these medications may be taken with food. • Constipation may occur and the physician may wish to suggest an appropriate laxative. • The patient should be cautious driving, operating machinery, and performing detailed tasks. • Federal law prohibits the patient from giving the medication to any other person. • After the course of therapy, any remaining drug should be destroyed.

NON-NARCOTIC ANALGESIC/ANTIPYRETIC/ ANTI-INFLAMMATORY AGENTS

Non-narcotic analgesics are used for the relief of pain and fever, and many of these drugs have anti-inflammatory effects as well and are therefore used for arthritis and gout. When used for arthritis and gout, these drugs are also called nonsteroidal anti-inflammatory drugs (NSAIDs).

The non-narcotic analgesics are classified as salicylates, pyrazolone derivatives, *para*-aminophenol derivatives, and ibuprofen.

Salicylates

- Acetylsalicylic acid (ASA) (OTC)
- Bayer (OTC)

℞ **Common Analgesics (generic name: Tradename, *Over-the-Counter*)**

Muscle Relaxants
  baclofen: Lioresal
  carisoprodol: Soma Rela
  chloroxazone: Parafon Forte
  cyclobenzaprine: Flexeril
  methocarbamol: Robasin
  orphenadrine: Norflex
Narcotic Analgesics
  codeine
  fentanyl: Sublimaze
  hydromorphone: Dilaudid
  meperidine: Demerol
  methadone: Dolophine
  morphine sulfate: MS Contin, Roxanol
  naloxone: Narcan
  oxycodone: Roxicodone
  pentazocine: Talwin
Narcotic Combinations
  Darvocet
  Darvon Compound
  Empirin w/Codeine
  Fioricet w/Codeine
  Fiorinal w/Codeine
  Percocet
  Percodan
  Soma w/Codeine
  Talwin Compound
  Tylenol w/Codeine
  Tylox
  Vicodin
Non-Narcotic Combinations
  Ascriptin
  Fioricet

Fiorinal
Norgesic
Robaxisal
Soma Compound
Non-Steroidal Anti-Inflammatory Drugs (NSAIDs)
  Salicylates
    aspirin: *Ecotrin, Empirin, Bayer, ASA*
    diflunisal: Dolobid
    salsalate: Salflex, Disalcid
  Propionic acids
    fenoprofen: Nalfon
    flurbiprofen: Ansaid
    ibuprofen: *Motrin, Advil, Nuprin, Rufen*
    ketoprofen: Orudis
    naproxen: *Naprosyn, Aleve*
    oxaprozin: Daypro
  Acetic acids
    diclofenac: Voltaren
    etodolac: Lodine
    indomethacin: Indocin
    ketorolac: Toradol
    nambumetone: Relafen
    sulindac: Clinoril
    tolmetin: Tolectin
  Fenamates
    meclofenamate: Meclomen
    mefanamic acid: Ponstel
  Oxicams
    piroxicam: Feldene
  Miscellaneous
    acetaminophen: *Tylenol, Panadol, Tempra*
    phenazopyridine: Pyridium (urinary tract)

- Ecotrin (OTC)
- Empirin (OTC)

Salicylates (e.g., aspirin) are analgesic, antipyretic, and anti-inflammatory agents. They are used for treating fever and pain, such as simple headache, dysmenorrhea, muscle ache, neuralgia, and minor arthralgia. Aspirin is also used prophylactically for reduction of myocardial infarction risk after previous heart attack and thromboembolic disorders.

Salicylates prolong bleeding time and can cause ringing in the ears, GI distress and bleeding, occult bleeding, skin rash, bronchospasm, and aspirin hypersensitivity and toxicity. Salicylates are contraindicated in patients with GI ulcers or bleeding, in those with an aspirin sensitivity, and in children with chickenpox or flulike illness owing to the risk of Reye's syndrome. Salicylates must be used with caution in patients with bleeding disorders, vitamin K deficiency, asthma with nasal polyps, or diabetes, as well as after surgery and in elderly patients and dehydrated children.

> **PATIENT EDUCATION:** • **Instruction includes warning patients that aspirin may interact with antacids, corticosteroids, and oral anticoagulants.** • **Patients should be instructed to watch for unusual bleeding; to counsel with the physician or pharmacist concerning OTC drugs; to administer aspirin with meals or milk; and that enteric-coated tablets may be better tolerated in the stomach.** • **Patients should also be told *not to* use aspirin when treating children for fever—acetaminophen (Tylenol) products should be used instead—as there is a possible association between aspirin and Reye's syndrome.** • **Aspirin should be kept out of reach of children, as aspirin is the leading cause of poisoning in children.**

Para-Aminophenol Derivatives

- Datril (OTC)
- Liquiprin (OTC)
- Panadol (OTC)
- Tylenol (OTC)

Para-aminophenol derivatives (e.g., acetaminophen) are analgesic and antipyretic agents that are used for treating fever and mild pain. These drugs have no significant anti-inflammatory effects. They are particularly useful for patients who are allergic to aspirin products.

Untoward reactions include liver toxicity, skin rash, and increased possibility of hemorrhage when used with anticoagulants. *Para*-aminophenol derivatives are contraindicated in patients with anemia and renal insufficiency. New studies show that the effects of these analgesics may be potentiated by concomitant use of alcohol, causing liver damage. Long-term use of *para*-aminophenol derivatives requires caution in patients with cardiac, pulmonary, or liver disease.

> **PATIENT EDUCATION:** • **Patients should be advised that they should be seen if fever persists for more than 3 days or is greater than 103.1°F (39.5°C).** • **Many other OTC drugs also contain acetaminophen, which would increase the prescribed daily dosage.** • **These drugs may color urine dark brown or wine.**

Ibuprofen

- Advil (OTC)
- Rufen (Rx)
- Motrin (Rx and OTC)
- Nuprin (OTC)

Ibuprofen is an analgesic and anti-inflammatory drug used for treating mild to moderate pain associated with arthritis, primary dysmenorrhea, gout, and postextraction dental pain. The untoward reactions of ibuprofen include prolonged bleeding times, drowsiness, dizziness, visual and hearing disturbances, GI distress, occult bleeding, bronchospasm, impaired renal and liver function, and skin rash.

Ibuprofen is used with caution in patients with hypersensitivity to other NSAIDs, cardiac complications, GI disorders or ulcers, hepatic or renal disease, or bleeding disorders. Ibuprofen is contraindicated in asthmatic patients with nasal polyps and in breast-feeding women.

> **PATIENT EDUCATION:** • **The patient should be instructed that these drugs should be taken with meals or milk.** • **Use with aspirin, alcohol, or corticosteroids may increase GI distress and bleeding.** • **Full therapeutic effects may take up to 2 weeks.** • **Self-medicating for extended periods should not be done without the consent of the physician.** • **Signs of GI bleeding, edema, visual disturbances, rashes, or weight gain should be reported.**

Anesthetics and Sedatives

Local infiltration anesthetics prevent the initiation and transmission of pain impulses to the brain. They most often are used to desensitize an area of the skin or mucous membranes in preparation for minor surgery or wound repair, but they may be used in combination with intramuscular injections to decrease pain at the injection site. (See Local Anesthetics under Common Skin/Topical Agents later in chapter.)

Small amounts of epinephrine may be used in conjunction with local anesthetics to decrease systemic absorption of the agent and to prolong the duration of the anesthetic action. Anesthetics with epinephrine are contraindicated, however, in patients with heart block and in cases of facial or cosmetic repair, where large amounts of anesthesia remaining at the wound site could prolong the swelling of the tissues and distort the wound closure. Some anesthetics may also contain preservatives, but only careful use of the product will ensure the sterility of the preparation.

Anesthetics may cause hypersensitivity in patients. Allergic reactions include swelling of the lips and oral tissues; CNS excitation with tremors, shivering, and convulsions; hypotension; and, in rare cases, cardiac and respiratory arrest. Epinephrine in anesthetic preparations may cause anginal pain, tachycardia, headache, restlessness, palpitations, dizziness, and hypertension.

As a precaution, store anesthetics with epinephrine separately from plain anesthetics. Make sure each order is specific as to which type to prepare for injection. Anesthetics that must remain sterile should be stored in an antiseptic with a dye as a solution to ensure that the solution is sterile. If there is a crack in the vial or cartridge, the dye will seep into the solution and change the solution's color. Discard preparations without preservatives following initial use.

Certain topical anesthetic preparations are specific to the skin, eye, nasopharynx, rectum, and anus. Topical anesthetics are applied to the skin for skin disorders; anesthetic eyedrops are used to anesthetize the eye for removal of foreign bodies, some methods of tonometry (measuring intraocular pressure), and to relieve pain following injuries to the cornea; anesthesia may be administered to the nasopharynx prior to instrumentation for examination; and rectal or anal anesthesia may be applied prior to proctoscopy, for control of pain due to hemorrhoids and other anal lesions.

ADVERSE REACTIONS TO LOCAL ANESTHESIA

Patients may react adversely to local anesthetics. A patient who is systemically stimulated by local anesthesia may become very talkative, anxious, and exhibit signs of rapid heart beat (tachycardia). Or a patient may experience systemic depression and exhibit sleepiness, slowing of the heart rate (bradycardia), and hypotension. Other reactions to anesthesia include cyanosis, perspiration (diaphoresis), feeling cold, and restlessness (signs of shock). Fainting, itching, nausea, or sudden headache may also occur. Proper monitoring of blood pressure, pulse, and heart rhythm is essential during any procedure requiring an anesthetic, even topical anesthesia.

Most reactions are caused when the patient receives too much anesthesia too fast. These complications are usually caused by a temporary overdose and follow accidental puncturing of an artery or vein during the administration of the anesthetic. The drug quickly travels to the brain, causing one or many of the variety of symptoms mentioned above. All surgical team members should be aware of the dangers of local anesthesia. Not all symptoms occur in all patients. To treat an adverse reaction, the anesthetic is immediately discontinued and oxygen is administered. Cardiopulmonary resuscitation (CPR) is immediately initiated, if needed.

GENERAL ANESTHESIA AND SEDATION

Some medical practices perform outpatient surgery under general anesthesia. General anesthesia involves the loss of consciousness and, used at its fullest, results in the total body absence of feeling, sensation, or pain. General anesthesia types can be varied, however, to produce a slight responsiveness in the patient or no response at all.

Balanced anesthesia is the term for using a combination of anesthetic agents to achieve a desired level of muscle relaxation and postoperative analgesia. There are four stages of general anesthesia.

Stage 1: Induction

This is the beginning of anesthesia. The first anesthetic agent used is usually administered intravenously (i.e., sodium pentothal). During this stage the patient becomes unconscious. The patient retains an exaggerated sense of hearing until the last moment of consciousness, however, so it is important to keep conversation in the operating room to a minimum. Once the patient is unconscious and intubated, other drugs are given intravenously or by inhalation to maintain the state of general anesthesia.

Stage 2: Excitement

During this stage, the patient is delirious and sensitive to external stimuli. There is involuntary muscle activity, and the patient may struggle. The patient's condition at this point is very unstable.

Stage 3: Relaxation (Surgical Plane)

This is the stage where surgery may be performed safely. The patient is relaxed, unconscious of pain, and stable. Breathing is steady and automatic. This stage ends at the deepest level of anesthesia, with respiratory paralysis.

Stage 4: Danger Stage

This stage begins when the amount of anesthesia begins to depress the central nervous system. The patient is in immediate danger of cardiopulmonary arrest.

℞ **Common Sedatives (generic name: Tradename)**

Antihistamines
  diphenhydramine: Benadryl
  promethazine: Phenergan

Barbiturates
  amobarbital: Amytal
  pentobarbitol: Nembutol
  phenobarbital: Luminal
  secobarbital: Seconal
  thiopental: Pentothal

Benzodiazepines
  alprazolam: Xanax

chlordiazepoxide: Librium
diazepam: Valium
lorazepam: Ativan
midazolam: Versed
oxazepam: Serax
triazolam: Halcion

Non-Benzodiazepine
  hydroxyzine: Atarax, Vistaril
  meprobamate: Equinil, Miltown

As mentioned previously, successful, *balanced* anesthesia requires three elements: unconsciousness, relaxation, and analgesia (absence of pain). No one anesthetic agent can produce all three goals.

NEUROMUSCULAR BLOCKING AGENTS

Because the action of most general anesthetics cannot cause sufficient muscle relaxation for surgery, neuromuscular blocking agents are commonly given during the operation.

The advantage of mixing a *neuromuscular* blockade with anesthesia is that the muscles become more relaxed in preparation for the surgical incision and are less likely to spasm during the operation. (Even in the unconscious state, smooth muscles may automatically react to the instrumentation.)

PREOPERATIVE MEDICATION

Preoperative medication is administered approximately one hour prior to surgery. Sedatives relax the patient psychologically and prepare the patient for a smoother induction. Sedatives also dry the mucous membranes, which is important to prevent aspiration of mouth secretions into the lungs during surgery. Barbiturates produce an hypnotic effect in addition to sedation; opiates produce narcosis and analgesia; belladonna derivatives inhibit mucous secretions; and tranquilizers relax and decrease apprehension.

Following preoperative sedation, the patient must be watched closely for any signs of respiratory or circulatory depression. Any unusual reaction must be reported immediately.

ANESTHESIA REVERSAL

Most patients emerge from balanced anesthesia on their own, before leaving the operating room. The patient cannot be extubated until he or she is able to breath unassisted. If the patient is not aroused before leaving the operating room, drugs can be administered to reverse the anesthesia/analgesia or to reverse the neuromuscular blockade.

Antimicrobial and Anti-Infective Agents

Originally, antimicrobials (commonly called antibiotics) were chemical byproducts produced by micro-organisms grown in laboratories. The early drugs were manufactured from common bacteria and fungi. Most antimicrobials in use today, however, are synthetically prepared.

Antimicrobials work by interfering with the metabolism of the infectious organisms. Some are bacteriostatic, which means they only inhibit the growth of micro-organisms, while others are bacteriocidal, which means they actually kill bacteria (Table 9–5).

Antimicrobials vary in their effectiveness. Many can be used to treat a wide variety of infectious agents and are called broad spectrum; others are used to treat a limited number of infections and are therefore called narrow-spectrum antimicrobials. Antimicrobials are used to treat infections caused by bacteria, some of the rickettsial organisms, and a few of the larger viruses. Antimicrobials are not effective against most viruses, especially those that cause the common cold, influenza, hepatitis, and the acquired immunodeficiency syndrome (AIDS) virus, also known as human immunodeficiency virus (HIV). Antiviral drugs are effective when treating herpes simplex infections, acute herpes zoster (shingles), some influenzas (Influenza A), and in managing patients with HIV infections and parkinsonism.

In addition to their curative effects, antimicrobials may be given prophylactically to protect patients who have been exposed to certain bacterial infections, to prevent secondary bacterial infections in the chronically ill patient, to decrease the chances of infection following an injury or surgery, or to decrease the chance of contracting rheumatic heart disease following oral surgery.

℞ Common Skin/Topical Agents (generic name: Tradename, *Over-the-Counter*)

Antimicrobial
  acyclovir: Zovirax
  amphotericin B: Fungizone
  bacitracin combinations: *Neosporin, Polysporin*
  chloramphenicol: Chloromycetin
  clotrimazole: *Lotrimin, Mycelex*
  econazole: *Spectazole*
  fluocinolone combinations
  gentamicin: *Garamycin*
  ketoconazole: Nizoral
  lindane: *Kwell, Scabene*
  Miconazole: *Monistat*
  neomycin combinations
  nystatin: *Mycostatin*
  polymixin combinations
  silver sulfadiazine: *Silvadene*
  tolnaftate: *Tinactin*

Local Anesthetics
  bupivacaine: Marcaine, Marcaine with epinephrine, Sensorcaine, Sensorcaine with epinephrine
  chloroprocaine: Nesacaine
  lidocaine: Xylocaine, Xylocaine with epinephrine
  mepivacaine: Carbocaine
  procaine: Novocain
  tetracaine: Pontocaine

Miscellaneous Agents
  calamine
  capsaicin: Zostrix
  coal tar: *Tegrin*
  hydroquinone: *Melanex*
  masoprocol: *Actinex*
  minoxidil: *Rogaine*
  oatmeal: *Aveeno*
  selenium sulfide: *Selsun*
  tretinoin: *Retin-A*

℞ Common Antimicrobials (generic name: Tradename)

Cephalosporins—1st generation
  cefadroxil: Duricef, Ultracef
  cefazolin: Ancef, Kefzol
  cephalexin: Keflex
  cephalothin: Keflin
  cephradine: Valosef

Cephalosporins—2nd generation
  cefaclor: Ceclor
  cefamandole: Mandol
  cefpodoxime: Vantin
  cefprozil: Cefzil
  cefuroxime: Zinacef, Ceftin
  loracarbef: Lorabid

Cephalosporins—3rd generation
  cefixime: Suprax
  ceftriaxone: Rocephin

Fluoroquinolone
  ciprofloxacin: Cipro
  enoxacin: Penetrex
  lomefloxacin: Maxaquin
  norfloxacin: Noroxin
  ofloxacin: Floxin

Macrolides
  azithromycin: Zithromax
  clarithromycin: Biaxin
  erythromycin: Eryc, E-mycin, Ilosone, EES, Pediazole, Ery-Tab, Erythrocin

Penicillin (natural)—1st generation
  benzathine penicillin: Bicillin L-A, Bicillin CR
  penicillin G
  penicillin V: Pen-Vee K, Veetids
  procaine penicillin: Wycillin

Penicillin (penicillinase-resistant)—2nd generation
  cloxacillin: Cloxapen
  dicloxacillin: Dynapen
  nafcillin: Nafcil, Unipen
  oxacillin

Penicillin (aminopenicillin)—3rd generation
  amoxicillin: Amoxil, Polymox, Trimox, Wymox

amoxicillin clavulanate: Augmentin
ampicillin: Principen, Omnipen, Polycillin
ampicillin sulbactam: Unasyn

Penicillin (extended-spectrum)—4th generation
  carbenicillin: Geocillin

Sulfonamides
  cotrimoxazole: Bactrim, Septra, Cotrim, Sulfatrim
  sulfamethoxazole: Gantanol
  sulfisoxazole: Gantrisin

Tetracyclines
  demeclocycline: Declomycin
  doxycycline: Vibramycin
  oxytetracycline: Terramycin
  tetracycline: Achromycin

Antiparasitic
  mebendazile: Vermox
  metronidazole: Flagyl
  pyrantel: Antiminth

Antitubercular
  isoniazid: INH
  pyrazinamide
  rifabutin: Mycobutin
  rifampin: Rimactane

Antiviral
  acyclovir: Zovirax
  amantadine: Symmetrel
  didanosine: Videx
  famciclovir: Famvir
  indinavir (new drug)
  lamivudine
  nevirapine (new drug)
  rimantadine: Flumadine
  ritonavir (new drug)
  saquinavir mesylate
  stavudine: Zerif
  zalcitabine: Hivid
  zidovudine: Retrovir, AZT, azidothymidine

TABLE 9–5. **Commonly Used Antibiotics (Antimicrobials)**

Type	Source	Action	Sites	Routes	Spectrum
Penicillins (Penicillin G, Penicillin V, penicillinase-resistant, ampicillin, and extended-spectrum)	Penicillium mold, semisynthetic	Bacteriostatic or bacteriocidal	Most of the body tissues; passes placental barrier; passes into synovial, pleural, pericardial, intraperitoneal, spinal, and eye fluids; will be absorbed into inflamed meninges	Oral and parenteral	Narrow and broad spectrum
Erythromycins	Streptomyces erythraeus	Bacteriostatic, occasionally bacteriocidal	Body tissues, peritoneal, pleural, ascitic, and amniotic fluids, saliva, passes the placental barrier, and mucous membranes of the upper respiratory system	Oral	Broad spectrum
Tetracyclines	Streptomyces aureofaciens and S. rimosus	Bacteriostatic	Most of the body tissues, passes placental barrier, and all body fluids; will be absorbed into noninflamed meninges	Oral	Broad spectrum
Cephalosporins (1st, 2nd, and 3rd generation)	Semisynthetic derived from cultures of Cephalosporium acremonium	Bacteriocidal	Respiratory, GI, and urinary tracts except in patients with pernicious anemia or obstructive jaundice	Oral and parenteral (can cause pain and damage at the site of injection)	Broad spectrum
Chloramphenicol	Synthetic; Streptomyces Venezuelae	Bacteriostatic	Most of the body tissues, passes the placental barrier, and all body fluids; will be absorbed into noninflamed meninges; reserved for treating serious infections; has serious side effects	Oral and parenteral	Broad spectrum

---

℞ **Miscellaneous Antibiotics (generic name: Tradename)**

chloramphenicol: Chloromycetin

clindamycin: Cleocin

furazolidone: Furoxone

lincomycin: Lincocin

methenamine madelate: Mandelamine

mitrofurantoin: Macrodantin, Macrobid

rifampin: Rimactane

vancomycin: Vancomycin

℞ **Common Hematologic Drugs (generic name: Tradename)**

Anticoagulants
  heparin
  warfarin: Coumadin, Panwarfin

Antiplatelet Drugs
  abciximab: ReoPro

Thrombolytics
  alteplase: tPA, Activase, plasminogen activator
  streptokinase: Streptase, Kabikinase
  urokinase: Abbokinase

Certain precautions must be taken with antimicrobial therapy:

1. The patient must be carefully assessed for hypersensitivity. Allergic reactions to antimicrobials are common and may be quite severe.

2. Patients must be taught to complete the entire course of therapy prescribed for them. Most antimicrobials are dispensed for a 5-, 7-, or 10-day course. Patients must be cautioned to take the entire prescription, even though they feel better. Incomplete therapy could mean incomplete eradication of the infectious agent. The infectious agent could then become resistant to the particular drug, or a more serious infection could occur. That particular drug would then be ineffective for the patient.

3. Antimicrobial therapy also destroys the normal flora of the body. Normal flora is the helpful bacteria always present on and in our bodies. It is useful in keeping certain pathogenic organisms in check. If levels of normal flora are decreased, a *superinfection* may occur. Superinfections are new infections that complicate the course of antibiotic therapy for an existing infection; they are usually due to bacteria and fungi normally present in the body. Superinfections include such conditions as diarrhea, monilial vaginitis, enteritis, and urinary tract infections.

4. Antimicrobials must not be used for inappropriate infections (e.g., viral) or to treat infections when the causative agent is resistant. Whenever possible, infected areas should be cultured before beginning treatment with a specific antimicrobial drug.

Drugs Used for Cardiovascular Disease and Hypertension

Coronary artery disease (CAD) is one of the leading causes of death in the United States. In patients with CAD, the coronary arteries become narrowed and blood flow becomes insufficient (ischemia) to carry the needed amount of oxygen to the heart muscle (myocardium). The most common cause of CAD is *atherosclerosis*, the buildup of fatty deposits inside the coronary arteries. In addition to atherosclerosis, the coronary arteries become hardened and lose their elasticity, a condition known as *arteriosclerosis*. Both conditions result in a decreased amount of oxygen reaching the tissues of the heart.

The main symptom of myocardial ischemia is chest pain. Based on the degree of seriousness, CAD may be classified as either *angina pectoris* or *acute myocardial infarction*. Drugs used to treat these conditions both improve the flow of oxygenated blood to the heart and reduce the work of the heart, thereby reducing the heart's need for oxygen.

PATIENT EDUCATION: In general, patient support and teaching are important in all aspects of CAD. A teaching plan should be established that includes dealing with stress and emotional and physical factors that set off anginal attacks. The plan should include suggestions and assistance in helping the patient make certain lifestyle changes such as workload reduction, weight loss, avoidance of stimulants, and appropriate exercise.

ACE INHIBITORS

Angiotensin-converting enzyme (ACE) inhibitors block ACE in the lungs from converting certain enzymes into powerful vasoconstrictors. Blocking the production of vasoconstrictors keeps the blood vessels dilated, which lowers blood pressure. In addition to lowering blood pressure, there is a small increase in potassium levels and sodium and fluid loss. Used alone or with other antihypertensive diuretics, ACE inhibitors are effective in the treatment of hypertension, and with the addition of cardiotonics, for the treatment of congestive heart failure in patients who do not respond to the more conventional therapy. These drugs can have serious side effects, such as bone marrow depression and kidney disease.

> PATIENT EDUCATION: • Patients may feel dizzy when standing from a lying or sitting position. • Nausea, vomiting, and diarrhea could indicate serious dehydration and should be reported immediately. • Beware of overexertion, even though the patient's chest pain may lessen or disappear. • Patients should not drive or perform activities that require alertness when first starting therapy. • Alcohol should be avoided. • Surgery should not be performed without a surgeon's knowledge that the patient is taking this drug. • Over-the-counter drugs could cause serious interactions. • Patients should keep the physician informed of all other drugs being taken.

ANTIARRHYTHMICS

Antiarrhythmics interfere with the electrical impulses. Their use is to slow the heart rate and stabilize irregular heartbeat. They are used with continual cardiac monitoring (BP, heart rate, and rhythm) for the treatment of tachycardia and atrial arrhythmias. They are usually reserved for emergency use in the acute care setting. In the outpatient setting, antiarrhythmics are prescribed only when irregular heart rates cannot be controlled by safer drugs. Since there is a narrow range between therapeutic and toxic amounts, patients should be cautioned to take the drug exactly as prescribed and followed carefully. Older adults are especially sensitive to the harmful effects of these drugs. Adverse effects include mental changes, dry mouth, constipation, difficulty urinating, blurred vision, increased body temperature and decreased perspiration, and worsening of glaucoma.

> PATIENT EDUCATION: • Patients may feel dizzy when standing from a lying or sitting position. • Patients should not drive or perform activities that require alertness when first starting therapy. • Alcohol should be avoided. • Surgery should not be performed without a surgeon's knowledge that the patient is taking this drug. • Over-the-counter drugs could cause serious interactions. • Patients should keep the physician informed of all other drugs being taken. • Patients should wear a medical identification bracelet or carry a card saying they are taking antiarrhythmics. • Regular appointments are necessary for potassium and glucose level testing.

ANTICOAGULANTS

Oral anticoagulants decrease the production of vitamin K-dependent clotting factors in the liver, causing a prolongation of clotting times. Injectable anticoagulants do not affect the manufacture of clotting factors in the liver, but interfere with the conversion of prothrombin to thrombin, blocking the final step in clot formation in the circulating blood. Oral anticoagulants are used to prevent blood clots from re-forming in patients who have had a myocardial infarction (MI), deep leg thrombosis, or any other thrombotic condition or embolic event. Patients must be closely monitored for unusual bleeding and frequent blood tests should be undertaken to evaluate drug effects. Patients over the age of 60 should take less than the usual dose, to lower the risk of serious bleeding. Vitamin K is the antidote in case of overdose.

PATIENT EDUCATION: • Patient should not take double doses if a dose is missed. Missed doses should be recorded and reported to the physician at the next visit. • Patients should wear a medical identification bracelet or carry a card saying they are taking anticoagulants. • When using this drug, a normal balanced diet is recommended. Consult the physician before making any changes in diet or taking nutritional supplements or vitamins that may increase the chance of bleeding. • Over-the-counter drugs could cause serious interactions, especially aspirin products, antacids, and laxatives (which may cause bleeding). • Patients should keep the physician informed of all other drugs being taken. • Regular appointments are necessary for blood clotting testing. • Surgery should not be performed without a surgeon's knowledge that the patient is taking this drug. • The patient should avoid activities that may cause cuts or bleeding.

BETA-ADRENERGIC BLOCKING AGENTS

Beta-blocking agents are used to treat cardiac arrhythmias, angina pectoris, postmyocardial infarction, hypertension, and migraine headaches. Beta blockers prevent norepinephrine from producing the excitatory response that increases the heart's rate and force of contraction. Beta blockers also prevent epinephrine and epinephrinelike drugs from producing their characteristic effects.

Beta blockers have several untoward reactions such as bradycardia, congestive heart failure, hypotension, bronchospasm, weakness, fatigue, and mental depression, and GI distress. Beta blockers are contraindicated in patients with CAD and vascular conditions in whom a sudden change in blood pressure would be dangerous. Beta blockers must be used with caution in patients with asthma, respiratory disease, or peptic ulcer.

PATIENT EDUCATION: Most importantly the patients should be taught about the disease itself and that the abrupt withdrawal of the drug may precipitate hypertensive crisis or myocardial infarction.

CALCIUM CHANNEL BLOCKERS

Calcium channel blockers selectively block the flow of calcium ions in the heart and are used to treat angina pectoris and some arrhythmias. These drugs control arrhythmias by slowing the rate of sinoatrial (SA) node discharge and the conduction rate of the discharge through the atrioventricular (AV) node. They control angina by relaxing and preventing coronary artery spasm.

Patients taking these drugs usually need concurrent sublingual nitrate (see farther on), and some patients benefit from concurrent beta-blocker therapy (see previous section). Untoward reactions include hypotension, bradycardia, dizziness, weakness, nausea, and headache. Calcium blockers are contraindicated in pregnancy and lactation and in patients with head trauma or cerebral hemorrhage. They are used with caution in patients with hepatic or renal impairment and recent cerebral hemorrhage.

PATIENT EDUCATION: • The patient should be told to report to the physician immediately any blurred vision, severe headache, skin rash, more frequent or more severe angina attacks, or fainting. • Do not use OTC drugs without the physician's approval. • Report the use of the medication to any other medical personnel and dentist treating him or her. • Do not use stimulants with the medication. • Do not discontinue the use of the drug without notifying the physician.

CARDIAC GLYCOSIDES

Cardiac glycosides (digoxin) are used to treat heart failure, a condition in which the heart cannot pump enough blood through the body. The symptoms of heart failure are fatigue, difficulty breathing, swelling of the lower extremities, and a rapid, galloping heart rate. Cardiac glycosides are also used to slow certain kinds of tachycardia and to stabilize certain kinds of arrhythmias.

Anyone taking digoxin is at risk of toxic effects (digitalis toxicity). Patients taking digoxin should have blood drawn regularly to check the levels of the drug in the blood. Toxicity symptoms include fatigue, loss of appetite, nausea and vomiting, vision problems, nightmares, nervousness, drowsiness, and hallucinations. Other signs of toxicity include changes in heart rhythm, slowing of the pulse, and lethargy. Since there is a narrow range between therapeutic and toxic amounts, patients should be cautioned to take the drug exactly as prescribed and should be followed carefully.

> **PATIENT EDUCATION:** • **Teach patients to take their own pulse, and seek immediate medical help if the heart rate slows to 60 beats or fewer per minute.** • **Suddenly discontinuing the drug could cause serious heart changes.** • **Patients must be withdrawn from drug use slowly by gradually reducing the dosage.** • **Patients should wear a medical identification bracelet or carry a card saying they are taking digoxin.** • **When using this drug, the patient's diet should be rich in potassium, adequate in magnesium, and low in sodium.** • **Over-the-counter drugs could cause serious interactions.** • **Patients should keep the physician informed of all other drugs being taken.** • **Regular appointments are necessary for digoxin blood level testing.** • **Surgery should not be performed without a surgeon's knowledge that the patient is taking this drug.**

DIURETICS

Diuretics, commonly called "water pills," are used to treat hypertension, congestive heart failure, and other conditions in which the body retains too much fluid. All types of diuretics have potential side effects, including loss of potassium and sodium from the body, harmful interactions with other drugs, and allergic reactions.

Thiazide diuretics are mild, which reduces the risk of dizziness, falling, and other side effects when the body suddenly loses too much fluid. Loop diuretics are much stronger with more side effects. Potassium-sparing diuretics remove less of the mineral potassium from the body than other diuretics, but can cause serious side effects such as kidney stones, kidney failure, retention of too much potassium, and bone marrow depression.

> **PATIENT EDUCATION:** • **Patients should make certain their fluid intake is adequate to offset water loss and dehydration.** • **Diuretics may make patients sensitive to the sun.** • **Potassium loss is a harmful side effect of most diuretics; greater potassium depletion occurs when there is too much salt in the diet.** • **Patients may feel dizzy when standing from a lying or sitting position.** • **Surgery should not be performed without a surgeon's knowledge that the patient is taking this drug.** • **Over-the-counter drugs could cause serious interactions.** • **Patients should keep the physician informed of all other drugs being taken.** • **Regular appointments are necessary for potassium and sodium level testing.**

HMG CoA INHIBITORS

HMG CoA inhibitors are antihyperlipidemic drugs. They are manufactured from a fungal metabolite that inhibits the enzyme synthesis of cholesterol in humans, resulting in a decrease in serum cholesterol, serum low-density lipoproteins (LDLs; associated with an increased risk of CAD) and either an increase or no change in serum high-density lipoproteins (HDLs; associated with a decreased risk of CAD). These drugs are used as an adjunct to diet in the treatment of elevated total and LDL cholesterol in patients for whom dietary restriction of saturated fat and cholesterol alone has not been successful. Common side effects include headache, blurred vision, GI upset, and muscle and joint pains.

> **PATIENT EDUCATION:** • **Instruct patients to take the drug at bedtime.** • **The patient should continue low-cholesterol diet and regular exercise.** • **Regular ap-**

℞ **Common Antihypertensive Drugs (generic name: Tradename)**

ACE inhibitors
  benazepril: Lotensin
  captopril: Capoten
Anti-Adrenergic—Central Acting
  clonidime: Catapres
Anti-Adrenergic—Peripherally Acting
  doxazosin: Cardura
  prazosin: Minipress
  reserpine: Serpasil
Beta-Blockers
  atenolol: Tenormin
  labetalol: Trandate, Normodyne
  metoprolol: Lopressor
  naldol: Corgard

penbutolol: Levatol
propanolol: Inderal
Calcium Channel Blockers
  amlodipine besylate: Norvasc
  bepridril: Vascor
  diltiazem HCl: Calcicard, Cardizem
  nifedipine: Procardia
  nimodipine: Nimotop
  verapamil HCl: Calan
Diuretics
  acetazolamide: Diamox
  methazolamide: Neptazane
Diuretics—Loop
  furosemide: Lasix

℞ **Common Cardiovascular Drugs (generic name: Tradename)**

Antihyperlipidemic Drugs
  cholestyramine: Questran
  colestipol: Colestid
  fluvastatin: Lescol
  lovastatin: Mevacor
  pravastin: Pravachol
  simvastin: Zocor
Nitrites (Vasodilators)
  nitroglycerin: Tridil, NitroBid, Nitrol, Nitrostat

Antidysrhythmics/Cardiac Arrest
  atropine
  bicarbonate sodium
  digitoxin: Crystogin
  digoxin: Lanoxin
  disopyramide: Norpace
  epinephrine
  isoproterenol: Isuprel
  lidocaine: Xylocaine

pointments are necessary for cataract examinations and liver-function tests. • Severe GI upset, vision changes, unusual bleeding or bruising, dark urine, and light-colored stools should be reported immediately.

NITRATES

Nitrates relax the smooth muscles of the coronary arteries by directly depressing muscle tone rather than blocking the nerve impulses that cause these muscles to contract. Nitrate-induced relaxation causes vasodilation and, in turn, an increase of blood flow and oxygenation to the heart. In addition to increased blood flow to the heart, nitrates also dilate the peripheral vessels of the lower extremities, and blood tends to pool in the legs and other areas of the body. This decreases the amount of blood returning to the heart, which, in turn, lessens the heart's work demand and need for oxygenation. By increasing the oxygen to the heart and, at the same time, decreasing its workload, nitrates relieve or prevent angina attacks.

Nitrates are used to treat acute attacks of angina pectoris and, as prophylactic therapy, to reduce the number and severity of such attacks. Adverse reactions include headaches, fainting spells, nausea, vomiting, dizziness, weakness, skin rash, and tolerance.

Nitrates are contraindicated in patients with hypersensitivity to nitrites. They are used with caution in patients with glaucoma, head injuries, anemia, or cerebral hemorrhage (stroke).

PATIENT EDUCATION: • The patient should keep track of the drug's expiration date. • Take the medication (sublingually or by inhalation) while sitting or lying. • Watch for lack of response to the drug (which would indicate tolerance). • Do not drink alcohol. • Notify the physician before taking other drugs and of adverse effects or signs of hypersensitivity. • The patient should learn to take the least amount of medication needed to relieve the chest pains: once relieved, the patient may spit out any undissolved medication. • Because chest pain not relieved

by ordinary doses may indicate acute myocardial infarction, the patient should be instructed to notify the physician immediately of any changes in response to treatment. • Instruct the patient to keep nitrates in their original containers, which should be closed tightly at all times.

Insulin Initiation

Diabetes mellitus is the most common of the metabolic diseases. There are more than 3 million known individuals with diabetes, with almost as many not yet diagnosed. As the majority of the population shifts to middle and old age during the 1990s, the number of patients with diabetes is expected to double.

Diabetes results from a lack of effective insulin activity. Some patients with diabetes control their condition through diet and weight control; others are able to use oral hypoglycemic agents. For those patients who cannot control their conditions with oral hypoglycemic agents or dietary changes, however, the way to replace the insulin needed by the body is by regular injections of insulin, usually for life.

Insulin therapy has improved greatly over the past decade. New equipment has been developed and recombinant DNA technology has made the synthesis of human insulin possible. Recombinant drugs are made by taking the genes from one organism and inserting them into the DNA of another to make a new cell (recombination). The process is also called gene splicing. Human insulin is made by genetically altering bacteria to produce synthetic human insulin. Human insulin has replaced the older forms of insulin made from the pancreases of beef and pork.

There are four types of insulin, each based on its rapidity of onset. The type of insulin or combination of insulins to initiate treatment and for long-term maintenance depends on the severity of the condition and various other conditions of the diagnosis. The four types are *rapid-acting, intermediate acting*, a mixture of *rapid-acting and intermediate-acting*, and *long-acting*. These forms are listed in Table 9–6.

Because insulin is now available in 100 units/ml, the amount of insulin measured is the same in the 0.5-ml (50 units), and 1-ml (100 units) syringes and in the tuberculin syringe. Because insulin quantities are so small, every effort should be made to use the correctly calibrated syringe. Only in an emergency should the regular 3-ml hypodermic syringe be used.

Insulin is injected subcutaneously, using a 5/8-in needle. Because insulin is not effectively absorbed in fatty tissue, a longer needle may be needed for overweight patients. In an emergency, insulin may be ordered given intramuscularly (IM) for a more rapid action. In that case, a longer IM needle is used.

New, automatic insulin delivery devices are now available for administering insulin—the MediJector EZ (Fig. 9–2) and the NovolinPen (Fig. 9–3). These newer devices attach either to a vial of insulin or to a cartridge, and remain attached until the containers are empty. They both have mechanisms for presetting the doses of insulin. These features reduce the chances for contamination and errors in dosage.

Insulin injections must be rotated. The patient must be taught to alternate injections among the preferred injection sites, to prevent hypertrophy of the tissues at the injection sites. The preferred sites are the deltoid muscle area at the back of the arms, the front of the thigh, the skin of the fronts and sides of the abdomen, and the buttocks (Fig. 9–4).

PATIENT EDUCATION: Patient teaching must emphasize how to inject insulin and care for the equipment; how to perform urine or blood tests to check that the treatment is controlling the diabetes; how to balance insulin dosage with food intake and exercise; and how to prevent infections of the skin, feet, upper respiratory tract, and urinary tract, which could become serious complications in patients with diabetes.

Careful reading of insulin labels is essential for correct identification. The origin (human or animal) and type of insulin are printed on every label. The different types of insulin

TABLE 9–6. **Types of Insulin Available in 1991**

Product	Manufacturer	Form	Strength
Rapid-Acting (Onset 1/2–4 Hr)			
Humulin Regular	Lilly	Human	U-100
Humulin BR (for external insulin pumps only)	Lilly	Human	U-100
Novolin R (Regular)	Novo Nordisk	Human	U-100
Novolin R Penfill (Regular)	Novo Nordisk	Human	U-100
Velosulin Human (Regular)	Novo Nordisk	Human	U-100
Iletin II Regular	Lilly	Beef	U-100
Iletin II Regular	Lilly	Pork	U-100, U-500
Purified Pork R (Regular)	Novo Nordisk	Pork	U-100
Velosulin (Regular)	Novo Nordisk	Pork	U-100
Iletin I Regular	Lilly	Beef/Pork	U-100
Regular	Novo Nordisk	Pork	U-100
Iletin I Semilente	Lilly	Beef/Pork	U-100
Semilente	Novo Nordisk	Beef	U-100
Intermediate-Acting (Onset 2–4 Hr)			
Humulin L (Lente)	Lilly	Human	U-100
Humulin N (NPH)	Lilly	Human	U-100
Insulatard Human NPH	Novo Nordisk	Human	U-100
Novolin L (Lente)	Novo Nordisk	Human	U-100
Novolin N (NPH)	Novo Nordisk	Human	U-100
Novolin N Penfill (NPH)	Novo Nordisk	Human	U-100
Iletin II Lente	Lilly	Beef	U-100
Iletin II NPH	Lilly	Beef	U-100
Iletin II Lente	Lilly	Pork	U-100
Iletin II NPH	Lilly	Pork	U-100
Insulatard NPH	Novo Nordisk	Pork	U-100
Purified Pork Lente	Novo Nordisk	Pork	U-100
Purified Pork N (NPH)	Novo Nordisk	Pork	U-100
Iletin I Lente	Lilly	Beef/Pork	U-100
Iletin I NPH	Lilly	Beef/Pork	U-100
Lente	Novo Nordisk	Beef	U-100
NPH	Novo Nordisk	Beef	U-100
Long-Acting (Onset 4–6 Hr)			
Humulin U (Ultralente)	Lilly	Human	U-100
Iletin I Ultralente	Lilly	Beef/Pork	U-100
Ultralente	Novo Nordisk	Beef	U-100
Mixtures			
Mixtard (70% NPH, 30% Regular)	Novo Nordisk	Pork	U-100
Mixtard Human 70/30 (70% NPH, 30% Regular)	Novo Nordisk	Human	U-100
Novolin 70/30 (70% NPH, 30% Regular)	Novo Nordisk	Human	U-100
Novolin 70/30 Penfill (70% NPH, 30% Regular)	Novo Nordisk	Human	U-100
Humulin 70/30 (70% NPH, 30% Regular)	Lilly	Human	U-100

Source: Reprinted with permission from Diabetes Forecast, October 1991. Copyright © 1991 American Diabetes
Association, Inc.

identify the times to the first effect (onset) of the insulin and the duration of the effect. *Regular* and *Semilente* have a rapid onset, usually 1/2 hour, peaking in 2-1/2 to 5 hours, and lasting about 8 hours. The intermediate-acting, *Lente (L)* and *NPH* insulins, take effect in 1-1/2 to 2-1/2 hours, peak in 4 to 15 hours, and last about 16 to 24 hours. The long-acting insulins include *Ultralente (U)*, the effects of which occur in 4 hours, peak in 10 to 30 hours, and last about 36 hours. Insulin types and dosages are prescribed based not only on the severity of the patient's diabetes but also on the patient's lifestyle, diet, and activity schedule.

Insulin-dependent people must have at least one, sometimes several, subcutaneous injections of insulin each day. It is common to combine two insulins, intermediate and long-acting, for example, in a single syringe to reduce the number of injections required. Rapid-acting insulin is more often used in emergencies or when insulin levels in the blood fall below normal values.

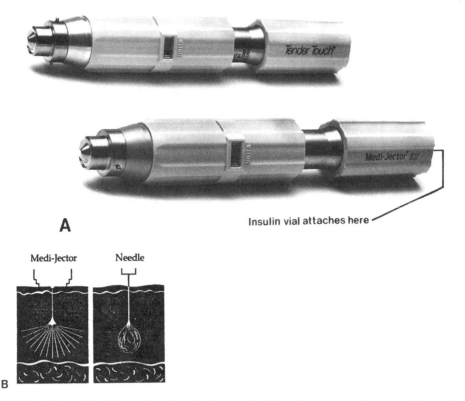

A

Insulin vial attaches here

Medi-Jector   Needle

B

FIGURE 9–2. *A*, Derata Medi-Jector EZ syringe. *B*, Comparative dispersion patterns. (Courtesy of Derata Corporation, Minneapolis, MN.)

Regular insulin does not need to be mixed before withdrawing it into a syringe. The other types settle, forming a precipitate, and must be mixed by gentle rotation before withdrawal from a vial. When insulin types are combined in one syringe, the Regular (shortest-acting) insulin is drawn up first.

The smallest possible capacity (0.5 ml or 1 ml) syringe is selected. This ensures the most accurate measurement and facilitates the reading of the syringe contents. The actual steps are as follows:

Example: The physician orders 10 U of Regular insulin and 50 U of NPH insulin.

1. Choose the 1 ml U-100 syringe.

   Rationale: the total amount (60 U) is greater than the U-50 syringe.

2. Draw up 6 U of air into the syringe.

   Rationale: Injecting amounts of air into vials prior to withdrawing solutions equalizes the pressures inside the vials.

3. Rotate the NPH insulin vial.

   Rationale: To mix the contents thoroughly.

4. Cleanse both vial tops with alcohol.

5. Draw up 50 U of air and inject the air into the NPH vial, being careful to keep the needle tip out of the solution.

   Rationale: To avoid contamination of the Regular vial during the next step.

6. Draw up 10 U of air and inject the air into the Regular insulin.

7. Draw up 10 U of Regular insulin.

8. Insert the needle back into the NPH vial and draw the plunger up to the 60 U of NPH insulin.

   Rationale: 10 U + 50 U = 60.

9. Administer the medication promptly.

   Rationale: To avoid precipitation (settling) of the NPH insulin.

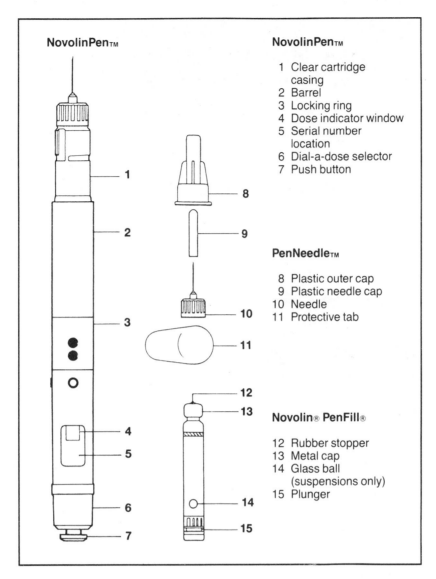

NovolinPen™

NovolinPen™

1 Clear cartridge casing
2 Barrel
3 Locking ring
4 Dose indicator window
5 Serial number location
6 Dial-a-dose selector
7 Push button

PenNeedle™

8 Plastic outer cap
9 Plastic needle cap
10 Needle
11 Protective tab

Novolin® PenFill®

12 Rubber stopper
13 Metal cap
14 Glass ball (suspensions only)
15 Plunger

FIGURE 9–3. The NovolinPen. (Courtesy of Squibb-Novo, Princeton, NJ.)

Pulmonary and Upper Respiratory Preparations

Upper respiratory medications usually refer to those prescribed for diseases of the lungs and bronchi (pulmonary drugs) as well as those used to treat diseases of the nose, throat, larynx, and trachea. Infections cause the most common acute lung diseases. They may be local infections (abscess, tracheitis) or generalized (pneumonia). The most universal ailment, of course, is the common cold. This can be caused by bacteria, viruses, or fungi. Tuberculosis, once thought eradicated, has made a come-back, and is an important disease of the lungs because it is both destructive and treatable. Cancer of the lungs is common in smokers. The diagnosis of cancer usually comes too late, when the cancerous tissue has already obstructed the bronchus or metastasized elsewhere. The lungs are also a frequent site of metastasis (secondary cancer) from cancers originating in other areas of the body.

Vascular disease of the lung is caused by increased pulmonary arteriolar resistance and can cause heart failure. Pulmonary emboli are blood clots that travel to the lungs from other sites and lodge in the arterioles of the lung. Emboli are a frequent cause of death in postoperative, disabled, or chronically ill patients. Other chronic and acute conditions include asthma, chronic obstructive pulmonary disease (COPD), emphysema, and seasonal allergies.

Setting Up An Easy Rotation Cycle

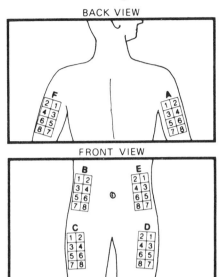

Injection Log

SITE		1	2	3	4	5	6	7	8
right arm	**A**								
right abdomen	**B**								
right thigh	**C**								
left thigh	**D**								
left abdomen	**E**								
left arm	**F**								

FIGURE 9–4. Rotation pattern for varying insulin injection sites. The right arm is marked *A*, the right side of the abdomen is *B*, and the right thigh is *C*. Crossing to the left side of the body, the left thigh is marked *D*, the abdomen is *E*, and the left arm *F*.

Each of these areas can be thought of as a rectangle that can be divided into 8 different squares measuring more than 1 in on each side. These squares are numbered starting from the upper and outside corner, which is number 1, to the lowest corner, which is number 8, with all even numbers toward the middle of the body.

If square 1 is selected and injected into at each of the 6 areas *A* through *F*, it will take 6 days to return again to area *A*. Then, by selecting square 2 and injecting into it at each of the 6 areas again, rotation around the body continues, returning in 6 days to area *A*. Square 3 is next, and so forth.

This procedure provides 48 different places in which to make the injections. If one injection is made daily, it will take that many days to return to square *A*1—almost 7 weeks. (Courtesy of Becton Dickinson and Co., Franklin Lakes, NJ.)

Bronchitis and emphysema are common diseases of the lungs related to air pollution (smoke, industrial pollution).

The main classes of drugs used to treat chronic and acute episodes of pulmonary disease are bronchodilators and corticosteroids. Antibotics are used to treat most types of respiratory infections. Tuberculosis requires the use of special drugs. Antihistamines, antitussives, decongestants, and expectorants are used to treat allergies, some symptoms accompanying bronchitis, and as remedies for the common cold. The limits of this book make it impossible to discuss all the brands and combinations of these last-mentioned drugs, but brief mention is made about their major considerations and uses. Antihistamines, antitussives, decongestants, and expectorants are overused and often useless for the conditions being treated.

The common cold cannot be "cured." This infection is caused by a virus that no drug will kill. It is best treated by time, rest, plenty of fluids, and not smoking.

ANTIHISTAMINES

Antihistamines block the effects of histamine (H_1) receptor sites, and have anticholinergic (atropinelike) and antipruritic effects. Antihistamines are used to prevent or relieve the symptoms of allergy (such as hay fever). Histamines are chemicals made by the body especially during an allergic reaction. Histamines produce dilation of small blood vessels producing redness, localized swelling, and often itching; lower blood pressure; and increase secretions from the stomach, salivary glands, and other organs. Antihistamines also are used to treat coughs, insomnia, motion sickness, and Parkinson's disease, and as adjunct treatment in anaphylactic reactions, blood transfusions, and to dry mouth secretions during anesthesia. *Contrary to belief, antihistamines should not be used to treat the common cold.* In fact, their use can thicken nasal secretions and dry mucous membranes, making a cold worse. Side effects include confusion, dizziness, fainting, painful urination, nightmares, unusual excitement, nervousness, and irritability. Because they cause drowsiness, they are contraindicated for anyone who must remain alert.

> **PATIENT EDUCATION:** • **The drug should be taken with food if GI upset occurs.** • **Avoid excessive dosage.** • **A humidifier can be used if nasal dryness becomes bothersome.** • **Drink plenty of fluids.** • **Avoid alcohol.** • **Report difficulty breathing, hallucinations, tremors, loss of coordination, unusual bleeding or bruising, irregular heart rate, visual disturbances.**

Newer antihistamines that do not cause drowsiness have been developed. These newer drugs (Hismanal, Claritin) cannot cross the blood–brain barrier to produce the effects of sedation. However, in certain individuals, even these newer drugs can cause sedation, drowsiness, or impair judgment and coordination.

ANTITUSSIVES AND EXPECTORANTS

Expectorants are used to thin the mucus in the airways, so that the mucus can be coughed up more easily. A productive cough is useful in helping the body clear material from the lungs. Expectorants may be used alone or in combination with antitussives. Antitussives (cough suppressants) are used to suppress the cough mechanism, and are used to treat a dry cough that brings up no mucus. Cough suppressants are most useful for a cough that prevents sleep or other activities. Cough suppressants may be narcotic or non-narcotic.

BRONCHODILATORS

Bronchodilators are used to open the bronchial tubes of the lungs to increase the flow of air in patients who have asthma, chronic bronchitis, or emphysema. Temporary narrowing of the bronchial tubes is known as bronchospasm. Inhaled beta agonists, such as albuterol and terbutaline, are the first-choice drugs for mild bronchospasms. Patients can inhale these drugs before exercise or before being exposed to allergens (cutting the grass, for instance).

℞ **Common Pulmonary–Asthma Medications (generic name: Tradename)**

Asthma

Beta agonists
    albuterol: Ventolin, Proventil
    bitolterol: Tornalate
    isoetharine: Bronkosol, Bronkometer
    metaproterenol: Alupent, Metaprel

Inhaled steroids
    beclomethasone: Vanceril, Beclovent

Methylxanthines
    aminophylline
    theophylline: Theo-Dur, Slo-bid

Other Pulmonary
    epinephrine (anaphylaxis, allergy): Ana-Kit,
        Epipen, Sus-Phrine
    dexamethasone (croup): Decadron

Inhaled corticosteroids are also prescribed as an adjunct treatment for patients who need regular, long-term steroid treatment to control their symptoms. Corticosteroids cannot provide bronchodilation but only reduce inflammation and tissue edema. For this reason, inhaled corticosteroids are not effective during acute attacks of bronchospasm. Steroids also suppress the immune system, which lowers defenses against disease, making patients more vulnerable to infections. Patients should be followed carefully.

PATIENT EDUCATION: • **Patients should wear a medical identification bracelet or carry a card stating the severity of asthma and which drugs are necessary for treatment. • Inhaled drugs should not be stored in the bathroom, exposed to heat, moisture, or strong light, or frozen. • To prevent dryness of the mouth and throat, the mouth should be rinsed with water after each inhaled dose. • Inhalants contain chemicals called chlorofluorocarbons and should be inhaled at least 15 minutes apart. • The eyes should be protected from aerosol medications. • Missed doses should be taken as soon as remembered and skipped if it is almost time for the next dose.**

Methylxanthine-derived drugs are taken orally. These drugs are used to treat the symptoms of *chronic* asthma, bronchitis, and emphysema. Since these drugs are slow acting, they must not be depended on in acute situations. There is a narrow range between helpful and harmful amounts of methylxanthine in the bloodstream, so it is important for patients to take these medications exactly as prescribed. Patient dosage and blood serum levels must be monitored closely.

℞ **Common Upper Respiratory ("Cough and Cold") Preparations (generic name: Tradename, *Over-the-Counter*)**

Antihistamines
    brompheniramine: *Dimetane*
    chlorpheniramine: *Chlor-Trimeton*
    clemastine: *Tavist*
    cyproheptadine: *Periactin*
    dimenhydrinate: *Dramamine*
    ephenhydramine: *Benadryl*
    hydroxyzine: Atarax, Vistiril
    promethazine: *Phenergan*

Antihistamine without Sedating Effects
    astemizole: Hismanal
    loratidine: Claritin
    terfenadine: Seldane (recently withdrawn from
        use due to safety issues)

Antitussive—DEA Controlled Substances
    Codeine
    Hydrocodone: Hycodan

Antitussive
    dextromethorphan: *Benylin, Robitussin
        combinations*
    guaifenesin: *Robitussin*

Expectorants
    terpin hydrate

Decongestants
    phenylpropanolamine (combinations):
        Dimetapp, Naldecon
    pseudoephedrine: *Actifed (combination), Afrin,
        Drixoral, PediaCare Infant's Decongestant,
        Sudafed*

Decongestants–Nasal
    beclomethasone: Beconase, Vancenase
    dexamethasone: *Decadron*
    oxymetazoline: *Afrin*
    phenylephrine: *Neo-Synephrine*
    saline nasal spray
    triamcinolone: *Nasacort*

Ear Preparations
    acetic acid 2%: *Domeboro Otic, VoSol Otic*
    carbamide peroxide: *Debrox, Murine Ear*
    hydrocortisone/antibiotic combination:
        Cortisporin otic
    isopropanolol: *Swim Ear*
    triethanolamine: *Cerumenex*

PATIENT EDUCATION: • Patients should take these drugs exactly as prescribed. • Dietary restrictions include a decrease in the intake of charcoal-broiled foods and caffeine, such as coffee, chocolate, cocoa, tea, and colas. • Notify the physician of any fever, flu, or diarrhea, since these conditions increase the chances of drug side effects. • Inform the physician of any planned surgery, including dental surgery. • Patients should make regular appointments for blood testing.

DECONGESTANTS

Decongestants constrict the small blood vessels, which reduces blood flow to swollen tissues in the nose, sinuses, and throat. This action decreases the swelling of the mucous membranes, relieves nasal stuffiness, promotes drainage of secretions, and opens the eustachian tubes. Decongestants are administered orally for a systemic effect or may be administered topically as nose drops or nasal sprays. Decongestants act as stimulants, whereas most antihistamines cause drowsiness; therefore, decongestants are preferred over antihistamines during activity, since they do not usually cause drowsiness, and antihistamines are preferred over decongestants at bedtime.

Newer spray forms of corticosteroids are also prescribed as an adjunct in the treatment of severe allergies and hay fever and sometimes polyps in the nose. Steroids, however, suppress the immune system, lowering defenses against disease, making patients more vulnerable to infections.

Gastrointestinal Drugs

Digestion begins in the mouth and continues in the stomach and upper portion of the small intestine. The absorption of nutrients takes place throughout the small intestine, and the absorption of water and elimination of feces takes place in the large intestine. Gastrointestinal diseases make up a large percentage of conditions for which drugs are prescribed, and sometimes overused or abused by patients.

The common diseases of the mouth, esophagus, and stomach are inflammation and tumors. The diseases of the small and large intestines are more numerous. Diarrhea is the most common symptom of bowel disease. Diarrhea may be caused by infections, inflammatory diseases, such as ulcerative colitis and regional ileitis, infiltrates, tumors, and obstruction of bile ducts. Complications of bowel inflammation include obstruction, perforation, and peritonitis. Vascular diseases, due to arterial occlusions, emboli, or venous obstruction may lead to gangrene of the bowel. Malabsorption syndromes can be caused by food allergies, liver disease, endocrine and metabolic disorders, enzyme deficiencies, or mechanical abnormalities, such as abnormal intestinal pathways or following intestinal surgery. Tumors of the colon are the most common tumor in humans, with the majority of these occurring within 6 inches of the anus.

Diarrhea is the change in the frequency and consistency of bowel movements, characterized by abnormally frequent passage of loose or watery stools. Simple diarrhea lasts only a few days and typically improves with or without medication. It is often caused by a viral infection, food poisoning, anxiety, or a reaction to medication, food, or alcohol. Drugs that commonly cause diarrhea include antibiotics, antacids containing magnesium (*Maalox*, *Mylanta*), drugs for high blood pressure, laxatives, and drugs taken to control arrhythmias.

ANTACIDS

Antacids neutralize acidity in the stomach and duodenum, and for many years were the only available treatment for peptic ulcers. Antacids contain aluminum, magnesium, calcium, sodium, or a combination of these ingredients. Older adults with metabolic bone diseases should not take aluminum antacids. Anyone with kidney disease should not take antacids containing magnesium. Patients on sodium-restricted diets should choose an antacid without sodium. The use of calcium antacids may have an additional benefit for women as a dietary calcium supplement.

> PATIENT EDUCATION: • **Aluminum products may cause constipation. Magnesium products may cause diarrhea.** • **Antacids should be taken 1 to 3 hours after meals and at bedtime with plenty of fluids.** • **Other drugs should not be taken for at least 1 to 2 hours after taking aluminum hydroxide.** • **Medical attention should be sought if there are any signs of bleeding ulcers, such as black tarry stools.** • **Avoid antacids with simethicone, since it is not proven that this product is effective in treating so-called excess gas.**

ANTIDIARRHEAL DRUGS

Antidiarrheal drugs may be over-the-counter or by prescription. They produce their effects by slowing peristalsis or by absorbing additional water in loose stools and forming a gel. Kaolin (microscopic clay particles) and pectin (derived from apples) absorb water and make up the most common non-narcotic, antidiarrheal products. Narcotic drugs containing opium work as antispasmodics as well as to relieve pain. Narcotics may be dispensed as controlled substances because of their addictive nature.

> PATIENT EDUCATION: • **Diarrhea often results in severe dehydration characterized by dizziness while standing, confusion, and unresponsiveness.** • **Avoid milk and dairy products, fresh vegetables and fruits, coffee, spicy foods.** • **Call the physician if diarrhea lasts more than 3 days, there is evidence of blood in the stools or black tarry stools, other medications are suspected as the cause of the diarrhea, or diarrhea is accompanied by severe, incapacitating abdominal pain.** • **To prevent constipation, discontinue antidiarrheal drugs as soon as the diarrhea stops.** • **Some antidiarrheal drugs may cause drowsiness, which may impair judgment when driving or performing tasks that require alertness.**

ANTIEMETIC DRUGS

Antiemetics are used to control nausea and vomiting, which may be caused by infections, other drugs, chemotherapy, radiation therapy, anesthesia, vertigo, or motion sickness. Vomiting results from irritation to vomiting centers either in the GI tract or in the brain. Most antiemetics block dopamine from activating vomiting centers in the GI tract and brain. Some patients may be able to tolerate oral administration of these drugs but most often antiemetic drugs are given by injection or rectal suppository.

> PATIENT EDUCATION: • **Patients may feel dizzy when standing from a lying or sitting position.** • **Patients should not drive or perform activities that require alertness when first starting therapy.** • **Alcohol should be avoided.** • **Surgery should not be performed without a surgeon's knowledge that the patient is taking this drug.** • **Over-the-counter drugs could cause serious interactions.** • **Patients should keep the physician informed of all other drugs being taken.**

ANTIULCER BETA-HISTAMINE (H$_2$) BLOCKERS

Histamine is a chemical made by the body that produces dilation of small blood vessels, lowers the blood pressure, and increases secretions from the stomach, salivary glands, and other organs. H$_2$ blockers block the release of stomach acid and are used to treat ulcers and conditions caused by excess stomach acid. Histamine$_2$ (H$_2$) antagonists inhibit the secretion of histamine receptor sites in the stomach, inhibiting gastric acid secretion and reducing the output of pepcin. This decrease in acid permits the healing of ulcerated areas.

> PATIENT EDUCATION: • **The drug should be taken with meals and at bedtime.** • **Cigarette smoking decreases the effectiveness of these drugs.** • **Report to the doctor any unusual bleeding or bruising, sore throat, fever, tarry stools, confu-**

℞ Common Gastrointestinal Drugs (generic name: Tradename, *Over-the-Counter*)

Antidiarrheals
  attapulgite: *Kaopectate*
  bismuth subsalicylate: *Pepto-Bismol*
  diphenoxylate/atropine: Lomotil
  loperamide: *Imodium*

Antiemetics
  dimenhydrinate: *Dramamine*
  ondansetrol: Zofran
  phosphorated carbohydrates: *Emetrol*
  prochlorperazine: Compazine
  promethazine: Phenergan
  scopolamine: Transdermal Scop
  trimethobenzamide: Tigan

Antacids
  aluminum hydroxide
  aluminum and magnesium hydroxide: *Maalox, Mylanta*
  calcium carbonate: *Tums*
  magaldrate: *Riopan*

Antiulcer Beta-Histamine Blocker
  cimetidine: *Tagamet*
  famotidine: *Pepcid*
  nizatidine: *Axid*
  ranitidine: *Zantac*

Antiulcer—Other
  cisapride: Propulsid
  dicyclomine: Bentyl

lansoprazole: Prevacid
omeprazole: Prilosec
propantheline: Pro-Banthine
simethicone: *Mylicon, Gas-X, Phazyme*
sucralfate: Carafate

Heliobacter pylori Treatment Combinations
  bismuth subsalicylate, metronidazole, amoxicillin
  bismuth subsalicylate, metronidazole, tetracycline
  clarithromycin, omeprazole

Laxatives
  bisacodyl: *Dulcolax*
  cascara
  docusate: *Colace, Peri-Colace*
  glycerin
  magnesium hydroxide: *Milk of Magnesia*
  mineral oil
  phenolphthalein: *Ex-Lax*
  polyethelene glycol
  psyllium: *Metamucil, Fiberall*
  senna: *Senokot*
  sodium biphosphate: *Fleet Enema*

Perineal Care
  Anusol
  witch hazel: *Tucks*

---

sion, hallucinations, dizziness, or joint or muscle pain. • Medical attention should be sought if there are any signs of bleeding ulcers, such as black tarry stools. • Alcohol and tobacco products should be avoided. • These medications should be taken with meals and at bedtime. • Tablets have an odor, which is normal. • These drugs should not be taken for minor digestive complaints, such as upset stomach, nausea, or heartburn. • H$_2$ blockers should be taken at least 1 hour apart from antacids.

HELICOBACTER PYLORI TREATMENTS

Gastritis has been associated with the presence of a spiral-shaped bacillus called *Helicobacter pylori*. This organism not only enjoys the hostile low pH of the stomach, but also can degrade the overlying mucus. *Helicobacter* is also thought to be associated with peptic ulcer disease and gastric carcinoma. Two or three drugs are used in combination to treat this condition: (1) Antibiotics specific for killing amebae and protozoa, (2) broad-spectrum antibiotics, and (3) bismuth subsalicylate (*Pepto-Bismol*).

LAXATIVES

Laxatives are used to encourage bowel movements. Laxatives work by softening stools or by stimulating the muscle contractions of the bowel. Many people take laxatives more often than they need to. Laxatives should not be taken to "clean out the system" or to "achieve normal regularity." Healthy people may have up to three bowel movements per day or as few as three bowel movements per week. It is untrue that everyone should have one bowel movement per day.

It is better not to take laxatives at all. If bowel movement frequency decreases or stools become difficult to pass, it is better to treat simple, occasional constipation without drugs, by eating a high-fiber diet, drinking plenty of water, and exercising regularly. Taking laxatives over a long period can cause serious health problems. Overuse of laxatives can gradually reduce the intestine's ability to work efficiently. This causes increased constipation and a disease of the large colon known as cathartic colon, in which the intestine becomes enlarged and will not move without chemical stimulation.

> **PATIENT EDUCATION:** • **Check with the physician to make sure fluid intake is adequate and appropriate. With too little fluids, laxatives may dry and harden stool, clogging the intestine. • Do not use laxatives for more than 1 week.**

Neurologic Drugs

The diseases of the central nervous system include both mental disorders and structural disorders of the brain, spinal cord, and peripheral nerves. The causes of structural disorders usually are easily determined; mental disorders may be explainable but often explanations can be difficult to determine. Structural diseases may be due to obstructions to the circulation of the cerebrospinal fluid, or vascular diseases such as aneurysms, hemorrhage, thrombosis or infarctions caused by embolizations, and, perhaps, migraine headaches. Infections of the nervous system are most commonly caused by pyogenic bacteria, tuberculosis, syphilis, or viruses. Demyelinating diseases (e.g., multiple sclerosis) are of unknown cause, but recent advances point toward "slow viruses" as a causative factor. Epilepsy and other seizure disorders may be due to tumors, scar tissue, or progressive neurologic diseases. In a great majority of cases, however, no pathologic basis for the seizures is evident. Tumors of the central nervous system are most commonly metastatic from the lung or other organs. Primary cancer sites arise from glial cells or from the meninges.

Mental disorders include organic syndromes, such as arteriosclerosis; Alzheimer's disease; Parkinson's disease; senile dementia; delirium tremens; toxic psychoses from alcohol, drugs, and other poisons; migraine headaches; and slow virus diseases. Functional disorders include schizophrenia, manic–depressive psychosis, neuroses, and personality disorders. As an introduction to neurologic drugs, only those drugs more frequently prescribed in the primary care setting will be considered here.

ALZHEIMER'S AGENTS

To date, there is no treatment for Alzheimer's dementia. The term dementia describes a collection of symptoms caused by more than 60 disorders. Alzheimer's dementia is not reversible and accounts for more than 50 percent of the cases of dementia. If all other efforts to improve the mental and physical state fail, drug treatment with ergoloid mesylates may be of some benefit. The drug, however, must be started at the earliest stages of the disease, as it has not been shown to be of any benefit in more severe cases. Even in the earliest stages, the benefits are minimal. The drug usually is discontinued unless the patient shows noticeable improvement.

> **PATIENT EDUCATION:** • **Patients may feel dizzy when standing from a lying or sitting position. • Tobacco and alcohol should be avoided. • The drug can affect the body's ability to adjust to heat, causing dizziness, lightheadedness, fainting, and an increase in body temperature. • Fluid intake should be increased to offset fluid loss.**

ANTICONVULSANTS

Seizures occur when a group of neurons emit electrical impulses in an abnormal, uncontrolled way. Symptoms may be almost imperceptible up to the loss of consciousness and convulsions. No single drug available can treat all types of seizures. Some drugs may prevent one type of seizure yet provoke another. Antiseizure drugs include barbiturates, hydantoins (phenytoin), and succinimides. Phenytoin (Dilantin) is the drug of choice for treating adults with tonic–clonic seizures, while barbiturates (penobarbital) are the drug of choice for treating children. Phenytoin is also used to treat excruciating face pain, called trigeminal neuralgia or tic douloureux.

PATIENT EDUCATION: • **Patients should not drive or perform activities that require alertness when first starting therapy.** • **Patients should avoid alcohol.** • **Patients should have frequent dental check-ups to prevent gum tenderness and bleeding.** • **Patients may feel dizzy, drowsy, have blurred vision, and lack muscle coordination.** • **Patients should wear a medical identification bracelet or carry a medical alert card.** • **Suddenly discontinuing the drug may cause severe convulsions.** • **Surgery should not be performed without a surgeon's knowledge that the patient is taking this drug.** • **Regular medical visits are necessary for testing blood levels of phenytoin.**

ANTIMIGRAINE DRUGS

Migraine headaches are thought to be the result of vasodilation of extracerebral cranial arteries. The best therapy is avoidance of conditions that bring on an attack. Treatments include prescribing a variety of pain-relieving drugs, such as aspirin, codeine, Demerol, and propanolol (Inderol). Another drug used for the treatment of migraine is ergot, a fungus that grows parasitically on rye. Ergotamine tartrate induces vasoconstriction and is used in combination with caffeine and barbiturates. Symptoms of ergot overdose include vomiting, burning, abdominal cramping, diarrhea, extreme weakness, slow or weak pulse, and tingling of the extremities. Untreated, the patient may lapse into a coma and die. Generalized gangrene of the extremities is a common complication in patients who survive.

PATIENT EDUCATION: • **Notify the physician of vomiting, burning, abdominal cramping, diarrhea, extreme weakness, slow or weak pulse, and tingling of the extremities.**

ANTIPSYCHOTIC DRUGS

Psychotic symptoms may be partly based on the overactivity of the neurotransmitter dopamine or from hypersensitivity of dopamine receptors. Antipsychotic drugs are used in

---

℞ **Common Neurologic Drugs (generic name: Tradename)**

Anticonvulsants
  carbamazepine: Tegretol
  clonazepam: Klonopin
  diazepam: Valium
  phenobarbital: Luminal
  phenytoin: Dilantin
  valproic acid: Depakene, Depakote

Antimigraine
  ergotamine/caffeine: Cafergot
  ergotamine/caffeine/pentobarbital: Cafergot PB

Parkinsonian Agents
  levodopa
  procyclidine: Kemadrin

Alzheimer's Agents
  ergoloid mesylates: Hydergine
  tacrine: Cognex

℞ **Common Antipsychotics (generic name: Tradename)**

chlorpromazine: Thorazine

halperidol: Haldol

lithium carbonate: Eskalith, Lithane, Lithobid

risperidone: Risperdal

thioridazine: Mellaril

℞ **Common Antidepressants (generic name: Tradename)**

Cyclic
  Amitriptyline: Elavil, Triavil
  imipramine: Tofranil
  nortriptyline: Aventyl, Pamelor

Monoamine Oxidase (MAO) Inhibitors
  phenelzine (Nardil)

Serotonin Reuptake Inhibitors
  fluoxetine: Prozac
  fluvozamine: Luvox
  paroxetine: Paxil
  sertraline: Zoloft

the treatment of psychoses. They are also classified as *major tranquilizers* or *neuroleptics*. These drugs block dopamine receptors in the limbic system of the brain, which controls emotions. The patient becomes less hostile, agitated, and paranoic without the side effects of sedation and confusion.

ANTIDEPRESSANTS

Antidepressants are similar to yet different from the antipsychotic drugs; they are used to relieve the symptoms of depression. Depression is associated with the levels of circulating amines norepinephrine and serotonin. Tricyclic antidepressants (TCAs) inhibit the reuptake of the norepinephrine and serotonin (both neurotransmitters). This prolongs the action of norepinephrine in the brain, which corrects the low levels associated with depression. Monoamine oxidase (MAO) inhibitors irreversibly inhibit MAO, an enzyme that breaks down epinephrine, norepinephrine and serotonin, leaving these amines to accumulate in neuronal storage sites. The newest drugs (Prozac, Paxil, Zoloft) act as antidepressants by inhibiting the neuronal uptake of serotonin, with little effect on norepinephrine.

PARKINSONIAN AGENTS

Parkinson's disease is a disorder of the nervous system marked by tremor, muscular rigidity, slow movements, stooped posture, salivation, and an immobile facial expression. Most drugs are used to combat muscle rigidity and lethargy. Drugs used include anticholinergics, antidepressants, antihistamines, dopa inhibitors combined with levodopa, dopamine antagonists, and MAO inhibitors.

> PATIENT EDUCATION: • **Avoid foods and vitamins that contain vitamin B6, since this vitamin can destroy the drug's effectiveness. • Levodopa may interfere with urine tests for sugar and ketones. • Patients may feel dizzy when standing from a lying or sitting position. • Patients should not drive or perform activities that require alertness when first starting therapy. • Alcohol should be avoided. • Surgery should not be performed without a surgeon's knowledge that the patient is taking this drug. • Over-the-counter drugs could cause serious interactions. • Patients should keep the physician informed of all other drugs being taken.**

Written Competency 9–1

Performance Objective: Using the information and a PDR, answer the following 10 questions by applying drug information to the assessment of the patient in the clinical setting, with 100 percent accuracy and within 30 minutes. Do not give yourself credit for incorrect or omitted answers.

1. A patient with diabetes is self-injecting insulin for the first time and suddenly appears pale and anxious. Vital signs reveal a drop in blood pressure (to 102/60) from when it was taken 15 minutes ago, shortness of breath, and tachycardia. Initial treatment for this condition should consist of:
   a. Placing the patient's head lower than the body.
   b. Preparing Benadryl (oral antihistamine).
   c. Preparing glucagon (antihypoglycemic agent).
   d. Preparing Phenergan (antihistamine injection).
   e. Administering spirits of ammonia.

2. Which of the following is recommended for fever for patients with GI ulcers?
   a. Ecotrin.
   b. Tylenol.
   c. Butazolidin.
   d. Motrin.
   e. Codeine.

3. For the second time, a patient develops marked redness and swelling at the injection site following an injection of 0.8 ml of a 1 : 10 allergy solution. The next dose administered should be:
   a. 0.9 ml 1 : 10.
   b. 0.8 ml 1 : 10.
   c. 0.8 ml 1 : 100.
   d. 0.7 ml 1 : 10.
   e. 0.6 ml 1 : 10.

4. The antacid aluminum hydroxide may be administered with:
   a. Tetracycline.
   b. Milk.
   c. Laxatives.
   d. Water.
   e. Simethicone.

5. Epinephrine added to local anesthesia:
   a. Prolongs numbness.
   b. Decreases swelling at the site caused by anesthesia.
   c. Both a and b.
   d. Decreases systemic absorption of the anesthesia.
   e. Both a and d.

6. A patient is prescribed a narcotic analgesic following minor surgery. Common side effects to expect from short-term narcotic analgesics include:
   a. Constipation.
   b. Drowsiness.
   c. Both a and b.
   d. Skin itching.
   e. Both a and d.

7. ASA is contraindicated in:
   a. Patients with chickenpox.
   b. Children with flulike symptoms.
   c. Both a and b.

d. Patients with a history of heart attack.

e. Both a and d.

8. Which of the following vaccines is given as early as 2 months of age?

a. Orimune.

b. Influenza vaccine.

c. DPT.

d. M-M-R II.

e. all of the above

9. Which of the following vaccine administrations would be questionable for a 2-month-old infant living in a household with an AIDS patient?

a. Tetanus Toxoid (adsorbed).

b. DTP.

c. Tetanus Toxoid (fluid).

d. Oral Polio Virus vaccine.

e. all of the above

10. Match the following descriptions to their correct terms:

a. Giant hives erupting on the face following the ingestion of tomatoes.

b. Generalized itching, swelling, and asthmalike breathing following an injection of penicillin.

c. Severe drop in blood pressure, fever, rash, and a 2-week history of a bacterial infection.

d. Vaginal discharge and severe diarrhea following a 2-week therapy of antibiotics.

(1) Serum sickness.

(2) Angioedema.

(3) Hypovolemic shock.

(4) Anaphylaxis.

(5) Superinfection.

(6) Septic shock.

Score: _____

See Appendix B for answers.

Terminal Performance Objective/Competency

Procedure 9–1: Teach a Patient to Administer Insulin

EQUIPMENT

Audio cassette and tape recorder
Insulin syringes, 30-unit, 50-unit, and 100-unit
Prescribed insulin(s)
Cottonball
Alcohol
Gloves
Rigid sharps container
Written patient teaching guide (handout)
Chart of rotation sites (handout)
Medical record with order: Rx: Novolin R

(regular insulin): Initial dose 10 units injected before breakfast and followed by similar doses ac and hs, depending on the results of blood and urine tests performed before each meal and at bedtime. Dosage may be increased 2 to 4 units every other day until blood glucose or urine glucose levels are within acceptable limits. To report in test results each day at the same hour.

REVIEW

Techniques to be followed (with rationales) for subcutaneous injections, Chapter 8.

Terminal Performance Objective: Teach a patient to administer insulin by completing each step accurately, safely, and in the correct order, without a break in sterile technique and within reasonable job production time. Tape-record the training session.

	V	S	U*

PROCEDURAL STEPS

Care of Equipment and Insulin

1. Wash hands.
2. Read the product information brochure included in the package.
3. Check expiration dates.
4. Discard open vials that have not been used for several weeks.
5. Store insulin vial in use at room temperature. Store stock supply in refrigerator. Do not freeze.
6. Gently rotate the vial between your palms. Do not shake, as shaking may inactivate the drug. (*Note:* Rapid-acting and globulin insulins do not have a precipitate.)
7. Discard any vial that appears clumped or granular.
8. Keep syringe units sterile.
9. Dispose of syringe units appropriately.

Procedure for Preparing a Rapid-Acting Insulin

1. Clean the vial with antiseptic.
2. Open the syringe unit with sterile technique.

*V = Value, to fill in if assigning points or other specific values to each step, or if designating a critical step.
S = Satisfactory completion of the step.
U = Unsatisfactory completion of the step, or step incomplete; needs more practice.

3. Inject an amount of air into the vial of rapid-acting insulin equal to the amount of rapid-acting insulin that is to be withdrawn.   ☐ ☐ ☐

4. Withdraw the correct amount of rapid-acting insulin into the syringe.   ☐ ☐ ☐

5. Withdraw the needle and make a final check for correct amount and no air bubbles.   ☐ ☐ ☐

Procedure for Mixing an Intermediate Insulin with a Rapid-Acting Insulin

1. Clean both vials with antiseptic.   ☐ ☐ ☐

2. Open the syringe unit with sterile technique.   ☐ ☐ ☐

3. Inject an amount of air into the vial of rapid-acting insulin equal to the amount of rapid-acting insulin that is to be withdrawn.   ☐ ☐ ☐

4. Inject an amount of air into the vial of intermediate insulin equal to the amount of intermediate insulin to be withdrawn.   ☐ ☐ ☐

5. Remove the needle, then withdraw the dose of rapid-acting insulin *first*.
   RATIONALE: When preparing a mixture of rapid-acting and intermediate insulins, avoid transferring intermediate insulin into the rapid-acting insulin vial.   ☐ ☐ ☐

6. Withdraw the needle and make sure the amount withdrawn is correct and no air bubbles are present.   ☐ ☐ ☐

7. Turn the intermediate insulin vial upside down and gently rotate to mix.   ☐ ☐ ☐

8. Insert the needle into the intermediate vial and withdraw the correct amount of insulin.   ☐ ☐ ☐

9. Withdraw the needle and make a final check for correct amount and no air bubbles.   ☐ ☐ ☐

Administration

1. Rotate sites and chart injection sites.   ☐ ☐ ☐

2. Allow 3 to 4 cm between injection sites.   ☐ ☐ ☐

3. Do not use the same site within a 1-month period.   ☐ ☐ ☐

4. Avoid the umbilicus.
   RATIONALE: The umbilical site is very vascular.   ☐ ☐ ☐

5. Avoid the waistline.
   RATIONALE: This site is sensitive.   ☐ ☐ ☐

6. Brace arm or leg to be injected against a hard surface.   ☐ ☐ ☐

7. Use a 90-degree angle when using a 1/2-in needle; a 45-degree angle with a 5/8-in needle.   ☐ ☐ ☐

8. Apply pressure for 1 minute after injection. Do not massage.
   RATIONALE: Massage may interfere with insulin absorption rate.   ☐ ☐ ☐

9. Delay administration of insulin if breakfast is to be delayed for tests.   ☐ ☐ ☐

10. Have a second vial of rapid-acting insulin on hand for emergency use.   ☐ ☐ ☐

11. Have extra insulin and equipment on hand at all times.   ☐ ☐ ☐

Signs and Symptoms of Hypoglycemia (Too Much Insulin)

1. Watch for nervousness, anxiety, sweating, pale and cool skin, headache, nausea, hunger, shakiness. ☐ ☐ ☐

2. If these occur, eat candy, honey, or sugar or drink orange juice. ☐ ☐ ☐

3. Hypoglycemia may occur if you skip a meal, exercise too much, or experience too much stress. ☐ ☐ ☐

4. During the initiation of insulin therapy, notify the physician each and every time this occurs. ☐ ☐ ☐

5. After your condition is stabilized, notify the physician should these symptoms happen very often. ☐ ☐ ☐

Additional Instructions

1. If an insulin injection must be skipped, decrease food intake by one third and drink plenty of fluids. ☐ ☐ ☐

2. Notify the physician of any illness and test urine glucose frequently. ☐ ☐ ☐

3. Avoid the use of OTC drugs. ☐ ☐ ☐

4. Avoid the use of alcohol. ☐ ☐ ☐

5. Follow prescribed diets. ☐ ☐ ☐

6. Monitor blood and glucose levels. ☐ ☐ ☐

7. Tell any physician, dentist, or other medical personnel that you are taking insulin. ☐ ☐ ☐

8. Wear a medical identification tag. ☐ ☐ ☐

9. Schedule regular visits for examination. ☐ ☐ ☐

10. Keep medication and equipment out of the reach of children. ☐ ☐ ☐

11. Notify the physician of any of the following: loss of appetite, blurred vision, fruity breath odor, increased urination, increased thirst, nausea, or vomiting. ☐ ☐ ☐

12. Strenuous, unusual exercise is undesirable. If this type of activity occurs, extra sugary snacks can make up for the carbohydrates lost in exercise. It may be necessary to reduce the next insulin dose. ☐ ☐ ☐

13. Care must be taken to prevent infections of the skin of the feet, upper respiratory infections, and urinary tract infections. ☐ ☐ ☐

14. Record the patient teaching session on the patient's chart. ☐ ☐ ☐

Date: _____ Competency achieved: Y _____ N _____

Designated reasonable time standard: _____

Actual completion time: _____

Fifty Most Commonly Prescribed Drugs

The decision to include or exclude particular drugs in this appendix is based on the 1997 report of the *The Pharmacy Times*, "Top 200 Drugs of 1997," published February, 1997. Included are the 50 most commonly prescribed (new and refill) trade name drugs in 1997. Although some of these drugs may shift in their ranking and a few drop below the rank of the top 50 by the time of your reading, the trend of drug treatment should remain, on average, the same for some years to come.

This textbook contains five assigned projects (beginning with Chapter 4) based on the information contained in this appendix. By the completion of Chapter 9, you will have 50 *drug guides* (drug information cards) for each of the top 50 drugs in Table A–1. It is assumed that you will check the manufacturer's product information insert contained in the packaging of each drug and use the PDR or other drug administration handbook for the specific details about each drug. A *drug guide* example is provided in Chapter 4.

The names of the drugs also appear in the general index at the back of the book. The generic names are in lowercase letters, and the trade (brand) names are in capitals. For each of the drugs listed, the pregnancy risk category (see Table 5–1), published by the Food and Drug Administration (FDA), is included. Table A–1 lists the top 50 drugs by *rank*. Tables A–2 through A–4 are included as a cross-reference, listing drugs by alphabetic order of *brand name*, *therapeutic classification*, and *pregnancy risk*.

TABLE A–1. **Top 50 Drugs by Rank**

Rank	Brand Name	Generic Name	Classification	Pregnancy Risk	General Use
01	PREMARIN	Conjugated estrogen	Hormone	X	Hormone imbalance/breast and prostate cancer/menopausal symptoms
02	SYNTHROID	Levothyroxine sodium	Hormone	A	Hypothyroidism/cretinism/myxedema coma
03	TRIMOX	Amoxicillin trihydrate	Antimicrobial/penicillin	NR	Systemic infections, acute and chronic
04	LANOXIN	Digoxin	Cardiac glycoside	C	CHF/atrial fibrillation and flutter/supraventricular tachycardia
05	HYDROCODONE/APAP	Hydrocodone/APAP	Narcotic analgesic	Not established	Moderate to severe pain relief
06	PROZAC	Fluoxetine hydrochloride	Antidepressant	B	Depression/obsessive-compulsive disorder/bulimia nervosa
07	ALBUTEROL	Albuterol	Bronchodilator	C	COLD/asthma/pre-term labor/bronchospasm
08	PRILOSEC	Omeprazole	Ulcer medication	C	Gastric and duodenal ulcers/GERD
09	VASOTEC	Enalapril maleate	Antihypertensive/Ace inhibitor	C/D	Hypertension/renal impairment or hyponatremia
10	NORVASC	Amlodipine besylate	Antihypertensive/antianginal/Ca channel blocker	C	Hypertension/angina
11	COUMADIN	Warfarin sodium	Anticoagulant	X	Clotting disorders/MI/chronic atrial fibrillation
12	ZOLOFT	Sertraline hydrochloride	Antidepressant	B	Depression/obsessive compulsive disorder
13	CLARITIN	Loratadine	Antihistamine	B	Allergic rhinitis
14	ZOCOR	Simvastatin	Antihyperlipidemic	X	Cholesterol-lowering agent
15	PAXIL	Paroxetine hydrochloride	Antidepressant	B	Depression/panic disorder
16	PROCARDIA XL	Nifedipine	Antihypertensive/antianginal/Ca channel blocker	C	Hypertension/angina
17	ZANTAC	Ranitidine hydrochloride	Ulcer medication/HO$_2$ inhibitor	B	Duodenal and gastric and ulcer/pathologic hypersecretory conditions
18	ZESTRIL	Lisinopril	Antihypertensive/Ace inhibitor	C/D	Hypertension
19	FUROSEMIDE	Furosemide	Diuretic	C	Hypertension/edema/pulmonary edema
20	CARDIZEM CD	Diltiazem hydrochloride	Antihypertensive/antianginal/Ca channel broker	C	Hypertension/angina

TABLE A–1. **Top 50 Drugs by Rank** (*Continued*)

Rank	Brand Name	Generic Name	Classification	Pregnancy Risk	General Use
21	AUGMENTIN	Amoxicillin/ clavulanic acid	Antimicrobial/ penicillin	B	Moderate to severe bacterial infections
22	BIAXIN	Clarithromycin	Antimicrobial/ macrolide	C	Mild to moderate infections
23	PREMPRO	Conjugated estrogen/medroxy- progesterone acetate	Hormone	X	Relieve postmenopausal symptoms
24	GLUCOPHAGE	Metformin hydrochloride	Antidiabetic agent, oral	B	Noninsulin- dependent (Type II) diabetes
25	TRIMETHOPRIM SULFA	Trimethoprim Sulfa	Antimicrobial, urinary	C	Uncomplicated urinary tract infection
26	AMOXIL	Amoxicillin trihydrate	Antimicrobial/ penicillin	NR	Systemic infections, acute and chronic
27	CIPRO	Ciprofloxacin	Antimicrobial/ fluroquinolone	C	Moderate to severe bacterial infections
28	TRIAMTERENE/ HCTZ	Triamterene/ HCTZ	Diuretic/ antihypertensive	D	Hypertension/edema
29	K-DUR	Potassium chloride	Mineral/potassium supplement	C	Hypokalemia
30	PRAVACHOL	Pravastatin sodium	Antihyperlipidemic	X	Reduce cholesterol levels
31	CEPHALEXIN	Cephalexin monohydrate	Antimicrobial/ cephalosporin	B	Moderate to severe infections
32	PROPOXY- PHENE N/APAP	Propoxyphene with aspirin	Narcotic analgesic	Not estab- lished	Relieve moderate pain
33	AMOXICILLIN	Amoxicillin trihydrate	Antimicrobial	B	Systemic infections, acute and chronic
34	ULTRAM	Tramadol hydrochloride	Narcotic analgesic	C	Relieve moderate pain
35	ZITHROMAX Z-PAK	Azithromycin	Antimicrobial/ macrolide	B	Mild to moderate infections
36	ACETAMINO- PHEN/ CODEINE	Acetaminophen/ codeine	Analgesic/narcotic	C	Relieve moderate pain
37	HYTRIN	Terazosin	Antihypertensive	C	Hypertension and symptoms of benign prostatic hypertrophy
38	DILANTIN	Phenytoin	Anticonvulsant	NR	Control tonic- clonic and complex partial seizures
39	PEPCID	Famotidine	Ulcer medication/H2 inhibitor	B	Gastric and duodenal ulcers and heartburn
40	AMBIEN	Zolpidem tartrate	Sedative/ hypnotic	B	Insomnia
41	VEETIDS	Penicillin V potassium	Antimicrobial/ penicillin	B	Mild to moderate systemic infections
42	PRINIVIL	Lisinopril	Antihypertensive/ Ca channel blocker	C/D	Hypertension
43	PROPACET 100	Propoxyphene and acetaminophen	Narcotic analgesic	Not estab- lished	Relieve moderate pain
44	LEVOXYL	Levothyroxine sodium	Hormone	A	Hypothyroidism/ cretinism/ myxedema coma
45	HUMULIN N INSULIN	Isophane insulin, human, rDNA	Hormone/ hypoglycemic agent	B	Hyperglycemia

TABLE A–1. **Top 50 Drugs by Rank** (*Continued*)

Rank	Brand Name	Generic Name	Classification	Pregnancy Risk	General Use
46	ACCUPRIL	quinipril hydrochloride	Antihypertensive/ ACE inhibitor	C	Hypertension/CHF
47	RELAFEN	Nabumetone	Non-steroidal anti-inflammatory	C	Arthritis and moderate pain
48	LIPITOR	atorvastatin calcium	Antihyperlipidemic	X	Reduce cholesterol levels
49	GLUCOTROL XL	glipizide	Antidiabetic agent, oral	C	Noninsulin dependent (Type II) diabetes
50	IBUPROFEN	ibuprofen	Nonsteroidal anti-inflammatory	NR	Arthritis/moderate pain

TABLE A–2. **Top 50 Drugs by Brand Name**

Brand Name	Generic Name	Classification	Rank	Pregnancy Risk	General Use
ACCUPRIL	quinipril hydrochloride	Antihypertensive/ACE inhibitor	46	C	Hypertension/CHF
ACETAMINOPHEN/CODEINE	Acetaminophen/codeine	Analgesic/narcotic	36	C	Relieve moderate pain
ALBUTEROL	Albuterol	Bronchodilator	07	C	COLD/asthma/pre-term labor/ bronchospasm
AMBIEN	Zolpidem tartrate	Sedative/ hypnotic	40	B	Insomnia
AMOXICILLIN	Amoxicillin trihydrate	Antimicrobial	33	B	Systemic infections, acute and chronic
AMOXIL	Amoxicillin trihydrate	Antimicrobial/penicillin	26	NR	Systemic infections, acute and chronic
AUGMENTIN	Amoxicillin/clavulanic acid	Antimicrobial/penicillin	21	B	Moderate to severe bacterial infections
BIAXIN	Clarithromycin	Antimicrobial/macrolide	22	C	Mild to moderate infections
CARDIZEM CD	Diltiazem hydrochloride	Antihypertensive/antianginal/ Ca channel blocker	20	C	Hypertension/angina
CEPHALEXIN	Cephalexin monohydrate	Antimicrobial/cephalosporin	31	B	Moderate to severe infections
CIPRO	Ciprofloxacin	Antimicrobial/fluroquinolone	27	C	Moderate to severe bacterial infections
CLARITIN	Loratadine	Antihistamine	13	B	Allergic rhinitis
COUMADIN	Warfarin sodium	Anticoagulant	11	X	Clotting disorders/MI/chronic atrial fibrillation
Dilantin	Phenytoin	Anticonvulsant	38	NR	Control tonic-clonic and complex partial seizures
FUROSEMIDE	Furosemide	Diuretic	19	C	Hypertension/edema/ pulmonary edema
GLUCATROL XL	glipizide	Antidiabetic agent, oral	49	C	Noninsulin dependent (Type II) diabetes
GLUCOPHAGE	Metformin hydrochloride	Antidiabetic agent, oral	24	B	Noninsulin-dependent (Type II) diabetes
HUMULIN N INSULIN	Isophane insulin, human, rDNA	Hormone/hypoglycemic agent	45	B	Hyperglycemia
HYDROCODONE/APAP	Hydrocodone/APAP	Narcotic analgesic	05	Not established	Moderate to severe pain relief
HYTRIN	Terazosin	Antihypertensive	37	C	Hypertension and symptoms of benign prostatic hypertrophy
IBUPROFEN	ibuprofen	Nonsteroidal anti-inflammatory	50	No rating	Arthritis/moderate pain
K-DUR	Potassium chloride	Mineral/potassium supplement	29	C	Hypokalemia

TABLE A–2. **Top 50 Drugs by Brand Name** (*Continued*)

Brand Name	Generic Name	Classification	Rank	Pregnancy Risk	General Use
LANOXIN	Digoxin	Cardiac glycoside	04	C	CHF/atrial fibrillation and flutter/ supraventricular tachycardia
LEVOXYL	Levothyroxine sodium	Hormone	44	A	Hypothyroidism/cretinism/ myxedema coma
LIPITOR	atorvastatin calcium	Antihyperlipidemic	48	X	Reduce cholesterol levels
NORVASC	Amlodipine besylate	Antihypertensive/antianginal/ Ca channel blocker	10	C	Hypertension/angina
PAXIL	Paroxetine hydrochloride	Antidepressant	15	B	Depression/panic disorder
PEPCID	Famotidine	Ulcer medication/H2 inhibitor	39	B	Gastric and duodenal ulcers and heartburn
PRAVACHOL	Pravastatin sodium	Antihyperlipidemic	30	X	Reduce cholesterol levels
PREMARIN	Conjugated estrogen	Hormone	01	X	Hormone imbalance/breast and prostate cancer/menopausal symptoms
PREMPRO	Conjugated estrogen/ medroxyprogesterone acetate	Hormone	23	X	Relieve postmenopausal symptoms
PRILOSEC	Omeprazole	Ulcer medication	08	C	Gastric and duodenal ulcers/GERD
PRINIVIL	Lisinopril	Antihypertensive/ Ca channel blocker	42	C/D	Hypertension
PROCARDIA XL	Nifedipine	Antihypertensive/ antianginal/Ca channel blocker	16	C	Hypertension/angina
PROPACET 100	Propoxyphene and acetaminophen	Narcotic analgesic	43	Not established	Relieve moderate pain
PROPOXYPHENE N/APAP	Propoxyphene with aspirin	Narcotic analgesic	32	Not established	Relieve moderate pain
PROZAC	Fluoxetine hydrochloride	Antidepressant	06	B	Depression/obsessive-compulsive disorder/bulimia nervosa
RELAFEN	Nabumetone	Non-steroidal anti-inflammatory	47	C	Arthritis and moderate pain
SYNTHROID	Levothyroxine sodium	Hormone	02	A	Hypothyroidism/cretinism/ myxedema coma
TRIAMTERENE/HCTZ	Triamterence/HCTZ	Diuretic/antihypertensive	28	D	Hypertension/edema
TRIMETHOPRIM/SULFA	Trimethoprim sulfa	Antimicrobial, urinary	25	C	Uncomplicated urinary tract infections

TABLE A–2. **Top 50 Drugs by Brand Name** (*Continued*)

Brand Name	Generic Name	Classification	Rank	Pregnancy Risk	General Use
TRIMOX	Amoxicillin trihydrate	Antimicrobial/penicillin	03	NR	Systemic infections, acute and chronic
ULTRAM	Tramadol hydrochloride	Narcotic analgesic	34	C	Relieve moderate pain
VASOTEC	Enalapril maleate	Antihypertensive/ Ace inhibitor	09	C/D	Hypertension/renal impairment or hyponatremia
VEETIDS	Penicillin V potassium	Antimicrobial/penicillin	41	B	Mild to moderate systemic infections
ZANTAC	Ranitidine hydrochloride	Ulcer medication/H2 inhibitor	17	B	Duodenal and gastric and ulcer/ pathologic hypersecretory conditions
ZESTRIL	Lisinopril	Antihypertensive/ Ace inhibitor	18	C/D	Hypertension
ZITHROMAX Z-PAK	Azithromycin	Antimicrobial/macrolide	35	B	Mild to moderate infections
ZOCOR	Simvastatin	Antihyperlipidemic	14	X	Cholesterol-lowering agent
ZOLOFT	Sertraline hydrochloride	Antidepressant	12	B	Depression/obsessive compulsive disorder

TABLE A–3. Generic Names of the Top 50 Drugs Listed in This Appendix

Generic Name	Brand Name	Classification	Rank	Pregnancy Risk	General Use
Acetaminophen/codeine	ACETAMINOPHEN/CODEINE	Analgesic/narcotic	36	C	Relieve moderate pain
Albuterol	ALBUTEROL	Bronchodilator	07	C	COLD/asthma/pre-term labor/bronchospasm
Amlodipine besylate	NORVASC	Antihypertensive/antianginal/Ca channel blocker	10	C	Hypertension/angina
Amoxicillin trihydrate	AMOXICILLIN	Antimicrobial	33	B	Systemic infections, acute and chronic
Amoxicillin trihydrate	AMOXIL	Antimicrobial/penicillin	26	NR	Systemic infections, acute and chronic
Amoxicillin trihydrate	TRIMOX	Antimicrobial/penicillin	03	NR	Systemic infections, acute and chronic
Amoxicillin/clavulanic acid	AUGMENTIN	Antimicrobial/penicillin	21	B	Moderate to severe bacterial infections
Atorvastatin calcium	LIPITOR	Antihyperlipidemic	48	X	Reduce cholesterol levels
Azithromycin	ZITHROMAX Z-PAK	Antimicrobial/macrolide	35	B	Mild to moderate infections
Cephalexin monohydrate	CEPHALEXIN	Antimicrobial/cephalosporin	31	B	Moderate to severe infections
Ciprofloxacin	CIPRO	Antimicrobial/fluroquinolone	27	C	Moderate to severe bacterial infections
Clarithromycin	BIAXIN	Antimicrobial/macrolide	22	C	Mild to moderate infections
Conjugated estrogen	PREMARIN	Hormone	01	X	Hormone imbalance/breast and prostate cancer/menopausal symptoms
Conjugated estrogen/medroxyprogesterone acetate	PREMPRO	Hormone	23	X	Relieve post menopausal symptoms
Digoxin	LANOXIN	Cardiac glycoside	04	C	CHF/atrial fibrillation and flutter/supraventricular tachycardia
Diltiazem hydrochloride	CARDIZEM CD	Antihypertensive/antianginal/Ca channel blocker	20	C	Hypertension/angina
Enalapril maleate	VASOTEC	Antihypertensive/Ace inhibitor	09	C/D	Hypertension/renal impairment or hyponatremia
Famotidine	PEPCID	Ulcer medication/H2 inhibitor	39	B	Gastric and duodenal ulcers and heartburn
Fluoxetine hydrochloride	PROZAC	Antidepressant	06	B	Depression/obsessive-compulsive disorder/bulimia nervosa

TABLE A–3. Generic Names of the Top 50 Drugs Listed in This Appendix (*Continued*)

Generic Name	Brand Name	Classification	Rank	Pregnancy Risk	General Use
Furosemide	FUROSEMIDE	Diuretic	19	C	Hypertension/edema/ pulmonary edema
Glipizide	GLUCATROL XL	Antidiabetic agent, oral	49	C	Noninsulin dependent (Type II) diabetes
Hydrocodone/APAP	HYDROCODONE/APAP	Narcotic analgesic	05	Not established	Moderate to severe pain relief
Ibuprofen	IBUPROFEN	Nonsteroidal anti-inflammatory	50	No rating	Arthritis/moderate pain
Isophane insulin, human, rDNA	HUMULIN N INSULIN	Hormone/hypoglycemic agent	45	B	Hyperglycemia
Levothyroxine sodium	LEVOXYL	Hormone	44	A	Hypothyroidism/cretinism/ myxedema coma
Levothyroxine sodium	SYNTHROID	Hormone	02	A	Hypothyroidism/cretinism/ myxedema coma
Lisinopril	PRINIVIL	Antihypertensive/ Ca channel blocker	42	C/D	Hypertension
Lisinopril	ZESTRIL	Antihypertensive/ Ace inhibitor	18	C/D	Hypertension
Loratadine	CLARITIN	Antihistamine	13	B	Allergic rhinitis
Metformin hydrochloride	GLUCOPHAGE	Antidiabetic agent, oral	24	B	Noninsulin-dependent (Type II) diabetes
Nabumetone	RELAFEN	Non-steroidal anti-inflammatory	47	C	Arthritis and moderate pain
Nifedipine	PROCARDIA XL	Antihypertensive/antianginal/ Ca channel blocker	16	C	Hypertension/angina
Omeprazole	PRILOSEC	Ulcer medication	08	C	Gastric and duodenal ulcers/ GERD
Paroxetine hydrochloride	PAXIL	Antidepressant	15	B	Depression/panic disorder
Penicillin V potassium	VEETIDS	Antimicrobial/penicillin	41	B	Mild to moderate systemic infections
Phenytoin	DILANTIN	Anticonvulsant	38	NR	Control tonic-clonic and complex partial seizures
Potassium chloride	K-DUR	Mineral/potassium supplement	29	C	Hypokalemia
Pravastatin sodium	PRAVACHOL	Antihyperlipidemic	30	X	Reduce cholesterol levels
Propoxyphene and acetaminophen	PROPACET 100	Narcotic analgesic	43	Not established	Relieve moderate pain

TABLE A–3. **Generic Names of the Top 50 Drugs Listed in This Appendix** (*Continued*)

Generic Name	Brand Name	Classification	Rank	Pregnancy Risk	General Use
Propoxyphene with aspirin	PROPOXYPHENE N/APAP	Narcotic analgesic	32	Not established	Relieve moderate pain
Quinipril hydrochloride	ACCUPRIL	Antihypertensive/ACE inhibitor	46	C	Hypertension/CHF
Ranitidine hydrochloride	ZANTAC	Ulcer medication/ H2 inhibitor	17	B	Duodenal and gastric and ulcer/ pathologic hypersecretory conditions
Sertraline hydrochloride	ZOLOFT	Antidepressant	12	B	Depression/obsessive compulsive disorder
Simvastatin	ZOCOR	Antihyperlipidemic	14	X	Cholesterol-lowering agent
Terazosin	HYTRIN	Antihypertensive	37	C	Hypertension and symptoms of benign prostatic hypertrophy
Tramadol hydrochloride	ULTRAM	Narcotic analgesic	34	C	Relieve moderate pain
Triamterene/HCTZ	TRIAMTERENE/HCTZ	Diuretic/antihypertensive	28	D	Hypertension/edema
Trimethoprim sulfa	TRIMETHOPRIM/SULFA	Antimicrobial, urinary	25	C	Uncomplicated urinary tract infections
Warfarin sodium	COUMADIN	Anticoagulant	11	X	Clotting disorders/MI/chronic atrial fibrillation
Zolpidem tartrate	AMBIEN	Sedative/hypnotic	40	B	Insomnia

TABLE A–4. Top 50 Drugs Listed From Greatest to Least Pregnancy Risk (See Chapter 5, Table 5–1)

Pregnancy Risk	Generic Name	Brand Name	Classification	Rank	General Use
X	Conjugated estrogen	PREMARIN	Hormone	01	Hormone imbalance/breast and prostate cancer/menopausal symptoms
X	Conjugated estrogen/medroxyprogesterone acetate	PREMPRO	Hormone	23	Relieve post menopausal symptoms
X	Atorvastatin calcium	LIPITOR	Antihyperlipidemic	48	Reduce cholesterol levels
X	Pravastatin sodium	PRAVACHOL	Antihyperlipidemic	30	Reduce cholesterol levels
X	Simvastatin	ZOCOR	Antihyperlipidemic	14	Cholesterol-lowering agent
X	Warfarin sodium	COUMADIN	Anticoagulant	11	Clotting disorders/MI/chronic atrial fibrillation
No rating	Ibuprofen	IBUPROFEN	Nonsteroidal anti-inflammatory	50	Arthritis/moderate pain
No rating	Hydrocodone/APAP	HYDROCODONE/APAP	Narcotic analgesic	05	Moderate to severe pain relief
No rating	Propoxyphene and acetaminophen	PROPACET 100	Narcotic analgesic	43	Relieve moderate pain
No rating	Propoxyphene with aspirin	PROPOXYPHENE N/APAP	Narcotic analgesic	32	Relieve moderate pain
No rating	Amoxicillin trihydrate	AMOXIL	Antimicrobial/penicillin	26	Systemic infections, acute and chronic
No rating	Amoxicillin trihydrate	TRIMOX	Antimicrobial/penicillin	03	Systemic infections, acute and chronic
No rating	Phenytoin	DILANTIN	Anticonvulsant	38	Control tonic-clonic and complex partial seizures
D	Triamterene/HCTZ	TRIAMTERENE/HCTZ	Diuretic/antihypertensive	28	Hypertension/edema
C/D	Enalapril maleate	VASOTEC	Antihypertensive/Ace inhibitor	09	Hypertension/renal impairment or hyponatremia
C/D	Lisinopril	PRINIVIL	Antihypertensive/Ca channel blocker	42	Hypertension
C/D	Lisinopril	ZESTRIL	Antihypertensive/Ace inhibitor	18	Hypertension
C	Acetaminophen/codeine	ACETAMINOPHEN/CODEINE	Analgesic/narcotic	36	Relieve moderate pain
C	Albuterol	ALBUTEROL	Bronchodilator	07	COLD/asthma/pre-term labor/bronchospasm
C	Amlodipine besylate	NORVASC	Antihypertensive/antianginal/Ca channel blocker	10	Hypertension/angina
C	Quinipril hydrochloride	ACCUPRIL	Antihypertensive/ACE inhibitor	46	Hypertension/CHF

TABLE A–4. Top 50 Drugs Listed From Greatest to Least Pregnancy Risk (See Chapter 5, Table 5–1) (Continued)

Pregnancy Risk	Generic Name	Brand Name	Rank	Classification	General Use
C	Ciprofloxacin	CIPRO	27	Antimicrobial/ fluroquinolone	Moderate to severe bacterial infections
C	Clarithromycin	BIAXIN	22	Antimicrobial/macrolide	Mild to moderate infections
C	Digoxin	LANOXIN	04	Cardiac glycoside	CHF/atrial fibrillation and flutter/ supraventricular tachycardia
C	Diltiazem hydrochloride	CARDIZEM CD	20	Antihypertensive/ antianginal/Ca channel blocker	Hypertension/angina
C	Furosemide	FUROSEMIDE	19	Diuretic	Hypertension/edema/pulmonary edema
C	Glipizide	GLUCATROL XL	49	Antidiabetic agent, oral	Noninsulin dependent (Type II) diabetes
C	Nabumetone	RELAFEN	47	Non-steroidal anti-inflammatory	Arthritis and moderate pain
C	Nifedipine	PROCARDIA XL	16	Antihypertensive/ antianginal/Ca channel blocker	Hypertension/angina
C	Omeprazole	PRILOSEC	08	Ulcer medication	Gastric and duodenal ulcers/GERD
C	Potassium chloride	K-DUR	29	Mineral/potassium supplement	Hypokalemia
C	Terazosin	HYTRIN	37	Antihypertensive	Hypertension and symptoms of benign prostatic hypertrophy
C	Tramadol hydrochloride	ULTRAM	34	Narcotic analgesic	Relieve moderate pain
C	Trimethoprim sulfa	TRIMETHOPRIM/SULFA	25	Antimicrobial, urinary	Uncomplicated urinary tract infections
B	Amoxicillin trihydrate	AMOXICILLIN	33	Antimicrobial	Systemic infections, acute and chronic
B	Amoxicillin/clavulanic acid	AUGMENTIN	21	Antimicrobial/penicillin	Moderate to severe bacterial infections
B	Azithromycin	ZITHROMAX Z-PAK	35	Antimicrobial/macrolide	Mild to moderate infections
B	Cephalexin monohydrate	CEPHALEXIN	31	Antimicrobial/cephalosporin	Moderate to severe infections
B	Famotidine	PEPCID	39	Ulcer medication/ H2 inhibitor	Gastric and duodenal ulcers and heartburn
B	Fluoxetine hydrochloride	PROZAC	06	Antidepressant	Depression/obsessive-compulsive disorder/bulimia nervosa
B	Isophane insulin, human, rDNA	HUMULIN N INSULIN	45	Hormone/hypoglycemic agent	Hyperglycemia

TABLE A-4. **Top 50 Drugs Listed From Greatest to Least Pregnancy Risk (See Chapter 5, Table 5-1)** (*Continued*)

Pregnancy Risk	Generic Name	Brand Name	Classification	Rank	General Use
B	Loratadine	CLARITIN	Antihistamine	13	Allergic rhinitis
B	Metformin hydrochloride	GLUCOPHAGE	Antidiabetic agent, oral	24	Noninsulin-dependent (Type II) diabetes
B	Paroxetine hydrochloride	PAXIL	Antidepressant	15	Depression/panic disorder
B	Penicillin V potassium	VEETIDS	Antimicrobial/penicillin	41	Mild to moderate systemic infections
B	Ranitidine hydrochloride	ZANTAC	Ulcer medication/ H2 inhibitor	17	Duodenal and gastric and ulcer/ pathologic hypersecretory conditions
B	Sertraline hydrochloride	ZOLOFT	Antidepressant	12	Depression/obsessive compulsive disorder
B	Zolpidem tartrate	AMBIEN	Sedative/hypnotic	40	Insomnia
A	Levothyroxine sodium	LEVOXYL	Hormone	44	Hypothyroidism/cretinism/myxedema coma
A	Levothyroxine sodium	SYNTHROID	Hormone	02	Hypothyroidism/cretinism/myxedema coma

Answers to Written Competencies, Procedures, and Conversion Drills

CHAPTER 1

Written Competency 1–1

1. milli. 2. g or mg. 3. ml or cc. 4. same. 5. same. 6. greater than. 7. less than.
8. 0 (zero). 9. 0.1 ml. 10. 2 cc. 11. 0.1. 12. ml, cc, L. 13. area. 14. equivalent.
15. ten. 16. milli. 17. kilo. 18. micro. 19. centi. 20. deci.

Written Competency 1–2

1. grain; gr; minim; minim symbol. 2. 60; 60; equal to. 3. ʒ̅ʒ̅ʒ̅ʒ̅ʒ̅ 4. ℥̅℥̅℥̅℥̅℥̅ 5. Rx: ℥ iv Sig:
ʒ iss tid. 6. drop; gt; gtt. 7. 60. 8. c.; gal 9. 128℥. 10. liquid Tylenol Sig: 1 tsp qid.
11. before 12. ss 13. roman numerals 14. 1/150 15. ʒ iiss 16. ℳ vi 17. ʒ 1-2/3
18. gtt xx 19. gr v 20. gr 1/10

Written Competency 1–3

1. 1. 2. 1000. 3. 1. 4. 3. 5. 15 or 16. 6. 15 or 16. 7. 2. 8. 2. 9. 15.
10. 4 or 5. 11. 6. 12. 15. 13. 300, 320, 325, or 330. 14. 70. 15. 0.4. 16. 10.
17. 240 or 256. 18. 100. 19. 2. 20. 0.25. 21. 110. 22. 120. 23. 150 or 160.
24. 480 or 512. 25. 200. 26. 30, 32, or 33. 27. 1250. 28. 0.75. 29. 32 or 33.3.
30. 450, 480, 512.

Procedure 1–1

1. Yes. 2. 4 ml (cc). 3. 4 ml (using 15 gtt = ml); 4 to 5 ml (using 16 gtt = 1 ml). 4. Equal
to; 60 gtt; 4 to 5 ml. 5. 15 to 16 minims. 6a. 5 minims. 6b. More than 10 minims.
6c. Slightly more; using an angle less than 90 degrees to dispense an oily substance usually results in a greater amount of fluid being dispensed from a dropper opening. 7. A slightly greater
quantity of oil than water is dispensed. 8. (No answer required.) 9. 8 minims (using 16 minims = 1 ml). 10. 10 minims (0.66 = 2/3; 2/3 × 15 = 10).

CHAPTER 2

Written Competency 2–1

Completed calendar of duties and responsibilities.

1. Day 1: Conduct a first inventory of all controlled substances. If none on hand, enter 0.

2. Receipt of controlled substances from supplier: Enter date of receipt and quantity received on the invoice and/or in a log book.

3. Daily: Complete records by comparing the doses administered/dispensed against the end of day inventory.

4. Biennially: New inventory *required* by DEA.

5. Triennially: Renew physician registration with Form 224a within 45 days of the expiration date of the current registration.

6. Moving a practice: Notify the DEA and request modification of the Registration Certificate prior to the move.

7. Selling a practice: Call the DEA for guidance and further information. Return the Registration Certificate and any unused order forms. Follow DEA Office directions for disposal of controlled substances remaining in the office inventory.

Written Competency 2–2

1.

James Ho, M.D.
1 Main Street
Anywhere, USA 12345-6789
Tele: (111) 555-6666

DEA#: AD 000000   Fax: (111) 555-5555

Patient: John Doe   Age: _____

Address: _____ Date: _____

Rx   NO REFILL

SIG

Generic OK? ☐ Yes ☐ No   Refill: None 1x 2x 3x PRN

Copy 1 of 2   *James Ho* ,M.D.

2.

James Ho, M.D.
1 Main Street
Anywhere, USA 12345-6789
Tele: (111) 555-6666

DEA#: AD 000000   Fax: (111) 555-5555

Patient: Mary Jones   Age: 45

Address: 495 Elm Street   Date: 01/01/99

Rx   Darvocet-N 50 mg #60

SIG   2 tabs q4h, not to exceed 12 tabs per day

Generic OK? ☐ Yes ☑ No   Refill: None [1x] 2x 3x PRN

Copy 1 of 2   *James Ho* ,M.D.

3.

James Ho, M.D.
1 Main Street
Anywhere, USA 12345-6789
Tele: (111) 555-6666

DEA#: AD 000000   Fax: (111) 555-5555

Patient: Jerry Miller   Age: 65

Address: 10 E. 29th Street   Date: 01/01/99

Rx   Naprosyn 250 mg #100

SIG   3 tabs to start, then 1 tab q8h until attack subsides

Generic OK? ☐ Yes ☑ No   Refill: None 1x 2x 3x [PRN]

Copy 1 of 2   *James Ho* ,M.D.

4.

James Ho, M.D.
1 Main Street
Anywhere, USA 12345-6789
Tele: (111) 555-6666

DEA#: AD 000000   Fax: (111) 555-5555

Patient: Jane Wiggs   Age: 35

Address: 123 Main St.   Date: 01/01/99

Rx   Amoxil 250 mg #30

SIG   1 cap q8h x 10 days

Generic OK? ☑ Yes ☐ No   Refill: [None] 1x 2x 3x PRN

Copy 1 of 2   *James Ho* ,M.D.

5.

James Ho, M.D.
1 Main Street
Anywhere, USA 12345-6789
Tele: (111) 555-6666

DEA#: AD 000000   Fax: (111) 555-5555

Patient: Mary Smith   Age: 75

Address: 1 West St.   Date: 01/01/99

Rx   Premarin 0.625 mg #60

SIG   1 tablet daily

Generic OK? ☐ Yes ☑ No   Refill: None 1x 2x 3x PRN [6 x]

Copy 1 of 2   *James Ho* ,M.D.

6.

James Ho, M.D.
1 Main Street
Anywhere, USA 12345-6789
Tele: (111) 555-6666

DEA#: AD 000000   Fax: (111) 555-5555

Patient: Joe Baker   Age: 21

Address: 1512 North Ave.   Date: 01/01/99

Rx   Tylenol #3   #30

SIG   1 - 2 tabs prn for pain

Generic OK? ☑ Yes ☐ No   Refill: [None] 1x 2x 3x PRN

Copy 1 of 2   *James Ho* ,M.D.

7.

James Ho, M.D.
1 Main Street
Anywhere, USA 12345-6789
Tele: (111) 555-6666

DEA#: AD 000000   Fax: (111) 555-5555

Patient: Nancy Jones   Age: 67

Address: 550 Atlantic Ave.   Date: 01/01/99

Rx   Lanoxin 125 mcg. #30

SIG   1 q a.m. p. checking pulse. D/C & call MD if pulse >50

Generic OK? ☐ Yes ☑ No   Refill: None 1x 2x 3x PRN [12 x]

Copy 1 of 2   *James Ho* ,M.D.

8.

James Ho, M.D.
1 Main Street
Anywhere, USA 12345-6789
Tele: (111) 555-6666

DEA#: AD 000000   Fax: (111) 555-5555

Patient: Jack Smith   Age: 48

Address: 1531 South St.   Date: 01/01/99

Rx   Coumadin 1 mg #300

SIG   3 tabs q evening

Generic OK? ☐ Yes ☑ No   Refill: None 1x 2x [3x] PRN

Copy 1 of 2   *James Ho* ,M.D.

9.

James Ho, M.D.
1 Main Street
Anywhere, USA 12345-6789
Tele: (111) 555-6666

DEA#: AD 000000   Fax: (111) 555-5555

Patient: John Max   Age: 23

Address: 324 Main St.   Date: 01/01/99

Rx   Biaxin 500 mg

SIG   1 cap BID x 14 d

Generic OK? ☐ Yes ☑ No   Refill: None [1x] 2x 3x PRN

Copy 1 of 2   *James Ho* ,M.D.

10.

James Ho, M.D.
1 Main Street
Anywhere, USA 12345-6789
Tele: (111) 555-6666

DEA#: AD 000000   Fax: (111) 555-5555

Patient: Pat Reed   Age: 58

Address: 475 West St.   Date: 01/01/99

Rx   Furosemide 40 mg #30

SIG   1 q a.m.

Generic OK? ☑ Yes ☐ No   Refill: None 1x 2x 3x PRN [12 x]

Copy 1 of 2   *James Ho* ,M.D.

11.

James Ho, M.D.
1 Main Street
Anywhere, USA 12345-6789
Tele: (111) 555-6666

DEA#: AD 000000   Fax: (111) 555-5555

Patient: Denise Jones   Age: 19

Address: 980 Atlantic Ave,   Date: 01/01/99

Rx   Ortho-Novum 7/7/7-28

SIG   1 q a.m.

Generic OK? ☐ Yes ☑ No   Refill: None 1x 2x 3x PRN [12 x]

Copy 1 of 2   *James Ho* ,M.D.

12.

James Ho, M.D.
1 Main Street
Anywhere, USA 12345-6789
Tele: (111) 555-6666

DEA#: AD 000000   Fax: (111) 555-5555

Patient: Jack Jones   Age: 35

Address: 5934 Main St.   Date: 01/01/99

Rx   Prozac 20 mg #60

SIG   1 BID

Generic OK? ☑ Yes ☐ No   Refill: None 1x [2x] 3x PRN

Copy 1 of 2   *James Ho* ,M.D.

Conversion Drill 2–1

1. 1.   2. 0.00003.   3. 0.005.   4. 22.   5. 8 or 10.   6. 2.   7. 2.   8. 40.   9. 5 (use 60 mg = 1 gr).   10. 8.   11. 60.   12. 10.   13. 0.25.   14. 1.5.   15. 20.   16. 1.25.   17. 5. 18. 750.   19. 1.   20. 28 or 35.   21. 360 or 384.   22. 12.5.   23. 1/2.   24. 20. 25. 400.

Procedure 2–1

See Reverse of PURCHASER'S Copy for Instructions			No order form may be issued for Schedule I and II substances unless a completed application form has been received. (21 CFR 1305.04).			**OMB APPROVAL No. 1117-0010**		
TO: *(Name of Supplier)* ACME WHOLESALE DRUGS			STREET ADDRESS 600 NORTH AVE					
CITY and STATE ANYTOWN, USA		DATE TODAY'S DATE	NATIONAL DRUG CODE			**TO BE FILLED IN BY PURCHASER**		
L I N E No	No. of Packages	Size of Package	Name of Item				No. of Packages Received	Date Received
1	3	100	Sodium pentothal Capsules, 100 mg				3	0/0/9-
2	2	100	Secobarbital Capsules, 100 mg				2	0/0/9-
3	3	100	Desoxyn Tablets, 5 mg				3	0/0/9-
4	1	30 ml	Demerol, 50 mg/ml				1	0/0/9-
5	2	PINT	Robitussin A-C, 2 mg/ml				2	0/0/9-
6								
7								
8								
9								
10								

5 ◄ **NO. OF LINES COMPLETED**   SIGNATURE OF PURCHASER OR HIS ATTORNEY OR AGENT

Date Issued 12/31/82   DEA Registration No. AD.000000   Name and Address of Registrant

Schedules 2,2N,3,3N,4,5

Registered as a Practitioner   No. of this Order Form PO 123456

JAMES HO, M.D.
1 MAIN STREET
ANYWHERE, USA 55555-0000

DEA Form -222 (Aug 1990)   **U.S. OFFICIAL ORDER FORMS - SCHEDULES I & II DRUG ENFORCEMENT ADMINISTRATION PURCHASER'S Copy 3**

CHAPTER 3

Written Competency 3–1

1. d.   2. d.   3. e.   4. d.   5. a.   6. d.   7. b.   8. a.   9. b.   10. a.

Conversion Drill

1. 8 (not 7.5).   2. 10 (not 10.66).   3. 75 or 80.   4. 4.   5. 64.   6. 0.25.   7. 113.64. 8. 51.81.   9. 41.82.   10. 76.36.   11. 10.   12. 45.   13. 16 or 20.   14. 1.25.   15. 120. 16. 0.15.   17. 250.   18. 300.   19. 10.   20. 15.   21. 30,000.   22. 175.   23. 9. 24. 1.   25. 1.5.

CHAPTER 4

Written Competency 4–1

1. e.   2. a.   3. c.   4. b.   5. d.   6. e.   7. a.   8. d.   9. d.   10. a.

Written Competency 4–2

1. a.   2. e.   3. b.   4. d.   5. c.   6. e.   7. d.   8. b.   9. c.   10. a.

Written Competency 4–3

1. F.   2. F.   3. F.   4. F.   5. F.   6. F.   7. T.   8. T.   9. F.   10. T.

Written Competency 4–4

1. Aspirin. (Although the physician may reduce Coumadin dosage, the patient should not be advised to discontinue the anticoagulant therapy.)   2. increased.   3. potentiation.   4. adverse reaction.   5. prophylactic.   6. pathology.   7. contraindication.   8. OTC drugs.   9. brand name.   10. come into the office for laboratory tests and examination. (Prothrombin time and examination will be used to diagnose the fever.)

Written Competency 4–5

1. Slow-K, aspirin.   2. aspirin and Lasix.   3. Lasix.   4. Lasix, Lanoxin and aspirin.   5. aspirin.

Procedure 4–1

1. Squibb.   2. hydrochlorothiazide and triamterene.   3. Lasix.   4. X.   5. 250–500 mg q8h.
6. oral, IM, IV.   7. thyroid extract.   8. propranalol hydrochloride.   9. Round: 6 brown, 5 white,
10 yellow.   10. Round: 7 white, 7 light peach, 7 peach.

Conversion Drill

1. 10.91.   2. 28.18.   3. 39.09.   4. 47.73.   5. 65.   6. 13.2.   7. 22.   8. 10.   9. 88.
10. 220.   11. 10.91, 54.55, 27.3.   12. 28.18, 141, 70.5.   13. 39.09, 195.45, 97.7.
14. 47.73, 238.65, 119.3.   15. 65, 325, 162.5.   16. 10.   17. 0.5.   18. 0.175.   19. 4.
20. 8.   21. 32.   22. 12 or 15.   23. 1/6.   24. 1000.   25. 1.

CHAPTER 5

Written Competency 5–1

1. d.   2. e.   3. d.   4. a.   5. d.   6. c.   7. d.   8. e.   9. c.   10. b.

Procedure 5–3

PATIENT MEDICATION PLAN

Patient Name: _____ John Doe _____   Date: _____ 8/1/91 _____

FOR: Narcotic Analgesic DRUGS to TREAT: _____ Pain _____

This drug has been prescribed for your pain due to injury. It is a nonaspirin product and is considered a schedule II controlled substance narcotic. This drug will have many effects on the body. The drug will lower fever, decrease pain, and relieve signs and symptoms of inflammation.

Instructions:

The name of your drug is Tylenol with Codeine.

The dose ordered for you is 1 to 2 tablets.

Special storage needs are necessary to keep this medication out of the reach of children and others.

The drug should be taken <u>every 4 hours.</u>

The best times are when you get home and then every 4 hours after that, only if necessary and for no longer than 48 hours. Pain relief medication is more effective if taken before pain becomes severe.

This drug should be taken with food or milk to minimize stomach irritation.

This drug may cause nausea, vomiting, constipation, and dry mouth.

Some other side effects that you should be aware of include drowsiness, dizziness, visual changes, and light-headedness when suddenly standing or changing position. If any of these should occur, avoid driving and activities requiring alertness.

Do not use alcohol, over-the-counter drugs, or other medications with this medication, unless specifically ordered by your physician.

Tell any physician, nurse, dentist, and so on, who takes care of you that you are taking this medication.

Keep this and all medications out of the reach of children.

Notify your physician immediately if any of the following occur:

1. Your pain does not subside within 48 hours.

2. You have difficulty breathing.

3. You develop a rash.

Do not use this medication for any other illness or give this medication to any other person.

Conversion Drill

1. 8 or 10.   2. 300 or 320 or 325 or 330.   3. 15 or 16.   4. 63.63.   5. 8 or 10.   6. 1000. 7. 0.3.   8. 15.45.   9. 1.   10. 10.9.   11. 100.   12. 10.   13. 500.   14. 0.5.   15. 600, 640, 650, or 660.   16. 0.6.   17. 3.   18. 20 or 25.   19. 125.   20. 0.75.   21. 132. 22. 1/2.   23. 45 or 48.   24. 0.45.   25. 5.   26. 1,500.   27. 12 or 15.   28. 0.4.   29. 200.   30. 1,500.

CHAPTER 6

Written Competency 6–1

1. c.   2. a.   3. d.   4. e.   5. c.   6. b.   7. b.   8. d.   9. b.   10. b.

Written Competency 6–2

1. ml

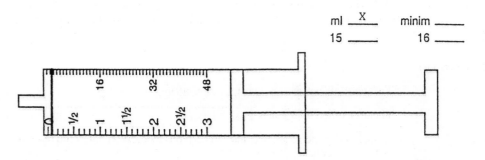

2. ml

ml $\underline{\quad X \quad}$ minim $\underline{\qquad}$
15 $\underline{\qquad}$ 16 $\underline{\qquad}$

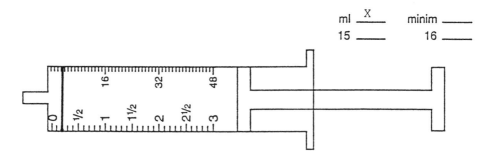

3. minim; 15

ml $\underline{\qquad}$ minim $\underline{\quad X \quad}$
15 $\underline{\quad X \quad}$ 16 $\underline{\qquad}$

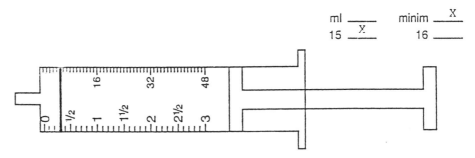

4. ml

ml $\underline{\quad X \quad}$ minim $\underline{\qquad}$
15 $\underline{\qquad}$ 16 $\underline{\qquad}$

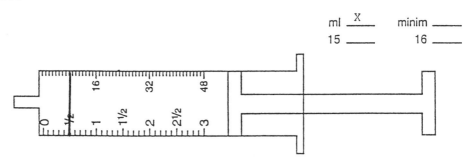

5. minim; 15

ml $\underline{\qquad}$ minim $\underline{\quad X \quad}$
15 $\underline{\quad X \quad}$ 16 $\underline{\qquad}$

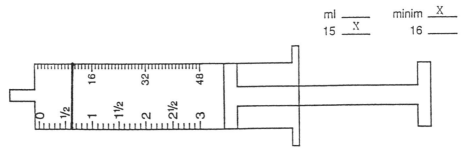

6. minim; 16

ml $\underline{\qquad}$ minim $\underline{\quad X \quad}$
15 $\underline{\qquad}$ 16 $\underline{\quad X \quad}$

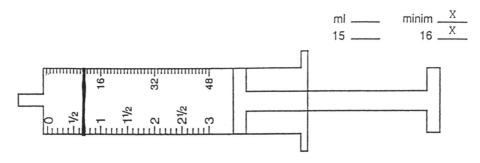

7. ml

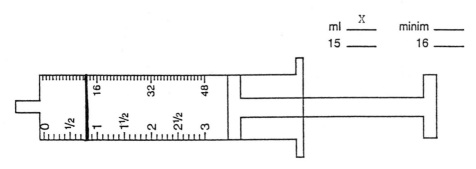

8. ml

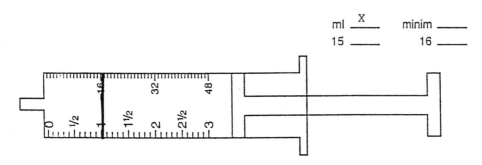

9. ml

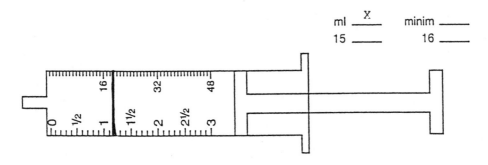

10. minim; 15

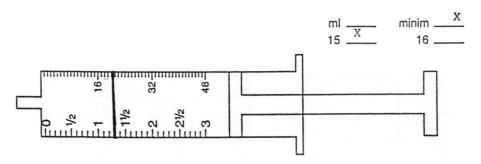

Written Competency 6–3

1.

   1. 0.1 ml

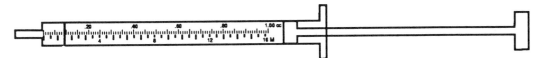

2.

   2. 0.15 ml

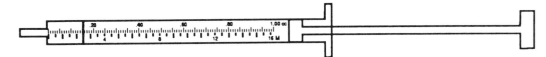

3.

   3. 0.2 ml

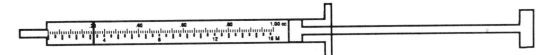

4.

   4. 0.25 ml

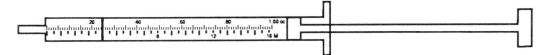

5.

   5. 0.33 ml

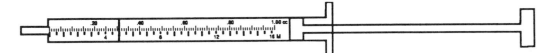

6.

   6. 0.5 ml

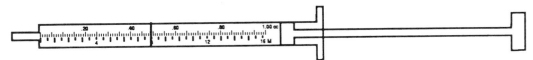

7.

   7. 0.66 ml

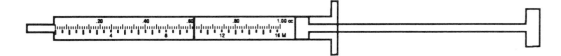

8.

8. 0.75 ml

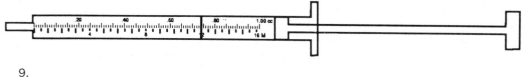

9.

9. 0.8 ml

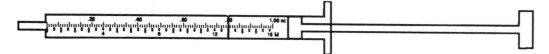

10.

10. 1.0 ml

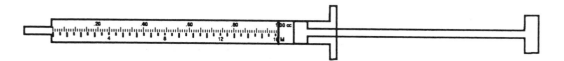

Conversion Drill

1. 250.   2. 250.   3. 125,000.   4. 0.125.   5. 0.00005.   6. 500,000.   7. 0.1.
8. 1.   9. 1.   10. 1.

CHAPTER 7

Appendix B: ANSWERS to Competency 7–1

1. A) Heparin sodium B) 10,000 U/ml C) solution for injection D) 4 ml   2. A) cephalexin B) 125 mg/ml C) oral suspension D) 200 ml   3. A) lidocaine hydrochloride B) 20 mg/ml (2%) C) solution for injection D) 5 ml   4. A) diphenylhydantoin B) 30 mg/capsule C) capsules D) 100 capsules 5. A) diphenylhydantoin B) 100 mg/capsule C) capsules D) 100 capsules   6. A) diphenylhydantoin B) 50 mg/ml C) solution for injection D) 5 ml   7. A) diphenylhydantoin B) 50 mg/ml C) solution for injection D) 20 ml   8. A) carbenicillin B) 1 gram/2.5 ml C) solution for injection D) 4.0 ml or A) carbenicillin B) 1 gram/3.0 ml C) solution for injection D) 5.0 ml or A) carbenicillin B) 1 gram/4.0 ml C) solution for injection D) 7.2.0 ml   9. A) 6/30/99 B) 6/30/99 C) 12/31/99 D) 12/31/99   10. A) Parke-Davis B) Roerig Pfizer C) Dista

Appendix B: Answers to Written Competency 7–2

1. 2.5 ml 2) 5.0 ml 3) 72 hours 4) 250 mg 5) 200 ml 6) after each 100 ml addition 7) room temperature 8) 14 days 9) 125 mg per teaspoon 10) four times per day

Written Competency 7–3

1. Measure 5 ml (1 tsp) in an oral syringe, or measure 1 tsp.   2. Measure 1-1/2 tsp (7.5 ml) in an oral syringe.   3. Fill the dropper to the half-full mark.   4. Because the quantity of 3.75 is greater than 3 ml, the dose may be rounded to the nearest 10th within the margin of safety (3.375 ml to 4.125 ml). Because 3.8 ml is measurable in the oral syringe and well within the

margin of safety, round off 3.75 to 3.8 ml and administer 3.8 ml.   5. Measure 6.25 ml. Because the margin of safety is 5.625 to 6.875, rounding to 6.2 (approximately 1-1/4 tsp) is considered a dose well within the safety range.   6. 15 to 16 ml or 3 tsp or 3 droppersful.   7. 5 ml. 8. 11.82 kg × 20 mg = 236.4 mg per day, divided into three doses of 78.8 mg each. BSA formula: (0.535/1.7) × 250 mcg = 78.68 mg per dose. Round down each dose to 75 mg (safety margin) and give 3 ml q8h.   9. Because the tablet is scored, cut at the score line and administer 1/2 tablet.   10. 1 tablet.   11. 3 tablets.   12. 250 mcg = 1/240 gr. Because the order is 96 percent of the amount available and within the 10 percent safety margin, it is considered safe to administer 1 tablet.   13. 3 tablets.   14. 1/2 tablet.   15. 2 tablets of No. 2 strength. 16. 1 tablet.   17. 1-1/2 tablets of 30-mg strength.   18. 3 tablets would equal 900 mg, and, although less than the 1000 mg ordered, this is within the 10 percent margin of safety.   19. 2 tablets.   20. 65 lb = BSA 1.05 = a safe dosage up to 46.32 mg per dose. Because the 12.5 mg is well below the BSA calculation, give 1/2 scored tablet.

Written Competency 7–4

1. 0.08 ml in a tuberculin syringe.

2. 0.5 ml.

3. 2.5 ml.

4. 0.75 ml.

5. 0.8 ml.

6. The amount of insulin ordered is the same as the amount measured into a syringe. The 50-unit syringe for dosages under 50 units and the 100-unit syringe for dosages greater than 50 units.

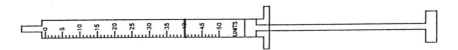

7. See answer 6 for explanation.

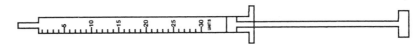

A

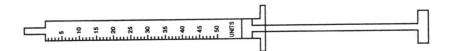

B

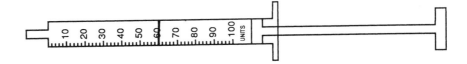

8. See answer 6 for explanation.

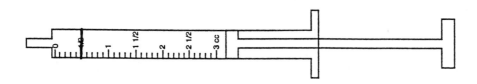

9. a. 0.2 ml.

   b. $\dfrac{44 \text{ lb}}{2.2}$ = 20 kg; 20 × 10 mcg = 200 mcg = 0.2 mg.

   Give 0.2 ml.

   c. Using the nomogram, the BSA = 0.8 m^2; 0.8 m^2 × 300 mcg = 240 mcg = 0.24 mg; give 0.24 ml.

   d. The 0.2 mg ordered stat is the same as the 0.2 mg recommended dosage using the mcg per kg method and slightly less than the 0.24 mg recommended dosage using the BSA guidelines.

10. 1.4 ml.

11. Add 10.0 ml diluent and give 0.5 ml of the drug.

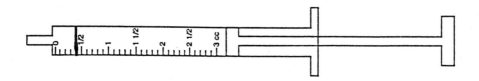

12. Add 1.8 ml diluent and give 0.4 ml *or* add 4 ml and give 0.8 ml. The first choice results in a smaller volume given to the neonate and is recommended.

13. Add 3.2 ml of diluent and administer 2.4 ml.

14. Use 2,400,000 units per 4.0-ml strength.

Round to 3.4 ml. Discard 0.6 ml and administer 3.4 ml.

15. 44 lb = 20 kg; 20 × 50 mg = 1000 mg per day, divided into two doses of 500 mg each.

$$0.25\text{-g vial} + 0.9 \text{ ml diluent} = 250 \text{ mg (0.25 g)/ml}$$
$$0.50\text{-g vial} + 1.8 \text{ ml diluent} = 500 \text{ mg (0.5 g)/2 ml}$$
$$1.0\text{-g vial} + 3.6 \text{ ml diluent} = 1000 \text{ mg (1 g)/4 ml}$$
$$2.0\text{-g vial} + 7.2 \text{ ml diluent} = 2000 \text{ mg (2 g)/8 ml}$$

Each reconstitution equals the same strength (250 mg)/ml. Add 7.2 ml of diluent to the 2-g vial and give 2 ml. The 2-g vial provides eight 250 mg per ml doses for multipatient use. As an alternative, the 1-g vial could be prepared to provide two 500 mg per 2 ml doses for this patient only.

16. There are 10 0.5-ml doses in each 5-ml vial. Fifteen doses will require the use of 1-1/2 vials.

17. 132 lb = 60 kg
    Give 2 ml Hepatavax-B and 3.6 ml Hepatitis B Immune Globulin.
18. 2.5 ml
19. 2.0 ml
20. Use the 50 mg vial.
    0.8 ml

Procedure 7–1

1.

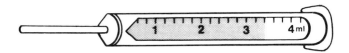

2.

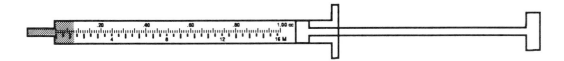

3.

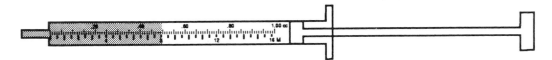

OR

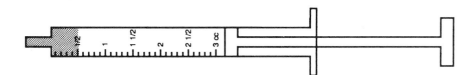

4.

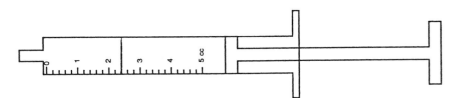

5.

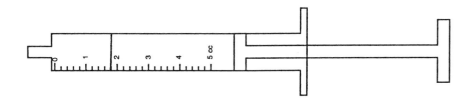

6.

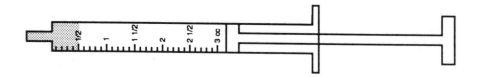

7.

Heptavax—B

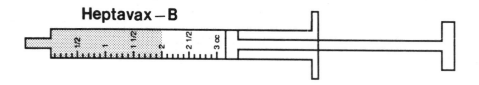

8.

Hepatitis B Immune Globulin

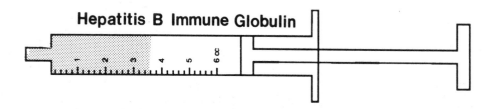

9.

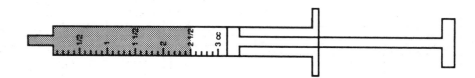

10.

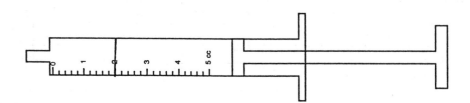

CHAPTER 8

....

Written Competency 8–1

1. e.   2. a.   3. e.   4. c.   5. d.   6. e.   7. a.   8. b.   9. b.   10. c.

Procedure 8–1

DATE			SUBSEQUENT VISITS AND FINDINGS	B.P.	WGT.
MO.	DAY	YR.			
8	1	91	R: Metaprel Inhalant Sol 5% (10 ml) Sig: 2-3 inhalations, undiluted, q 3-4 h, 5-15 (usually 10) inhalations/day.		
			Teaching Session: Pt instructed on use of medication and care of equipment. First self-administration observed as correctly administered. Directions handout given to pt and instructions verbally reviewed. Pt had no further questions. To call in one week. File in recall file for 8/9/91. KL		

Procedure 8–2

DATE			SUBSEQUENT VISITS AND FINDINGS	B.P.	WGT.
MO.	DAY	YR.			
7	7	91	Rx: (Name of sterile eye medication). Sig: gt ī both eyes. Pt tolerated treatment well and left the office after 10 minutes c̄ confirmed clear vision. KL		

Procedure 8–4

DATE			SUBSEQUENT VISITS AND FINDINGS	B.P.	WGT.
MO.	DAY	YR.			
5	23	91	Rx: Sodium chloride (isotonic). Sig: 0.5 mL SC (R) deltoid.		
			No adverse reaction. Pt left the office after 20 min.		
			Pt Instr: No special care, area may be slightly		
			reddened for 24 hours, no return visit necessary.		
			KL		

Procedure 8–5

DATE			SUBSEQUENT VISITS AND FINDINGS	B.P.	WGT.
MO.	DAY	YR.			
6	1	91	Rx: Sodium chloride (isotonic). Sig: 0.5 mL, IM, (L) vastus		
			lateralis. No adverse reactions. Pt left the office		
			after 20 min.		
			Pt Instr: area may be tender next 24 hours, no		
			covering required, no special care. Pt to return		
			in 5 days. Instructed to immediately notify		
			physician should any swelling, fever, or rash		
			occur. Medication handout given. Next appt.:		
			6/6/91. KL		

Procedure 8–6

DATE			SUBSEQUENT VISITS AND FINDINGS	B.P.	WGT.
MO.	DAY	YR.			
6	6	91	Rx: Sodium Chloride (isotonic) Sig: 0.5 mL, IM, Z-tract, Ⓡ VG. No adverse reactions. Pt left the office after 20 minutes		
			Pt instr: area may be tender for next 24 hours, no covering required, no special care. Pt to return in 5 days. Instructed to notify physician STAT should any swelling, fever, or rash occur. Pt given Medication Handout. No follow-up appt rec. KL		

Procedure 8–7

DATE			SUBSEQUENT VISITS AND FINDINGS	B.P.	WGT.
MO.	DAY	YR.			
6	6	91	Tine test Ⓡ forearm		
			Pt Instr: No local care of skin is necessary. Pt to return in 48-72 hours for reading. Testing info discussed and pamphlet given to pt. Appt for M.A. to read reaction made for 6/8/91 at 2pm KL		

CHAPTER 9

Written Competency 9–1

1a. Anxiety and other strong stimuli that overtax the nervous system may cause neurogenic shock and fainting. Place the patient's head lower than the body and keep the patient comfortable. In mild cases of fainting, drug therapy is usually contraindicated.   2b. Tylenol is the only drug used to treat fever that does not have undesirable gastrointestinal tract side effects, and would therefore be the drug of choice among these selections.   3d. Should a last dose cause marked swelling for a second time, it is necessary to return to the previous dose, which failed to give a reaction.   4d. Aluminum hydroxide may be administered with small amounts of water. Do not give activated charcoal (if needed) until after vomiting.   5e. Epinephrine, when added to local anesthesia, decreases systemic absorption of the anesthesia and therefore prolongs numbness. Its presence at the wound site increases swelling, which is one reason plain anesthesia may be used for facial and other cosmetic surgeries.   6c. Constipation and drowsiness may be commonly experienced by patients using narcotic analgesics, even if for just a few days.   7c. Evidence indicates a possible association between ASA (aspirin) and Reye's syndrome. Until further evidence suggests otherwise, the Academy of Pediatrics advises against the use of aspirin for proved or suspected cases of chickenpox and influenza.   8c. DPT. Check the product information insert and seek further instructions from the physician.   9d. Orimune is a live viral vaccine that could transmit an infection to an AIDS patient because AIDS patients' immune systems are compromised.   10a. (2)   10b. (4)   10c. (6)   10d. (5).

Index

Page numbers followed by "f" indicate figures; those followed by "t" indicate tables.